CRIMINAL INDIFFERENCE OF THE FDA TO CANCER PREVENTION

CRIMINAL INDIFFERENCE OF THE FDA TO CANCER PREVENTION

An Anthology of Citizen Petitions,
Newspaper Articles, Press Releases,
and Blogs 1994-2011

Samuel S. Epstein, M.D.

Emeritus Professor Environmental and Occupational Medicine,
University of Illinois at Chicago School of Public Health and
Chairman, the Cancer Prevention Coalition

To order additional copies of this book, contact:
Xlibris LLC
1-888-795-4274
www.Xlibris.com
Orders@Xlibris.com
139080

Contents

To the next generation: Ethan and Calvin

Citizen Petitions to the FDA

A. Mammography   May 12, 1995

B. Hormonal Milk   January 12, 2010

C. Hormonal Meat   April 25, 1995
                                                January 29, 2010

D. Cosmetics and Personal Care Products   November 17, 1994
                                                January 17, 1995
                                                October 22, 1996
                                                May 13, 2008

Acknowledgments

Warm commendations are due to Cong. John Conyers, Jr., former chairman of the House Judiciary Committee, for his longstanding public health policy initiatives, and also for his acceptance of my 1979 invitation to draft legislation on "white-collar crime" in relation to industry malpractice. This crime continues to expose millions of unsuspecting citizens and consumers to avoidable risks of cancer from a wide range of industrial chemicals and ingredients in consumer products. In 1981, Congressman Conyers warned that "Monsanto and the FDA have chosen to suppress and manipulate animal health test data in efforts to approve commercial use of rBGH, genetically engineered milk." Congressman Conyers also endorsed my 2006 book *What's in Your Milk?*

Thanks are also due to Dr. Quentin D. Young, former president of the American Public Health Association, Chairman of the Health and Medicine Policy Research Group, for his longstanding emphasis on the critical but infrequently exercised role of physicians in public health policy and cancer prevention.

It is a pleasure to acknowledge the over one hundred scientific experts in cancer prevention and public health and the several hundred representatives of consumer and citizen activist groups who endorsed my Cancer Prevention Coalition's February 2003 report, "Stop Cancer Before It Starts Campaign: How to Win the Losing War Against Cancer." It is also a pleasure to acknowledge the leading scientific experts who endorsed the 2007 Citizen Petition on the hormonal and cancer risks of milk to the

FDA and also my 1995 and 2010 Petitions on nitrite preservatives and hormonal meat to the FDA.

I would also like to thank my research assistant, Alessandra Gibson, MPH, for her creative support.

BIOGRAPHY OF THE AUTHOR

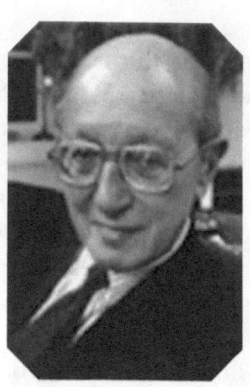

Samuel S. Epstein, M.D., is professor emeritus of Environmental and Occupational Medicine at the University of Illinois School of Public Health and chairman of the Cancer Prevention Coalition. He has published some 270 peer-reviewed articles, and authored twenty books.

Dr. Epstein is an internationally recognized authority on avoidable causes of cancer, particularly unknowing exposures to industrial carcinogens in air, water, the workplace, and consumer products—food, cosmetics and toiletries, and household products including pesticides—besides carcinogenic prescription drugs.

Dr. Epstein's past public policy activities include consultant to the U.S. Senate Committee on Public Works, drafting congressional legislation, frequently invited congressional testimony, membership of key federal committees including EPA's Health Effects Advisory Committee, and the Department of Labor's Advisory Committee on the Regulation of Occupational Carcinogens, and key expert on banning of hazardous products and pesticides including DDT, Aldrin, and Chlordane. He is the leading international expert on cancer risks of petrochemicals and of consumer products including rBGH milk, meat from cattle implanted with sex hormones in feedlots—on which he has testified for the EC at January 1997 WTO hearings, and irradiated food. In 1998, he presented "Legislative Proposals for Reversing the Cancer Epidemic" to the Swedish Parliament and in 1999 to the UK All Parliamentary Cancer Group. He has also submitted eight citizen petitions to the U.S. Food and Drug Administration on the undisclosed dangers of carcinogens and carcinogenic products. These include talc, lindane, nitrite-preserved foods, silicone gel and polyurethane implants, cosmetics containing DEA, genetically engineered milk (rBGH), and hormonal beef.

He is also the leading critic of the cancer establishment, the National Cancer Institute (NCI) and American Cancer Society (ACS), for fixation on damage control—screening, diagnosis and treatment, and genetic research—with indifference for cancer prevention, which for the ACS extends to hostility. This mind-set is compounded by ACS conflicts of interest with the cancer drug industry and also with the petrochemical and other industries. The ACS thus qualifies for Ralph Nader's 1975 adage, "Jail for crime in the streets, [but] bail for crime in the suites."

Dr. Epstein past professional society involvement includes founder of the Environmental Mutagen Society, president of the Society for Occupational and Environmental Health, president of the Rachel Carson Council, and advisor to environmental citizen activist and organized labor groups.

His honors include the 1969 Society of Toxicology Achievement Award, the 1977 National Wildlife Federation Conservancy Award, the 1989 Environmental Justice Award, the 1998 Right Livelihood Award (Alternative Nobel Prize) for international contributions to cancer prevention, the 1999 Bioneers Award, the 2000 Project Censored Award (Alternative Pulitzer Prize for investigative journalism) for an article critiquing the American Cancer Society and National Cancer Institute, the 2005 Albert Schweitzer Golden Grand Medal for Humanitarianism from the Polish Academy of Medicine, and the 2007 Dragonfly Award from Beyond Pesticides.

Dr. Epstein has extensive media experience with numerous regional and national radio programs, including NPR; major TV programs, including

Sixty Minutes, Face the Nation, Meet the Press, McNeil/Lehrer, Donohue, Good Morning, America, and the *Today Show;* Canadian, European, Australian, and Japanese TV. He has also contributed numerous editorials and letters to leading national newspapers and published about 150 press releases and forty Huffington Post blogs over the last two decades.

OTHER BOOKS BY THE AUTHOR

The Mutagenicity of Pesticides (MIT Press, 1971)

Drugs of Abuse: Their Genetic and Other Chronic Nonpsychiatric Hazards (MIT Press, 1971)

The Legislation of Consumer Product Safety (MIT Press, 1974)

The Politics of Cancer (Sierra Club Books, 1978)

Hazardous Wastes in America (Sierra Club Books, 1982)

Cancer in Britain: The Politics of Prevention (London: Pluto Press, 1983)

The Safe Shopper's Bible (MacMillan Publishing Company, 1995)

The Breast Cancer Prevention Program (MacMillan Publishing Company, 1997; Second Edition, 1998)

The Politics of Cancer, Revisited (East Ridge Press, 1998)

GOT (Genetically Engineered) MILK! The Monsanto rBGH/BST Milk Wars Handbook (Seven Stories Press, 2001)

The Stop Cancer before It Starts Campaign: How to Win the Losing War Against Cancer (2003)

Unreasonable Risk: How to Avoid Cancer from Cosmetics and Personal Care Products: The Neways Story (Environmental Toxicology, 2005)

Cancer-Gate: How to Win the Losing Cancer War (Baywood Publishing Company, Inc., 2005)

Shopper Beware: How to Avoid Cancer and Other Toxic Effects from Cosmetics and Personal Care Products (Japan: Lyon-sha Publishing, 2006)

What's In Your Milk? (Trafford Publishing, 2006)

Healthy Beauty (BenBella Books, 2009)
National Cancer Institute and American Cancer Society: Criminal Indifference to Cancer Prevention and Conflicts of Interest (Xlibris Publishing, 2011)
Good Clean Food (Skyhorse Publishing, 2013)
Stop Breast Cancer before It Starts (Seven Stories Press, 2013)
Avoidable Causes of Childhood Cancer (Xlibris Publishing, 2013)

FOREWORD[1]

"Americans count on this agency, [the FDA] to make sure that we have a steady stream of wonderful new pills that are potent and perfectly safe at the same time, as well as a supermarket full of goodies we can gobble up without worrying about food poisoning."

[1] Fran Hawthorne, *Inside the FDA: The Business and Politics behind the Drugs We Take and the Food We Eat* (John Wiley, 2005).

INTRODUCTION[2]

"The 1938 provisions of the Federal Food, Drug and Cosmetic Act charged the FDA with responsibility to regulate and warn the public of cancer risks from ingredients in their products. However, and with few exceptions, the FDA has failed to warn the public of such risks, for which it shares criminal liability with the responsible industries.

"The 1938 FDA Regulations (21 CFR Sec. 740/10) explicitly stipulate: 'Each ingredient used in a cosmetic product and each finished cosmetic product shall be adequately substantiated for safety prior to marketing. Any such ingredient or product whose safety is not adequately substantiated prior to marketing is misbranded unless it contains the following conspicuous statement on the principal display panel: WARNING. THE SAFETY OF THIS PRODUCT HAS NOT BEEN DETERMINED.'

"However, the FDA has rarely exercised these options since its founding, no matter how dangerous the product and its ingredients have been shown to be. The very few exceptions are the following nine prohibited ingredients in the 1938 Federal Food, Drug, and Cosmetic Act:

- Complexes containing zirconium, as ingredients in aerosol products, as they can induce granulomas in the lung.
- Hexachlorophene, because of its neurotoxicity. However, this ingredient may still be used in the absence of 'an alternative (effective) preservative.'

---

[2] S. S. Epstein and R. Fitzgerald, *Healthy Beauty: Your Guide to Ingredients to Avoid and Products You Can Trust* (BenBella Books, 2009).

- Mercury compounds, because of their neurotoxicity.
- Chlorofluorocarbon propellants, although they may still be exported. (The reason is not stated.)
- Bithionol, as it can cause photosensitivity.
- Halogenated salicylanilides, as they can induce photosensitivity.
- Chloroform, 'because of its animal carcinogenicity and likely hazard to human health.'
- Vinyl chloride, as an ingredient in aerosol products, because of its carcinogenic effects.
- Methylene chloride, 'because of its animal carcinogenicity and likely hazard to human health' (Epstein and Fitzgerald, 2009).

"In 1979, the FDA expressed concerns about significant nitrosamine contamination 'in a variety of cosmetic products.' The Agency asked 'for voluntary industry action' and left open the possibility of taking regulatory steps. Although the requested voluntary action was not forthcoming, the Agency still has not used its regulatory authority.

"As mentioned, it has been well known since 1978 that ethoxylate detergents are contaminated with 1,4-dioxane at levels as high as 100 parts per million. In 1985, the FDA requested that manufacturers limit the level of dioxane in cosmetic products to less than ten parts per million. A decade later, levels in some products were found to range up to eight parts per million, but the FDA still took no regulatory action against dioxane-contaminated detergents. A further example of the FDA's regulatory recklessness is its continued failure to require labeling of alpha-hydroxy acid 'skin peelers,' even though the Agency admitted in 1992 that these chemicals pose a serious risk to health (ibid.).

"As for the industry and its record of voluntary actions and compliance, it should be noted that manufacturers have only voluntarily discounted the use of three ingredients that are known to be toxic:

- Methylcoumarin (6-MC), as it can induce photosensitivity.
- Musk ambrette, because of its neurotoxicity and ability to induce photosensitivity.
- Acetylethyletetramethyltetraline (AETT), because of its serious neurotoxicity, in addition to its discoloration of internal organs (Epstein and Fitzgerald, 2009).

"If and when manufacturers do conduct safety testing of ingredients used in their products, the results become privileged information and there is no requirement that they be made public. Because safety testing is strictly voluntary, not even the FDA has access to this information.

"According to the guidelines, these ingredients, either individually or compositely, should be tested for primary skin, eye, and mucous membrane irritation; sensitizing potential; sensitization to light; oral toxicity; and inhalation toxicity. However, all these are short-term tests (the longest duration is only ninety days) and exclude testing for the effects of chronic use and for carcinogenicity. The word "carcinogenicity" is conspicuous in its absence from the guidelines. However, a section on 'Evaluation of Cosmetic Products' admits that the 'potential for chronic toxicity should be considered in the evaluation of safety.'

"The FDA was so impressed by the Council's guidelines that it decided to rely on them rather than formalize good manufacturing practice regulations on its own. In 1983, FDA Commissioner Arthur Hayes Jr. publicly enthused about the guidelines' publication in advance of the FDA requesting them, and about the guidelines' excellent quality. Unbelievably, the FDA's position and reliance on these guidelines remains unchanged despite a wealth of evidence showing their inadequacies (ibid.).

"The Council's Labeling Manual, last updated 1997, is also revealing of the association's lack of safety concern. This manual provided information on FDA's labeling requirements under the Fair Packaging and Labeling Act (FPLA) and the Federal Food, Drug, and Cosmetic Act (FFDCA). The manual states that the "industry takes pride in its reputation for providing safe products while requiring the minimum use of government resources (Epstein and Fitzgerald, 2009).

"Conspicuous in the manual, however, is the absence of any reference to the carcinogenicity of product ingredients. A meaningless exception is the reference to two carcinogenic coal tar dyes, which had already been banned in 1078. For other "coal tar" dyes, the manual relies on the Hair Dye Exemption clause of the FFDCA, which allows these dyes' use provided there is a trivializing warning to the effect that these dyes may "cause skin irritation in certain individuals.

"Most major industrialized nations now require ingredient labeling, even though this is minimally, if at all, informative in the absence of appropriate warnings. (Disturbingly, the Council noted that "disclosure of ingredients is still not required on the package of cosmetic products" in Canada, and also that "there is no requirement for full ingredient labeling" in Korea.) Products that appear in hotels, restaurants, condominiums, public washrooms, and schools are still generally unlabeled. Additionally, unlabeled products manufactured by small, unregistered "rogue" industries are commonplace (ibid.)."

FDA and Monsanto Massive Cover-Up[3]

"On July 27, 1989, the Los Angeles Times published an op-ed piece on rBGH by Dr. Samuel Epstein entitled, "Growth Hormones Would Endanger Milk." Epstein outlined "grave consumer health risks that have not been investigated by the industry or FDA.

"Epstein had accumulated significant evidence about the potential health dangers of the hormone. In September 1989, he submitted his findings to the commissioner of the FDA, urging the agency not to approve the drug. His report, which went unanswered, outlined many of the key criticism that the scientist at Health Canada were later to address. Epstein also received a box of secret FDA documents, sent to him anonymously. The information revealed that a high percentage of cows injected with rBGH had serious health problems and, according to Epstein, showed that Monsanto and the FDA were involved in a massive cover up."

---

[3] Jeffrey Smith, *Seeds of Deception: Exposing Industry and Government Lies about the Safety of the Genetically Engineered Foods You're Eating* (Yes! Books, 2003).

Explicit Conflicts of Interest and Failure of the FDA[4]

"The FDA has shown reckless failure to warn the public, the media, and Congress of explicit epidemiological evidence on a wide range of avoidable and involuntary risk factors or causes of cancer.

"These causes include:

- Exposure of the entire U.S. population, to varying degrees, to a wide range of industrial carcinogens, particularly dioxin, PCBs, and agricultural pesticides which have polluted the entire environment, food and water, besides air.
- Extensive use of the herbicide atrazine in the United States, although banned in most European nations. This is the commonest pollutant in rain and drinking water. A series of epidemiological studies over the last decade have incriminated atrazine as a cause of noon-Hodgkin's and Hodgkin's lymphoma and ovarian cancer.
- The common recycling of toxic wastes, including heavy metals, dioxins, and radionuclides, into plant foods and farm fertilizers. These wastes bioaccumulate in soil and contaminate food, water, and air.
- Unlabelled milk and other dairy products from cows injected with Monsanto's genetically engineered growth hormone (rBGH) are contaminated with high levels of IGF-1 and their consumption thus poses increased risks of breast, colon, and prostate cancers.
- High levels of estradiol and other natural and synthetic sex hormones in U.S. meant from cattle implanted with sex hormones to increase carcass weight, pose risks of breast and other hormonal cancers.
- As seriously, the FDA has ignored a wide range of exposures to carcinogens in food and drugs, besides also environmental contaminants.
- Prolonged use of estrogen and progesterone hormone replacement therapy; premenopausal mammography; and proximity of residence to Superfund sites.

---

4   S.S. Epstein, *CANCER-GATE: How to Win the Losing Cancer War* (Baywood Publishing, 2005).

- Exposure of some one million women to occupational carcinogens, particularly methylene chloride, benzene, ethylene oxide, and phenylenediamine dyes.
- The relationship between hormone replacement therapy and ovarian cancer.
- The relationship between perineal dusting with talcum powder by premenopausal women and ovarian cancer.
- The relationship between non-Hodgkin's lymphoma, multiple myeloma, and bladder and breast cancers and prolonged use by some 20 million women of permanent and semi-permanent black or dark brown hair dyes.
- The relationship between non-Hodgkin's lymphoma and exposure to herbicides, particularly, 2,4-D, in male agricultural workers.
- The relationship between frequent consumption of nitrite-dyed hot dogs and childhood leukemia and brain cancer (Epstein, 2005)."

"The granting by the FDA of an Investigative New Animal Drug (INAD) exemption for the synthetic hormones on the basis of allegedly confidential data and their allowing the sale of unlabeled hormonal milk and meat reflects the agency's highly relaxed view of its responsibilities. As stated in a recent FDA Talk Paper, and elsewhere, sponsors have not been required to measure the increase of bovine growth hormone (BGH) in milk of treated cattle over that in milk from untreated cattle. Rather, the safety of BGH is allegedly based on the limited quantity of the hormone administered on a daily basis and the fact that BGH is not biologically active in humans or other primates. Furthermore, in granting the INAD exemption, the FDA is in apparent violation of the 1968 FFDCA amendments mandating that the agency must have a "prescribed and approved" test method, which the industry is required to provide, for determining whether the drug is being improperly used, with resulting illegal residues in food (Epstein, 2005).

"Of additional concern is the fact that the FDA, has inappropriately relied on standard protocols that are largely irrelevant for the safety evaluation of biosynthetic milk hormones. In fact, the only reported evidence of adverse effects has emerged from incidental findings in efficacy trials based on Technical Advisory Document (TAD) protocols designed primarily for milk production trials. In particular, the agency has failed to require evaluation of the toxicological effects of the milk hormones in large-scale multigenerational and multilactational tests, and evaluation of the safety of milk and dairy products, with regard to a wide range of critical public health concerns (ibid.).

"The conduct of the regulatory agencies in the matter of milk hormones is consistent with their tract record. As evidenced in an extensive series of Government Accounting Office investigations and Congressional hearings, USDA and FDA regulation is in near total disarray, aggravated by denials and cover-ups. A 1986 Congressional report concluded: "FDA has consistently disregarded its responsibility, . . . repeatedly put what it perceives are interest of veterinarians and the livestock industry ahead of its legal obligation to protect consumers, . . . jeopardizing the health and safety of consumers of meat, milk, and poultry." Further illustrative is the April 1989 USDA proposal to end inspection of the nation's 6,300 meat and poultry processing plants and instead to rely on voluntary compliance. The proposed plan, originally entitled "Discretionary Inspections," and then euphemistically renamed "Improved Processing Inspection System," has met with a storm of criticism from sources including the American Meat Institute and major meat packers (Epstein, 2005).

"A noteworthy exception is the 1958 Delaney Amendment to the Federal Food, Drug, and Cosmetic Act, with its absolute prohibition against the deliberate introduction of any level of carcinogen into the food supply. Over the last three decades, this Amendment has been under repeated vigorous attacks by (FDA) and EPA. The latest such initiative is EPA's October 1988 proposal to scrap the Amendment for carcinogenic pesticides contaminating processed agricultural foods, and the substitute a "negligible [cancer] risk" regulation, based on manipulated numbers and unjustifiable assumptions. The FDA shares with EPA unwillingness to obey the Delaney law, and has been enthusiastic in developing a legal basis for exemptions for a wide range of carcinogenic coal-tar food dyes, and animal feed additives. Both FDA and EPA are planning to fling open the leaking flood gates o a wide range of carcinogens in the nations' food supplies (ibid).

Q: Has the FDA Center for Veterinary Medicine (CVM) conducted the BGH review process in compliance with the Federal Food drug and Cosmetic Act, the current regulations and requirements of 21 CFR 514.1, published guidelines, and unpolished policies, with regard to efficacy, veterinary safety, and human safety?

A: No. For details, see below.

Q: Does CVM have inappropriate contacts with the regulated industries, and is there evidence of inappropriate industry influence (ibid.)?

A: Yes. The CVM director has met regularly with personnel of the Animal Health Institute, a trade organization representing the regulated industries. There is, however, no evidence that the director met with consumer groups concerned with food safety. There are also allegations that donations to a national political party were requested of applicants for CVM directorship, and that such a donation was ultimately paid by the regulated industry. Growing evidence indicates that corporate lobbyists "enjoy almost unlimited access" to CVM officials, and that the review process is characterized by illegal gratuities, favoritism, and rigging of assignments to "cooperative" staff members.

Q: Has the FDA undertaken unprecedented and inappropriate actions in support of an INADA for rBGH?

A: Yes. High-ranking CVM and other senior agency personnel have spoken out in support of rBGH. It is unprecedented for the FDA to publically support or otherwise advertise an approved or unapproved animal drug.

Q: Is the FDA review process on rBGH consistent with its tract record for other animal drugs and feed additives?

A: Yes. It demonstrates reckless irresponsibility and regulatory abdication. This was fully recognized in a recent Congressional report which concluded that "FDA has consistently disregarded its responsibility . . . repeatedly put what it perceives are interests of veterinarians and the livestock industry ahead of its legal obligation to protect consumers . . . jeopardizing the health and safety of consumers of meat, milk and poultry." Confirmation of such regulatory abdication is provided by the FDA's admission, in a November 1988 consumer report, that "illegal use of veterinary drugs can be an even greater threat to the public health than the illegal use of human drugs." These concerns are still further emphasized by the results of recent investigations demonstrating that up to 38 percent of milk and sampled nationally is contaminated by illegal residues of antibiotics and animal drugs, posing grave potential public health hazards, including antibiotic resistance, carcinogenicity, and allergic reactions. In this connection, without public notification, the CVM has recently tripled the allowable residues in milk of new antibiotics used for treatment of bovine mastitis, a common complication in *srBGH-treated cows* (Epstein, 2005)."

Expert's Warning Letter to FDA Comissioner[5]

Dear Commissioner Young:

I am writing to you on an issue of critical national concern relating to the safety of U.S. agriculture, in general, and to serious potential threats to safety of milk and meat, in particular.

I enclose my report entitled, "Potential Public Health Hazards of Biosynthetic Milk Hormones." Apart from raising questions on their efficacy, the report documents growing evidence on adverse veterinary effects of these hormones whose significance has been minimized by the industry and apparently not adequately recognized by the FDA. More critically, the report raises a wide range of unresolved questions on the human safety of consumption of milk and meat from hormone treated cows.

These concerns are all the more pressing in view of the fact that over the last five years the general public has been consuming unlabeled milk and meat from hormone treated cattle, in view of the fact that the FDA has stated that such foods are safe, and in view of the fact that the FDA appears to be moving closer to approving these hormones.

I would appreciate a reply at your earliest convenience.

Sincerely yours,

Samuel S. Epstein, M.D.

cc: USDA Sec. C. Yeutter; W. Graham (Executive Office of the President); Sen. T. Daschle; Sen. W. Fowler, Jr.; Sen. A. Gore Jr.; Sen. H. Kohn; Sen. P. Leahy; Sen. H. Metzenbaum; Sen. P. Simon; Cong J. Conyers, Jr.; Cong. C. Hatcher; Cong. E. Madigan; Cong. J. Scheuler; Cong. M. Synar; Cong. H. Waxman, Cong. T. Weiss; Wisconsin State Sen. T. Winkle; Wisconsin State Sen. B. Feingold

---

[5]   S. S. Epstein, *What's in Your Milk?* (Trafford Publishing, 2006).

Current FDA Comissioner Delusions

As published in a February 25, 2011, *Science Insider* editorial, "Advancing Regulatory Science," Dr. Hamburg, claimed that FDA's regulation of food safety must be based on "better predictive models" based on "functional genomics, proteomics, and metabolomics," rather than "high dose animal [carcinogenicity] studies—unchanged for decades." She also stated that "FDA is prepared to lead the way in strengthening regulatory science and transforming toxicology." It should further be noted that the 2011 FDA website claims that extensive studies have shown that the residual hormone level in meat is "a safe level for human consumption" and that the drugs "do not harm the treated animal or the environment."

Dr. Hamburg's dismissal of standard carcinogenicity tests is bizarre. Their scientific validity is endorsed by other Federal regulatory agencies, the National Toxicology Program, the International Agency for Research on Cancer, and also the April 2010 President's Cancer Panel. Furthermore, as stipulated in the 1938 Federal Food Drug and Cosmetic Act, the FDA is charged with regulating food, drugs, and cosmetics based on standard toxicology and carcinogenicity tests. Moreover, the FDA is not charged with, let alone capable of developing irrelevant "tests that incorporate the mechanistic underpinnings of disease."

FDA Lose Regulations for Advisory Members[6]

"FDA is authorized by statute to grant waivers to allow individuals with potentially conflicting financial interests to participate in meetings where it concludes, after close scrutiny, that certain criteria are met. The Agency has also issued a guidance document describing our policy for considering eligibility for advisory committee participation.

"FDA does not intend to publicly disclose financial interest information if the information is exempt under the Freedom of Information Act or otherwise protected from disclosure by statute or regulation, other than due to the fact that it is personal financial information reported on a Confidential Financial Disclosure Report. For example, FDA would not disclose the name of a company or institution if doing so would reveal that company's confidential commercial information."

[6]   U.S. Department of Health and Human Services Food and Drug Administration, *Guidance for the Public, FDA Advisory Committee Members, and FDA staff: Public Availability of Advisory Committee Members' Financial Interest Information and Waivers* (March 2012).

Congress Battles with the FDA[7]

"More than two years after Congress passed a landmark law meant to prevent the importation of contaminated food that sickens Americans, the Food and Drug administration proposed rules on Friday that for the first time put the main onus on companies to police the food they import . . . The F.D.A. has tried to keep tabs on imports, but, in reality, manages to inspect only 1 to 2 percent of all imports at American ports and borders."

<hr>

[7]   Sabrina Tavernise, "F.D.A. Says Importers Must Audit Food Safety" (*New York Times*, July 27, 2013).

A.
Mammography

Mammography

Citizen Petition Seeking a Medical Alert for All Women with Silicone Gel and Polyurethane Breast Implants

May 12, 1995

David A. Kessler, M.D.
Commissioner
Food and Drug Administration, Room 1-23
12420 Parklawn Drive
Rockville, MD 20857

This Petition is based on scientific publications dating back to 1960 which clearly demonstrate the carcinogenicity of silicone gel and polyurethane foam (PUF) breast implants. This evidence is further supported by internal Food and Drug Administration (FDA) memoranda.

The undersigned submits this petition to request the Commissioner of Food and Drugs to issue a medical alert to all women who have had silicone gel breast implants with high priority to those with PUF implants, warning them of their risks of breast cancer and of the need for ongoing medical surveillance.

A. Agency Action Requested

This petition requests that FDA take the following action:

Immediately issue a medical alert to women who have received silicone gel and PUF breast implants, informing them of the risks of breast cancer.

B. Statement of Grounds

In April 1992, the FDA banned silicone gel breast implants except for use in controlled trials. This decision by the FDA was in response to serious questions raised concerning the health risks of implants. However, despite banning the general use of silicone implants, the agency failed to address the risks of cancer.

1. Carcinogenicity of Silicone Gel

An unpublished Dow Corning study discovered by the FDA in 1987, demonstrated that subcutaneous injection of silicone gel in rats induced highly malignant and metastatic fibrosarcomas. Commenting on these findings, FDA Task Force scientists excluded the possibility that these could be solid state tumors; it was further urged that "a medical alert be issued to warn the public of the possibility of malignancy development in humans following long-term implant of silicone breast prostheses." The carcinogenicity of silicone gel was subsequently confirmed following intraperitoneal injection in mice.

2. Carcinogenicity of Polyurethane Foam

In a series of publications from 1960 to 1964, Dr. Wilhelm Hueper (Chief of the Environmental Cancer Section at the National Cancer Institute) reported on the induction of carcinomas and/or sarcomas following intraperitoneal or subcutaneous injection of PUF in rats. Apart from the induction of carcinomas, the possibility that the sarcomas could have been "solid state tumors" was definitively excluded. Furthermore, Hueper demonstrated the rapid in vivo degradation of PUF.

On the basis of these findings, Hueper warned:

- Since polyurethane plastics have been used in cosmetic and orthopedic surgery during recent years, these observations are of distinct significance and practical importance,—(and) should caution against the indiscriminate use of polyurethane plastics in medical practice—
- against indiscriminate parenteral use of polyurethane plastics—in medical practice.
- It is premature—to conclude from the present absence of carcinogenic (human) responses—that the innocuousness of these materials—is established—(as) any cancerous reaction—might require an induction period of some 30 years or more.

On the basis of Hueper's studies, a senior FDA staff scientist concluded in 1991 that "PU[polyurethane] is acting as a straight-forward chemical carcinogen—and is not an appropriate material for use in breast implants."

The carcinogenicity of PUF was subsequently confirmed by the induction of fibrosarcomas and carcinomas in rats following intraperitoneal and intrapulmonary administration, respectively. The authors excluded the possibility that the sarcomas were "solid state tumors, "and emphasized that their findings were "consistent with a mechanism of biological degradation."

3. Carcinogenicity of Contaminants and Degradation Products of Polyurethane Foam

2,4 Diaminotoluene (TDA) and 2,4—Toluene diisocyanate (TDI) have been demonstrated to be carcinogenic contaminants and degradation products of PUF in both in vitro and in vivo studies. Additionally, TDA has been identified in both the urine and breast milk of women with silicone gel breast implants. It was accordingly concluded in 1994 that "TDA release from PU foam covers of—breast implants will undoubtedly produce delayed adverse health effects."

The carcinogenicity of TDI in mice and rats was first reported in 1983. Of particular interest was the induction of a statistically significant incidence of mammary fibroadenomas, besides malignant tumors in other sites in rats. On the basis of these data the International Agency for Research on Cancer (IARC) determined that there was "sufficient evidence" of TDI's carcinogenicity in mice and rats, including the induction of mammary tumors in female rats. These conclusions were subsequently reiterated by the National Toxicological Program. TDI is currently regulated by: the Environmental Protection Agency (EPA), under the Clean Air Act (CAA), Comprehensive Environmental, Response, Compensation and Liability Act (CERCLA), Resource Conservation and Recovery Act (RCRA), and Superfund Amendments and Reauthorization Act (SARA); the Occupational Safety and Health Administration (OSHA) under the Hazard Communication Standard and as a Chemical Hazard in laboratories; and by the FDA as an indirect food additive.

There is substantial evidence on the carcinogenicity of TDA dating back to 1955, when it was found that subcutaneous injection induced local sarcomas in rats. Invasive and metastatic liver cancer was subsequently induced in rats fed with TDA. It is worthy of note that on the basis of these data, the cosmetic industry voluntarily eliminated the use of TDA in hair dyes in 1971. A statistically significant incidence of benign and malignant mammary tumors was induced in rats fed with TDA; these tumors developed after only one month feeding. A statistically significant incidence of liver cancer and vascular tumors was induced in mice, and benign and malignant breast tumors, besides tumors in other sites, were induced in rats following feeding of TDA. On the basis of these data, IARC concluded that there was "sufficient evidence "of the carcinogenicity of TDA in mice and rats. These conclusions were reiterated by the National Toxicology Program, which further warned that "the presence of TDA, even as a trace contaminant, may be a cause of cancer."

TDA is currently regulated by EPA as a priority hazardous substance under SARA; OSHA under the Hazard Communication Standard as a Chemical Hazard in laboratories; and by the FDA which requires warning labels on coal tar hair dyes containing TDA under the Federal Food Drug, and Cosmetic Act.

An unpublished Congressionally-mandated NCI report emphasized that concerns on "a carcinogenic hazard were recently heightened by reports that the polyurethane foam coating that envelopes the silica gel—may dissolve and produce the chemical 2,4 diaminotoluene (TDA)—linked to increased rates of breast and hepatocellular carcinomas in rats and mice and possibly also sarcomas and lymphomas in mice."

4. Carcinogenicity of Ethylene Oxide

Ethylene oxide (ETO) has been routinely used to sterilize breast implants. A July 11, 1988, FDA audit of Cooper Surgical revealed a wide range of deficiencies in control procedures, including the absence of formalized procedures for methods for sterilization and aeration, and for failure to test for residues. These concerns are of particular significance as ETO residues are known to persist on medical products, including plastics, even after seven days aeration. ETO is a well-recognized carcinogen inducing breast cancer, malignant lymphomas and other cancers in mice, and leukemia, brain tumors and other cancers in rats following inhalation, and fibrosarcomas in mice following subcutaneous injection.

5. Epidemiological studies on Women with Silicone Breast Implants

Based on a cohort of 11,676 women in Alberta receiving silicone gel or saline implants from 1973 to 1986, with a mean follow-up of only 10.2 years, a deficit of breast cancer was reported. PU implants were not used in Alberta during the study period. In a subsequent study with a median follow-up of only 10.6 years, deficits of breast cancer in implanted women and of all other malignancies combines were reported. However, based on small numbers, an increased incidence of lung, vulva, and invasive cervical carcinomas, was reported.

However, as emphasized by an NCI report, these studies are seriously flawed and clearly not exculpatory. Furthermore, NCI urged longitudinal studies on women with various types of implants. NCI stated: "This call for further study reflects the paucity of available data on long-term effects of augmentation mammaplasty. Most studies evaluating breast cancer risk have lacked systematic case ascertainment and estimates of expected risk. In the two large-scale epidemiologic studies, only scant information on possible disease covariates was available, limiting the ability to evaluate observed relationships. In addition, the devices evaluated were for the most part markedly different in design and material from those currently in use. Thus, further follow-up of a large cohort of women is needed, with particular attention given to effects of specific types of implants. Senior FDA scientists have also confirmed that sufficient time has not elapsed to record epidemiologically significant increases in human malignancies involving silicone gel implants.

This petition, based on thirty-five scientific references, was submitted by:

Samuel S. Epstein, M.D.
Chairman, Cancer Prevention Coalition
Professor Occupational and Environmental Medicine
University of Illinois School of Public Health, Chicago

Michael Deutsch, Esq.
Legal Director, Center for Constitutional Rights, New York

February 4, 1992

The Push for Mammography May Be Off Target

The Breast Cancer Coalition, a grass-roots group of women's consumer-health and provider organizations and the American Cancer Society, is holding hearings in Washington Wednesday to focus on the breast cancer epidemic now striking one in nine women.

Last year, the coalition succeeded in increasing the National Cancer Institute's budget by $30 million for research into causes, screening and treatment of breast cancer. The coalition is now pressing for even more NCI funds, but it has been co-opted into supporting discredited policies of the lavishly funded cancer establishment.

The establishment—NCI and American Cancer Society—concentrates on basic research, diagnosis and treatment. Cancer cause and prevention net only about 5% of the $1.8 billion annual NCI budget. The establishment is also closely interlocked with giant pharmaceutical firms whose cancer-drug sales net $1 billion annually.

Neither the establishment nor the coalition has recognized that the increase in breast cancer incidence, 57% since 1950, is similar or less than increases for other cancers: 44% for all cancer, 60% for male colon cancer, 100% for testis, prostate and kidney cancer, and over 100% for other cancers.

Also unrecognized is mounting evidence relating cancer increased to avoidable contamination of food, air and water and the workplace presence of cancer-causing industrial chemicals and radiation.

The establishment, with coalition support, is pushing for more mammography facilities. But the General Accounting Office reports, "There are more than enough machines to meet screening needs."

The establishment is also pushing for annual mammograms over age 40. There is general agreement that mammography improves cancer detection and survival in postmenopausal women, especially in modern facilities. But there is no evidence of benefit for younger women in whom screening, especially with x-ray exposures common on the '70's, caused more cancers than detected.

These concerns are emphasized by a recent Canadian study reporting 50% increased breast cancer mortality in women over 40 given annual mammograms vs. those given physical examinations only. Other studies have confirmed the dangers of routine mammograms in pre-menopausal women.

In spite of evidence since the '60's, women have never been warned of mammography risks. The reasons may be explained by a confidential memo form an NCI physician in charge of large-scale NCI and ACS screening in 1973. These programs, he confided, "will gain [us] a great deal of favorable publicity—and will assist in obtaining more research funds."

The coalition needs to rethink its policies on mammograms. Screening young women should be abandoned. Obsolete high-dose equipment should be banned, as should untrained mammogram entrepreneurs. The role of past mammography in increasing cancer rates must be admitted and investigated. Women must be informed of their x-ray dosage from each screening and warned of the cancer risk.

Apart from physical examination, safe alternatives to mammography, particularly transillumination with infrared light scanning, should be developed and made available on a crash basis.

The cancer establishment insists that fatty diet itself is a major cause of breast cancer, although proof for this is minimal at best. There is, instead, growing evidence of the role of carcinogenic pesticides and other contaminants in fat, such as DDT and PCBs which accumulate in the breast and which mimic the hormonal effects of estrogens. A related risk is lifelong exposure to estrogenic contaminants in dietary fat from their unregulated use of growth-promoting cattle-feed additives.

Public health is too important to be left to self-interested establishment professional and politicized bureaucracies. But to be effective, grass-roots advocacy requires radical new thinking besides good intentions.

The Breast Cancer Coalition should heed today's Washington Press conference, representing 60-plus prominent scientists who demand a total overhaul of federal cancer policies and who charge the cancer establishment with disinterest in cancer prevention and with misleading the nation into believing that we are "winning the war against cancer" while the facts show the contrary to be the case.

March 28, 1992

Los Angeles Times

Mammography Radiates Doubt

It has been widely (and with reason) charged that the makers and marketers of silicone breast implants, and self-interested plastic surgeons, made women their guinea pigs. But what of that other, and greater, scourge of women, breast cancer? There is reason to believe that, women are equally ill-served by the cancer establishment, especially in its unrelenting promotion of mammography.

Breast cancer now strikes one in nine women, a dramatic increase from the one in 20 measured in 1950. This year, 180,000 new cases and 46,000 deaths are expected. Hearings scheduled Feb. 5 in Washington by the Breast Cancer Coalition, an advocacy group loosely modeled on AIDS activists, could not seem more timely.

The coalition wants more federal funding for the National Cancer Institute (NCI) to increase its research into the causes and treatment of breast cancer, and to improve delivery of breast health care—including diagnostic screening. In pursuing these goals, the coalition has been co-opted into supporting the policies of the cancer Establishment—NCI and the American Cancer Society—which is fixated on basic research, diagnosis and treatment. Cancer prevention receives only an estimated 5% of the annual $1.8 billion NCI budget.

Breast cancer is not the only cancer on the rise. While its incidence has increased 57% since 1950, overall cancer has increased 44%, now striking one in three people and killing one in four. Male colon cancer is up 60%, testis, prostate and kidney cancer up 100%, and other cancers, such as malignant melanoma and multiple myeloma, more than 100%. The cancer Establishment trivializes evidence linking these increasing rates with avoidable exposure to cancer-causing industrial chemicals and radiation that permeate our environment—food, water, air and workplace.

The cancer Establishment maintains, on tenuous evidence, that a fatty diet itself is a major cause of breast cancer, while ignoring contaminants in fat. Carcinogenic pesticides, such as the highly persistent chlordane and dieldrin, which concentrate in animals fats, are known to cause breast cancer in rodents. Elevated levels of DDT and PCBs are found in human breast cancer deaths in younger women recently dropped by 30%, despite a substantial increase in consumption of animal fat. This drop followed, and seems linked to, regulations that reduced previously high levels of DDT and related pesticides in dairy products. These pesticides act by mimicking the action of estrogens or by increasing estrogen production in the body, which in turn increases the risk of breast cancer. A related concern is lifelong exposure of all women to estrogenic contaminants in animal fat, because of their unregulated use as growth-promoting additives in cattle feed.

In 1977, NCI's director of endocrinology, Dr. Roy Hertz, warned, without effect, of breast cancer risks from these contaminants.

More ominous is the enthusiastic endorsement by the cancer Establishment of massive nationwide expansion of x-ray mammography, including routine annual screening. While there is a general consensus that mammography improves early cancer detection and survival in post-menopausal women, no such benefit is demonstrable for younger women.

Furthermore, there is clear evidence that the breast, particularly in premenopausal women, is highly sensitive to radiation, with estimates of increased risk of breast cancer of up to 1% for every rad (radiation absorbed dose) unit of x-ray exposure. This project up to a 20% increased cancer risk for a woman who, in the 1970s, received 10 annual mammograms of an average two rads each. In spite of this, up to 40% of women over 40 have had mammograms since the mid-1960s, some annually and some with exposures of 5 to 10 rads in a single screening from older, high-dose equipment.

Significant studies on radiation risks to the breast have been well known since the late 1960s, including evidence that mammography, especially in younger women, was likely to cause more cancers than could be detected. A confidential memo by Dr. Nathaniel Berlin, a senior NCI physician in charge of large scale mammography screening, in 1973 may explain why women were not warned of this risk: "Both the [American Cancer Society] and NCI will gain a great deal of favorable publicity [from screening, and] . . . this will assist I n obtaining more research funds for basic and clinical research which is sorely needed."

Thus, once again, suspect technology was applied to women on a large scale, in spite of clear warning signals and with insufficient knowledge of the likely consequences. (On a smaller scale, but even more ethically appalling, was the use until last April of industrial polyurethane foam to coat silicone breast inserts, despite clear evidence that its manufacturing contaminants and breakdown products were carcinogenic. As with mammography, no serious studies have been launched to find out what happened to women n whom the foam was implanted, or indeed to women carrying any type of silicone implant.)

The risks of mammography, especially for premenopausal women, persist with the lower radiation doses (about one-half rad per screening) found in modern facilities with dedicated equipment and licensed operators. A large Canadian study conducted from 1980 to 1988 found a 52% increase in early breast cancer deaths in women aged 40 to 50 who had 10 annual mammograms, compared to women given just physical examinations. More recent concern comes from evidence that 1% of women carry a gene that increases their breast cancer risk from radiation four-fold.

The coalition should insist that the NCI and American Cancer Society initiate an immediate, large-scale, well-publicized study to further investigate the role of past mammography in increasing breast cancer rates, and to investigate future cancer risk from mammography as currently conducted under widely varying conditions. Women should also be informed of their x-ray exposure and individual and cumulative risks each time they undergo mammography. The coalition should demand an immediate ban on obsolete high-dose x-ray equipment, and the abandonment of routine mammograms on premenopausal women.

The coalition should also encourage a crash program to develop and make available safe alternatives to mammography, apart from physical examination. Two that show the most promise are magnetic resonance imaging and trans-illumination with infrared light. The expansion of mammography should be put on hold, especially in view of the 1991 conclusion of the General Accounting Office that there are more than enough machines to meet the screening needs of American women.

The Breast Cancer Coalition represents a welcome trend toward active grass-roots involvement in public health. However, its current goals are too narrowly defined within the context of existing perspectives and institutional policies. The coalition needs broader and more radical strategies if it is to reverse the modern epidemic of breast cancer.

March 2, 1993

The Cancer Establishment Ignores Avoidable Causes of Breast Cancer: Need for Initiatives by the New York City Commission on the Status of Women and by Wedo

Despite expenditures of over $1 billion on breast cancer over the last two decades, "we must conclude that there has been no progress in preventing the disease." The cancer establishment, the National Cancer Institute (NCI) and American Cancer Society (ACS), has long been, and still is, fixated on diagnosis and treatment and indifferent to or ignorant of cancer prevention. Establishment programs on breast cancer prevention reflect myopia and questionable science, as illustrated by their unsupported emphasis on high fat diet as the major cause. This is compounded by neglect of or unfamiliarity with longstanding evidence incriminating a wide range of environmental causes, particularly avoidable exposures to chemical and radioactive carcinogens (notably large scale emissions and discharges from civilian nuclear reactors) in air, water, food, and the workplace. Equally alarming is the cancer establishment's exploitation of women as scientific guinea pigs as evidenced by: their deliberate exposure of some 300,000 women without warning to high dose mammography in the 1970's; their failure to warn against breast cancer risks of the injectable contraceptive Depo-Provera; and by the grave risks of their ill-conceived breast cancer prevention trial with the carcinogenic drug Tamoxifen.

Carcinogenic Dietary Contaminants

None of the cancer establishment's heavily funded nutritional studies claiming associations between dietary fat and breast cancer (besides colon and other cancers) have investigated or even considered the role of carcinogenic dietary contaminants. Evidence for their role has accumulated over the last two decades and includes the following:

- Carcinogenic organochlorine pesticides, such as DDT, chlordane and dieldrin, which concentrate in animal fats, induce breast cancer in rodents. This creates the strong presumption for a causal role of such dietary contaminants in human breast cancer, particularly as the sites of cancer induced by carcinogens are generally similar in experimental animals and humans.

- Promotion by DDT of breast cancers induced in rodents by the potent carcinogen acetamidophenanthrene.
- DDT and PCBs concentrate in human breast cancer itself in contrast to adjacent non-cancerous tissue, and also in breasts with cancer in contrast to those with fibrocystic disease.
- Breast cancer mortality in premenopausal Israeli women declined by 30 percent following regulations in the mid 1970's reducing levels of DDT and other carcinogenic organochlorine pesticides in dietary fat, in spite of increasing fat consumption and decreasing birth rates.
- In view of the known carcinogenicity of exogenous estrogens, lifelong exposure to estrogenic contaminants in meat due to their unregulated use as growth-promoting feed additives, is clearly a risk factor for breast cancer. Warnings of such risks, including by Dr. Roy Hertz NCI's former leading expert in endocrinology, have gone unheeded.
- Exogenous estrogens synergize the carcinogenic effects of irradiation, and also of polynuclear hydrocarbon carcinogens in the rodent breast.

It may be further noted that the cancer establishment remained silent while the Bush Administration revoked the 1958 Delaney law banning the deliberate contamination of processed foods with carcinogenic pesticides.

Mammography

While there is general consensus that mammography improves early cancer detection and survival in post menopausal women, no such benefits have been demonstrated for younger women. Additionally, there is clear evidence that the breast, particularly in pre-menopausal women, is highly sensitive to the carcinogenic effects of radiation. Although this was well known since the late 1960's, the NCI and ACS embarked on a large scale Breast Cancer Detection Demonstration Program using high radiation exposures which, as admitted by a senior NCI epidemiologist then involved in the program, were likely to cause more breast cancers than could be detected. These concerns persist today, even with lower level radiation exposure. This is evidenced by several studies which show excess breast cancer mortality in pre-menopausal women receiving repeated mammograms. Available scientific information justifies the following recommendations:

- Pressures for expansion of the mammography industry should be strongly resisted, especially in view of the conclusion that "there are more than enough machines to meet the screening needs of American women."
- Mammography should be restricted to post-menopausal women.
- Mammography should be conducted only in major medical centers with licensed technicians using dedicated equipment calibrated at regular intervals.
- Women should be provided with information on actual, not just estimated, radiation doses at each mammography.
- The use of mammography should be phased out. Crash programs should be developed to develop and make available safe and similarly effective screening procedures, particularly transillumination with infrared light scanning.

It should further be stressed that the carcinogenic effects of "low dose" radiation are disproportionately greater than those from a single cumulative equivalent large dose exposure, and also that a significant proportion of the general population have high genetic sensitivity to radiation-induced breast cancer.

Depo-Provera

Depo-Provera (DP) is synthetic progesterone given by injection for long term contraception. Its use was approved by the Bush administration's Food and Drug Administration (FDA) in June 1992 in spite of unequivocal evidence of its carcinogenicity. DP induces breast cancer in mice and dogs. This evidence has been confirmed by recent international epidemiological studies demonstration high risks of breast cancer, particularly when DP's use is started before the age of 20 and continued for over two years. Other complications, include osteoporosis, depression, loss of libido, and substantial weight gain. Incredibly, the NCI and ACS have remained silent while this new major breast cancer risk has been introduced in the U.S.

Based on experience abroad, there seems little doubt that this dangerous contraceptive will be selectively offered to low income ethnic minority groups, just those women with the least power and most easily coerced.

The Tamoxifen Trial

In spring 1992, the NCI embarked on a large scale breast cancer trial recruiting thousands of healthy women at increased risk of breast cancer, including those with close relatives with the disease and also anyone over 60. Half these women are being treated with Tamoxifen, a drug closely related to DES, while the rest receive a placebo. NCI claims that Tamoxifen can reduce breast cancer by 30%, while also reducing heart attacks and preventing osteoporosis.

Not only is there no scientific basis for the alleged benefits of Tamoxifen, but there is also substantial evidence of its grave risks of liver ad uterus cancer, besides a wide range of other toxic effects. Any oncologist or institute participating in these trials is at serious risk of future malpractice and punitive claims.

The Role of New York City Commission and Wedo

It is recommended that the Commission and WEDO set up a series of task forces to investigate the following: the failure of the cancer establishment to undertake programs on breast cancer prevention; their failure to warn of avoidable causes of breast cancer; their failure to support available non-hazardous alternatives to mammography; their silence on the carcinogenic hazards of Depo-Provera; and, the scientific and ethical travesty of their Tamoxifen trial.

It is further recommended that the Commission and WEDO widely disseminate information relating escalating breast cancer rates to the overall current cancer epidemic now striking one in three and killing one in four. The involvement of activist women's groups should be extended to even broader concerns on cancer prevention in general.

It is finally recommended, that the Commission and WEDO join with the Cancer Prevention Coalition in appropriate and aggressive action to reform the policies and priorities of the NCI and ACS.

December 28, 1993

New York Times

Radiation's Risks

To the Editor:

The debate on mammography reflects flawed science and misplaced emotionalism (front page, Dec. 27). Despite more than three decades of large-scale experience in the United States and elsewhere, no study has shown any benefit for mammography in premenopausal, as opposed to postmenopausal women.

But substantial documentation on radiation risks to the breast has accumulated since the late 1980's. This includes evidence that mammography, especially in younger women whose breasts are sensitive to radiation, is likely to cause more cancer than could be detected. These risks are greater in women who unknowingly carry the A-T gene, which substantially increases risks from radiation cancer.

There is also evidence that radiation can synergize the carcinogenic effects of estrogens from sources such as oral contraceptives.

As an editorial in The Lancet, the British medical journal, emphasizes, recent studies have shown excess breast cancer mortality in premenopausal women receiving repeated mammography. Rather than pressuring the Clinton Administration for ineffective and hazardous mammography in younger women, the American Cancer Society and its supporters would do well to encourage a program to develop and use safer alternatives, such as transillumination with infrared light scanning and magnetic resonance imaging, besides emphasis on training in regular breast self-examination. Meanwhile, there is no reason to extend insurance coverage for premenopausal mammography.

March 20, 1994

Los Angeles Times

A Needless New Risk of Breast Cancer

The Food and Drug Administration recently warned dairy producers, distributors and retailers against "hormone-free" labels on milk from cows that have not been given the biotech milk-production stimulant known as recombinant bovine growth hormone. The FDA states that such labeling could be "false or misleading" under federal law, as there is "no significant difference between milk from treated and untreated cows." Monsanto, maker of the hormone, is already suing one large Midwest milk producer for using the label.

The confusing FDA guidelines were, according to the consumer publication Daily Citizen, written by Deputy Commissioner Michael Taylor, a former counsel for Monsanto and a biotech umbrella organization. The guidelines are scientifically flawed and reckless and reflect flagrant disregard of consumers' right to know. Furthermore, the FDA ignores evidence linking milk from treated cows with increased risk of breast cancer. The concerns, based on published research:

- The biotech hormone induces a marked and sustained increase in levels of insulin-like growth factor-1, or IGF-1, in cow's milk.
- IGF-1 regulates cell growth, division and differentiation, particularly in infants. While human and normal bovine IGF-1 are identical, they are largely bound to protein and thus probably less biologically active than the unbound IGF-1 in treated milk.
- IGF-1 is not destroyed by pasteurization or digestion and is readily absorbed across the intestinal wall. In a 1990 FDA publication disclosing toxicity tests conducted by Monsanto, feeding the hormone (trade name Posilac) to mature rats for only two weeks resulted in statistically significant increases in body and liver weights and bone length. These effects were seen at a small fraction of injected doses given to control rats. But by gerrymandering these explicit data, the FDA alleged that IGF-1 "lacks oral toxicity."

- Neither the FDA nor Monsanto has investigated the effects of long-term feeding of IGF-1 and treated milk on growth, or on more sensitive sub-cellular effects in infant rats or infants of any other species.

Cows injected with the biotech hormone show heavy localization of IGF-1 in breast (udder) epithelial cells; this does not occur in untreated cows.

- IGF-1 induces rapid division and multiplication of normal human breast epithelial cells in tissue cultures.
- It is highly likely that IGF-1 promotes transformation of normal breast epithelium to breast cancer.
- IGF-1 maintains the malignancy of human breast-cancer cells, including their invasiveness and ability to spread to distant organs.
- The breast tissues of female fetuses and infants are sensitive to hormonal influences. Imprinting by IGF-1 may increase future breast-cancer risks and sensitivity of the breast to subsequent unrelated risks such as mammography and the carcinogenic and estrogen-like effects of pesticide residues in food, particularly in premenopausal women.

These concerns are not new. In a 1989 letter to the FDA, I warned that the effects of IGF-1 "could include premature growth stimulation in infants, [breast enlargement] in young children and breast cancer in adult females." More recently, the Council on Scientific Affairs of the American Medical Association stated: "Further studies will be required to determine whether the ingestion of higher-than-normal concentrations of bovine insulin-like growth factor is safe for children, adolescents, and adults." The opposite of "further study" is uncontrolled, unlabeled sales of treated milk to unwitting consumers.

Apart from risks of breast cancer and other IGF-1 effects, the FDA and industry have down-played additional differences between hormonal and non-hormonal milk. The FDA—approved label insert for Posilac, a pamphlet that only dairy farmers see, admits that its "use is associated with increased frequency of use of medication in cows for mastitis and other health problems." Monsanto's own data further show up to an 80% incidence of mastitis, an udder infection, in hormone-treated cattle and resulting contamination of milk with statistically significant levels of pus;

this will necessitate virtually routine use of antibiotics, with attendant risks of allergic reactions and antibiotic resistance.

Congress should insist that, at the very least, the FDA immediately revoke its restrictions on labeling of milk from untreated cows. More prudently, it should ban the use of these hormones.

September 8, 1994

Breast Cancer Deaths Linked to Nuclear Emissions

The Cancer Prevention Coalition today released a report revealing a significant increase in breast cancer mortality rates among U.S. women living near nuclear facilities. Commenting on these findings, the Coalition questioned the methodology used by National Cancer Institute (NCI) scientists in a similar study.

The report, by Drs. Jay Gould and Ernest Sternglass, is based on a nationwide ecological survey of breast cancer mortality rates in 268 counties within 50 miles of five military facilities and 46 civilian nuclear power plants. From 1950 to 1989, age-adjusted cancer mortality rates rose from 24 to 26.4 deaths per 100,000 women, a 10% increase compared with a 4% increase for the nation as a whole.

For the five military plants—Hanford (WA), Idaho (ID), Savannah River (SC), Brookhaven (NY), and Oak Ridge (TN—the rates of increase were even higher, from 20.7 to 29.2 deaths per 100,000 women, a 41% increase. For the seven counties within 40 miles of the Oak Ridge plant, the breast cancer mortality rates increased by 39% for women living in three downwind counties, in contrast to a 4% decrease among women living in four upwind counties. This is consistent with recently published findings of excess cancer mortality rates for both men and women living within a 100 mile radius of the Oak Ridge plant.

Based on these data, Dr. Gould concluded, "Nuclear emissions appear linked to increased breast cancer deaths among women living near these facilities. The public has not been informed of its risks."

In a 1991 Journal of the American Medical Association article, NCI scientists claimed "if . . . any excess cancer risk was present in U.S. counties with nuclear facilities, it was too small to be detected with the methods employed." The Gould/Sternglass study raises serious questions about the particular statistical methods by NCI in that they used inappropriate controls based on small populations that were also exposed to nuclear emissions.

CPC Chair, Dr. Samuel Epstein, stressed the importance of the questions raised by these findings and called for a Congressional investigation and also for further study of past and continuing risks associated with proximity of residents to nuclear plants.

ENDORSERS:

Dr. Jay M. Gould
Radiation and Public Health Project, Director
EPA Science Advisory Board

Dr. Ernest J. Sternglass
Professor emeritus Radiological Physics
University of Pittsburgh School of Medicine

September 9, 1994

Los Angeles Times

Women at Risk Are Still in the Dark

Last week's establishment of a $4.25-billion settlement fund seems to add finality to the breast-implant controversy, even though the judge in the case believes that the amount, contributed by manufacturers, will be insufficient for current claims. The settlement also is insufficient because it ignores the risk of breast cancers developing decades later.

The Food and Drug Administration has consistently downplayed any cancer risk from silicone gel implants. But the agency's sanguine position is contradicted by substantial research, including its own. Why is no one sounding an alarm? Why is no one informing women of their risk and offering all women with breast implants the option of removal?

Studies by manufacturer Dow Corning, discovered in 1987 FDA inspections, showed that silicone-gel injection induced malignant tumors in rats. Internal memoranda by FDA scientists concluded that "while there is no direct proof that silicone causes cancer in humans, there is considerable reason to suspect that it can do so" and urged that "a medical alert be issued to warn the public of the possibility of malignancy following long-term implant(ation)." The FDA's response was to reassign the report's writers. Another report, in the July, 1994, Journal of the National Cancer Institute, confirmed that silicone gel is carcinogenic in mice as well.

Supporting this experimental evidence, a 1989 FDA internal report stated: "A survey of the literature indicates numerous case reports of cancer" long after implantation and warned of the "possibility of worsened diagnosis" and prognosis when implanted women developed breast cancer. The report stressed that population studies claimed as proof of safety by industry and surgeons were too short-term and flawed to "negate the potential risk of cancer."

At known higher risk of breast cancer are 350,000 women with foam-wrapped implants. These consist of a silicone pouch wrapped in industrial polyurethane foam made from the carcinogenic synthetic petrochemical toluene diisocyanate (TDI). The foam is unstable in the body and breaks down into TDI and another carcinogen, TDA, which was removed from hair dyes in 1971 for that reason.

The foam-wrapped implants were developed to reduce scar-like hardening in some women following silicone implantation. However, their use beginning in the early 1980s ignored unequivocal evidence published two decades previously. Beginning in 1960, Wilhelm Hueper, the National Cancer Institute's leading carcinogenesis authority showed that foam degraded and induced malignant tumors in rats following injection and warned: "Since the polyurethane plastics have been used in cosmetic surgery . . . these observations are of practical importance . . . (and) should caution against indiscriminate use." He also noted that carcinogenic effects "might require an induction period of some 30 years or more," as with other carcinogens, notably asbestos. Hueper's finding have since been fully confirmed and extended by other independent studies.

Polyurethane-wrapped implants are thus carcinogen-impregnated sponges. These gradually disintegrate, releasing carcinogens to which the breast cells of premenopausal women are particularly sensitive.

Scientific publications apart, there is extensive documentation on industry's secret knowledge of cancer risks from implants, which were nevertheless aggressively marketed with assurances of safety. Dow Corning's carcinogenicity information on silicone implants is two decades old. Shortly after foam implants were first manufactured, the industry admitted that carcinogenicity data were "significant in those applications . . . for use inside the body." In 1985, Medical Engineering Corp., a Bristol-Myers Squibb subsidiary, admitted that "degradation products of polyurethane are toxic and in some cases carcinogenic . . . . Whether they are released in such low levels as to be no threat, only time will tell . . . . The breakdown products of the fuzzy implant material may well be carcinogenic. How would anyone defend himself in a malpractice suit if a patient developed a breast malignancy?" At industry-sponsored meetings in 1985, leading plastic surgeons cautioned that "foam could be a time bomb . . . (in view of its) carcinogenic potential. Surgeons should not go on implanting."

Without mentioning cancer risk, in April, 1992, the FDA banned all silicone implants except for controlled trials. This action was aggressively challenged by the American Society of Plastic and Reconstructive Surgery, the American College of Radiology and the American Medical Assn.

Responsibility for undisclosed cancer risks in 2 million implanted women, most seriously in the 350,000 with foam implants, is broadly shared among: the industry, for egregious conduct; plastic surgeons, for self-interested complicity; the FDA, for reckless unresponsiveness; the American Cancer Society, for silence, and the media, for minimal coverage of longstanding evidence. An immediate medical alert should be sent to all implanted women, with priority for those with foam implants. This should be followed by long-term surveillance with offers to remove the implants of any concerned women, at industry's but not taxpayers' expense. And all of this should be thoroughly apart from the inadequate $4.25-billion settlement.

September 13, 1994

$4.25 Billion Implant Settlement Ignores Risk of Breast Cancer

The recent $4.25 billion settlement to women with silicone breast implants ignores the risks of developing breast cancer for two million women. Cancer Prevention Coalition (CPC) Chair, Dr. Samuel Epstein said, "The Food and Drug Administration (FDA) and the implant industry have failed to warn women of serious cancer risks, although they have known of this information for decades." CPC urges that women immediately be informed of these risks.

Unpublished Dow Corning studies, from 1976 onwards and discovered in a 1987 FDA inspection, showed that silicone gel injection induced malignant tumors in rats. FDA scientists concluded in 1988 confidential memoranda that: "While there is no direct proof that silicone causes cancer in humans, there is considerable evidence that it can do so," and recommended that, "a medical alert be issued to warn the public of the possibility of malignancy following long term implant(ation)." FDA's only response was to reassign the concerned scientists. A report in the July 1994 Journal of the National Cancer Institute further confirmed gel's carcinogenicity in experiments in mice.

Supporting this experimental evidence, a 1989 confidential FDA report warned: "A survey of the literature indicates numerous case reports of (breast) cancer" long after implantation; that population studies, claimed as proof of safety by industry and plastic surgeons, are too short term and flawed to "negate the potential risk of cancer"; and the "possibility of worsened diagnosis" and prognosis when implanted women developed breast cancer. These criticisms have been confirmed in a 1993 National Cancer Institute (NCI) internal analysis.

At still higher risk are some 350,000 women with silicone implants wrapped in industrial polyurethane foam to reduce scarring. Polyurethane foam is manufactured from the carcinogenic petrochemical toluene diisocyanate (TDI) which breaks down into another carcinogen, TDA. TDI and TDA have also been identified in fresh implants, and TDA has been identified in milk and urine of women with foam implants. It should be further noted that TDA had been removed from hair dyes by the cosmetic industry in 1971 following discovery of its carcinogenicity.

Large scale use of foam-wrapped implants since the 1980s ignored evidence published two decades before by NCI's leading authority on carcinogenesis, the late Dr. Wilhelm Hueper. His studies showed that foam gradually degrades and induces malignant tumors in rats. He warned: "Since the polyurethane plastics have been used in cosmetic surgery, . . . these observations are of practical importance, . . . (and) should caution against (their) indiscriminate use." He also noted that carcinogenic effects "might require an induction period of some 30 years or more," as with other carcinogens such as asbestos.

Dr. Epstein emphasized, "There is extensive previously undisclosed documentation of industry's secret knowledge of cancer risks from implants, which were nevertheless marketed with assurances of safety. In fact, Dow Corning's carcinogenicity information on silicone implants is two decades old." Shortly after foam implants were first marketed on a large scale, a Bristol-Myers subsidiary admitted that: "Degradation products of polyurethane are toxic and in some cases carcinogenic . . . . The breakdown products of the fuzzy implant material may well be carcinogenic. How would anyone defend himself in a malpractice suit of a patient developed a breast malignancy." At a 1985 industry-sponsored conference, a leading plastic surgeon cautioned that "foam could be a time bomb . . . (in view of its) carcinogenic potential. Surgeons should not go on implanting." Following identification of TDA in foam, Bristol-Myers employee warned ". . . there is pretty solid evidence that (it) is a carcinogen. The question is does PU foam . . . release TDA in the human breast to an extent that causes an unacceptable risk of cancer." Of still further concern is the identification in 1987 of residues of the carcinogenic, sterilizing agent ethylene oxide in foam implants.

"Polyurethane implants are carcinogenic-impregnated sponges. The foam gradually disintegrates and releases carcinogens into sensitive breast cells," concluded Dr. Epstein.

CPC urges that an immediate medical alert be sent to all implanted women, with priority for those with foam implants. This should be followed by offers to remove the implants of concerned women at industry's expense, quite apart from the recent $4.25 billion dollar settlement. This should be followed by comprehensive surveillance of all implanted women.

October 14, 1994

Breast Cancer Unawareness Month

Commenting on the anniversary of National Breast Cancer Awareness month (NBCAM), Dr. Samuel Epstein, Chairman of the Cancer Prevention Coalition (CPC) stated, "A decade-old multi-million dollar deal between National Breast Cancer Awareness Month sponsors and Imperial Chemical Industries (ICI) has produced reckless misinformation on breast cancer." Dr. Epstein, a leading international authority on cancer causing effects of environmental pollutants, will be speaking on breast cancer prevention at a conference, "Women, Health, & the Environment" in Albuquerque, New Mexico on October 14-15. It is sponsored by CPC, in conjunction with Greenpeace and Women's Environmental and Development Organization (WEDO).

Zeneca Pharmaceutical, a U.S. subsidiary and recent spinoff of ICI, has been the sole funder of National Breast Cancer Awareness Month since 1984. ICI is one of the largest manufacturers of petrochemical and chlorinated organic products, such as acetochlor and vinyl chloride, and the sole manufacturer of Tamoxifen, the world's top-selling cancer drug used for breast cancer. Financial sponsorship by Zeneca/ICI gives them editorial control over every leaflet, poster, publication, and commercial produced by NBCAM. NBCAM is promoted by the cancer establishment, the National Cancer Institute (NCI) and the American Cancer Society (ACS) with their corporate sponsors.

ICI has supported the NCI/ACS blame-the-victim theory of the causes of breast and other cancers. This theory attributes escalating cancer rates to heredity and faulty lifestyle, rather than avoidable exposures to industrial carcinogens contaminating air, water, food, consumer products, and the workplace.

Dr. Epstein will summarize the evidence on avoidable environmental and other causes of breast cancer ignored in NBCAM promotional materials:

- **Since the 1950's scientific evidence has incriminated chlorinated organic pesticides as breast cancer risk** factors because of their carcinogenicity, estrogenic effects, and accumulation in body fat, particularly the breast.

- **The unregulated use of growth promoting hormonal cattle feed additives has resulted in near universal contamination of meat products.** This results in life-long exposure to carcinogenic estrogens, and poses a major avoidable risk of breast cancer.
- **Where you work increases your breast cancer risks.** Excess breast cancers were found in the 1970's in women working with vinyl chloride. There is similar evidence among petrochemical and electrical workers. In spite of more women working in such industries, NCI recently admitted that it has still not investigated these risks among working women.
- **Where you live increases risks of breast cancer.** Based on a review of 21 New Jersey counties, and more recently 339 nationwide counties, statistically significant associations were found between excess breast cancer mortality and residence in counties where hazardous waste sites are located.
- **Living near a nuclear facility increases your chances of dying from breast cancer.** Based on a nationwide survey of 268 counties within 50 miles of 51 military and civilian nuclear reactors, CPC member Dr. Jay Gould, showed that breast cancer mortality in these "nuclear counties" has increased at 10 times the national rate from 1950 to 1989. Counties near military reactors, such as Hanford, Oak Ridge and Savannah River, have registered the greatest increases, ranging from 27 to 200%. Dr. Gould charged NCI with "misrepresentation of such findings."
- **Premenopausal mammography increases your risk of breast cancer.** Increases in breast cancer mortality have been consistently reported following repeated mammograms in younger women in six randomized controlled clinical trials over the last decade. Based on this evidence, NCI has recently withdrawn recommendations for pre-menopausal mammography. ACS, with financial support from DuPont and General Electric (both heavily invested in mammography equipment), and self-interested radiologists are still promoting this dangerous practice.
- **Participation in the 1972 NCI/ACS reckless, high dose mammography experiments** has increased breast cancer risks for the 400,000 women involved.
- **Breast implants, particularly polyurethane foam, pose serious risks of breast cancer.** Evidence on the carcinogenicity of polyurethane foam dates back to the early 1960's. One breakdown product of polyurethane is 2,4-toluenediamine which was removed from hair dyes in 1971 following discovery of its

carcinogenicity. Frank admission of these risks is found in internal NCI, FDA and industry documents.

- **The Tamoxifen "chemoprevention" trial is a travesty!** Since 1992, the cancer establishment recruited 16,000 healthy women in a Tamoxifen "chemoprevention" trial. NCI and ACS claimed in their patient consent forms that Tamoxifen could substantially reduce breast cancer risks, while trivializing risks of drug complications. There is strong evidence of Tamoxifen's toxicity, including high risks of uterine, gastrointestinal and fatal liver cancer. "This trial is scientifically and ethically reckless, and participating institutions and clinicians are at serious risk of future malpractice claims," warned Dr. Epstein.

"The ICI/NBCAM public relations campaign has prevented women from knowing of avoidable causes of breast cancer," concluded Dr. Epstein.

ENDORSER:

Dr. Jay M. Gould
Radiation and Public Health Project, Director
EPA Science Advisory Board

October 18, 1994

National Mammoscam Day

Commenting on tomorrow's National Mammography Day, Dr. Samuel Epstein, Chairman of the Cancer Prevention Coalition (CPC), charged that "this is a recklessly misleading and self-interested promotional event, more aptly named NATIONAL MAMMOSCAM DAY."

National Mammography Day, October 19, is the flagship of October's National Breast Cancer Awareness Month (NBCAM). NBCAM was conceived and funded in 1984 by Imperial Chemical Industries (ICI) and its U.S. subsidiary and spinoff Zeneca Pharmaceuticals. NBCAM is a multimillion-dollar deal with the cancer establishment, the National Cancer Institute (NCI) and American Cancer Society (ACS) and its multiple corporate sponsors, and the American College of Radiology.

ICI is one of the largest manufacturers of petrochemical and organochlorines, and Zeneca is the sole manufacturer of Tamoxifen, the world's top selling cancer drug widely used for breast cancer. Zeneca/ICI's financial sponsorship gives them control over every leaflet, poster, publication, and commercial produced by NBCAM.

ICI supports the NBCAM blame-the-victim theory of cancer causation, which attributes escalating rates of breast (and other) cancers to heredity and faulty lifestyle. This theory diverts attention away from avoidable exposures to carcinogenic industrial contaminants of air, water, food, consumer products, and the workplace—the same products which ICI has manufactured for decades. Ignoring prevention of breast cancer, NBCAM promotes "early" detection by mammography.

There are a wide range of serious problems with mammography, particularly with premenopausal women:

- There is no evidence of the effectiveness or benefit of mammography in pre-menopausal women.
- By the time breast cancers can be detected by mammography, they are up to 8 years old. By then, some will have spread to local lymph nodes or to distant organs, especially in younger women.
- Missed cancers (false negatives) are commonplace among younger women, as their dense breast tissues limit penetration by x-rays.

33

- About 1 in every 4 "tumors" identified by mammography in pre-menopausal women turns out not to be cancer following biopsy (false positive). Apart from needless anxiety, repeated surgery can result in scarring, and delayed identification of early cancer that may subsequently develop.
- Regular mammography of younger women increases their cancer risks, particularly for women already at risk for familial reasons. Analysis of controlled trials over the last decade, has shown consistent increases in breast cancer mortality within a few years of commencing screening. This confirms evidence on the high sensitivity of the pre-menopausal breast, and on cumulative carcinogenic effects of radiation.
- Pre-menopausal women carrying the A-T gene, about 1.5 percent of women, are more radiation sensitive and at higher cancer risk from mammography. It has been estimated that up to 10,000 breast cancer cases each year are due to mammography of A-T carriers.
- Radiation, particularly from repeated pre-menopausal mammography, is likely to interact additively or synergistically with other avoidable causes of breast cancer, particularly estrogens (natural; medical; contaminants of meat from cattle feed additives; and estrogenic pesticides).
- Forceful compression of the breast during mammography, particularly in younger women, may cause the spread of small undetected cancers.

Pressured by this evidence on the ineffectiveness and risks of pre-menopausal mammography, NCI recently withdrew recommendations for such screening. This evidence is still ignored by NBCAM, supported by radiologists and giant mammography machine and film corporations, which has specifically targeted pre-menopausal women with high-pressured advertisements.

CPC urges the immediate phase-out of pre-menopausal mammography. Post-menopausal mammography should be restricted to major centers and exposure reduced to a minimum. Women should be provided with actual close measurements, rather than estimates. NCI and ACS should develop large-scale use of safe screening alternatives, including imaging techniques, and blood or urine tumor markers or immunologic tests.

Dr. Epstein urges that a medical alert should be sent to women subjected to the Breast Cancer Detection Demonstration Project high dose radiation experiments commencing in 1972. These experiments were conducted in spite of explicit prior warnings by a National Academy of Sciences committee, and also by former senior NCI staffer, and noted epidemiologist, Dr. John Bailar. He cautioned, "Such radiation in pre-menopausal women would be likely to cause more breast cancers than could be detected." Dr. Bailar now concludes, "This experiment could well account for an "immediate investigation of the cancer establishment's reckless conduct by the President's Committee on Human Radiation Experiments."

ENDORSER:

Dr. John Bailar
Professor of Epidemiology and Biostatistics at McGill University, Montreal, Quebec, Canada

May 11, 1995

Cancer Expert Calls Dow Breast Implant Ads Deceptive

Dr. Samuel Epstein, Professor of Environmental and Occupational Medicine at the University of Illinois (at Chicago) School of Public Health and internationally recognized authority on cancer prevention, will present evidence, including an unpublished Dow study, on the cancer risks of silicone breast implants at the May 13 Silicone Device Conference.

"Recent Dow Corning advertisements on the safety of breast implants are deceptive in the extreme and are highly unethical," commented Dr. Epstein.

Dr. Epstein will offer a detailed critique of the Dow ads, in addition to a wide range of other evidence on the cancer risks of breast implants, at the conference to be held at 9:00 a.m. at the Washington Renaissance Hotel, 999 9th St. N.W. Washington, DC. He will charge the implant industry and government with a cover-up of these risks to some two million women. Highlights will include:

Unpublished Dow Corning studies discovered in a 1987 FDA inspection showed that silicone gel injection induced highly malignant tumors in rats. FDA scientists concluded in a confidential memorandum that: "While there is no direct proof that silicone causes cancer in humans, there is considerable evidence that it can do so." Accordingly, it was recommended that "a medical alert be issued to warn the public of the possibility of malignancy following long term implant(ation)."

A 1994 report in the Journal of the National Cancer Institute confirmed the carcinogenicity of silicone gel in experiments with mice.

A 1989 confidential FDA report admitted "numerous case reports of (breast) cancer" long after implantation. The report concluded that population studies, claimed as proof of safety by industry and plastic surgeons, are too short term and flawed to "negate the potential risk of cancer." The report also warned of the "possibility of worsened diagnosis" and prognosis when implanted women developed breast cancer. These conclusions were fully confirmed in a 1993 congressionally-mandated report by the National Cancer Institute (NCI).

Large scale use of foam-wrapped implants ignored evidence published in the early 1960's by NCI's leading authority on carcinogenesis, the late Dr. Wilhelm Hueper. Hueper's studies showed that foam gradually degrades and induces malignant tumors in rats. He warned: "Since the polyurethane plastics have been used in cosmetic surgery . . . these observations are of practical importance . . . (and) should caution against (their) indiscriminate use."

Over 350,000 women with silicone implants wrapped in industrial polyurethane foam to reduce scarring are at higher risk of cancer. Polyurethane foam is manufactured from the carcinogenic toluene diisocyanate (TDI) which breaks down into another carcinogen, TDA. It should be further noted that TDA was removed from hair dyes by the cosmetic industry in 1971 following discovery of its carcinogenicity.

In 1985, a Bristol-Myers subsidiary admitted that: "Degradation products of polyurethane are toxic and in some cases carcinogenic . . . The breakdown products of the fuzzy implant material may well be carcinogenic. How would anyone defend himself in a malpractice suit of a patient developed a breast malignancy."

At a 1985 industry-sponsored conference, a leading plastic surgeon cautioned that "foam could be a time bomb . . . (in view of its) carcinogenic potential. Surgeons should not go on implanting." Following identification of TDA in foam, a Bristol-Myers employee warned ". . . there is pretty solid evidence that (it) is a carcinogen. The question is does PU foam . . . release TDA in the human breast to an extent that causes an unacceptable risk of cancer."

Dr. Epstein will urge that the FDA issue a medical alert to all implanted women, with priority for those with foam implants. He also will urge that these women should be offered a program of comprehensive medical surveillance and be given the option of having their implants removed, both at industry's expense. "Dow Corning and other implant makers should be responsible for all costs," Dr. Epstein said.

ENDORSER:

Jill Stone
Founder
Triad Silicone Network

October 18, 1995

National Mammography Day

Commenting on tomorrow's National Mammography Day, Dr. Samuel Epstein, Chairman of the Cancer Prevention Coalition (CPC), charged that "this is a recklessly misleading and self-interested promotional event, more aptly named NATIONAL MAMMOSCAM DAY."

National Mammography Day, October 19, is the flagship of October's National Breast Cancer Awareness Month (NBCAM). NBCAM was conceived and funded in 1984 by Imperial Chemical Industries (ICI) and its U.S. subsidiary and spinoff Zeneca Pharmaceuticals. NBCAM is a multimillion-dollar deal with the cancer establishment, the National Cancer Institute (NCI) and American Cancer Society (ACS) and its multiple corporate sponsors, and the American College of Radiology.

ICI is one of the largest manufacturers of petrochemical and organochlorines, and Zeneca is the sole manufacturer of Tamoxifen, the world's top-selling cancer drug widely used for breast cancer. Zeneca/ICI's financial sponsorship gives them control over every leaflet, poster, publication, and commercial produced by NBCAM.

ICI supports the NBCAM blame-the-victim theory of cancer causation, which attributes escalating rates of breast (and other) cancers to heredity and faulty lifestyle. This theory diverts attention away from avoidable exposures to carcinogenic industrial contaminants of air, water, food, consumer products, and the workplace—the same products which ICI has manufactured for decades. Ignoring prevention of breast cancer, NBCAM promotes "early" detection by mammography.

There are a wide range of serious problems with mammography, particularly with premenopausal women:

- There is no evidence of the effectiveness or benefit of mammography in pre-menopausal women.
- By the time breast cancers can be detected by mammography, they are up to 8 years old. By then, some will have spread to local lymph nodes or to distant organs, especially in younger women.
- Missed cancers (false negatives) are commonplace among younger women, as their dense breast tissues limit penetration by x-rays.

- About 1 in every 4 "tumors" identified by mammography in pre-menopausal women turns out not to be cancer following biopsy (false positive). Apart from needless anxiety, repeated surgery can result in scarring, and delayed identification of early cancer that may subsequently develop.
- Regular mammography of younger women increases their cancer risks, particularly for women already at risk for familial reasons. Analysis of controlled trials over the last decade, has shown consistent increases in breast cancer mortality within a few years of commencing screening. This confirms evidence on the high sensitivity of the pre-menopausal breast, and on cumulative carcinogenic effects of radiation.
- Pre-menopausal women carrying the A-T gene, about 1.5 percent of women, are more radiation sensitive and at higher cancer risk from mammography. It has been estimated that up to 10,000 breast cancer cases each year are due to mammography of A-T carriers.
- Radiation, particularly from repeated pre-menopausal mammography, is likely to interact additively or synergistically with other avoidable causes of breast cancer, particularly estrogens (natural; medical; contaminants of meat from cattle feed additives; and estrogenic pesticides).
- Forceful compression of the breast during mammography, particularly in younger women, may cause the spread of small undetected cancers.

Pressured by this evidence on the ineffectiveness and risks of pre-menopausal mammography, NCI recently withdrew recommendations for such screening. This evidence is still ignored by NBCAM, supported by radiologists and giant mammography machine and film corporations, which has specifically targeted pre-menopausal women with high-pressured advertisements.

CPC urges the immediate phase-out of pre-menopausal mammography. Post-menopausal mammography should be restricted to major centers and exposure reduced to a minimum. Women should be provided with actual close measurements, rather than estimates. NCI and ACS should develop large-scale use of safe screening alternatives, including imaging techniques, and blood or urine tumor markers or immunologic tests.

Dr. Epstein urges that a medical alert should be sent to women subjected to the Breast Cancer Detection Demonstration Project high dose radiation experiments commencing in 1972. These experiments were conducted in spite of explicit prior warnings by a National Academy of Sciences committee. Finally, Dr. Epstein calls for an "immediate investigation of the cancer establishment's reckless conduct by the President's Committee on Human Radiation Experiments."

November 8, 1995

New Study Warns Implants Pose Risk of Breast Cancer

In the first comprehensive review of the scientific literature, internationally recognized cancer expert, Samuel Epstein M.D., concludes that implants pose significant risks of breast cancer. The study will appear in the November issue of the peer-reviewed International Journal of Occupational Medicine and Toxicology.

The review presents a detailed analysis of the scientific literature and confidential industry and government documents on the carcinogenicity of silicone and polyurethane breast implants.

"Risks of breast cancer have been ignored in the current controversy over implants," stated Dr. Epstein, Chair of the Cancer Prevention Coalition and pathology expert at the School of Public Health, University of Illinois-Chicago. "Evidence on the carcinogenicity of implants, particularly polyurethane, is strong. Recent epidemiological studies claimed as proof of safety are grossly flawed. Such studies would have even given a clean bill of health to asbestos."

Dr. Epstein continued, "Both industry and the Food and Drug Administration (FDA) have suppressed evidence on the cancer risk of silicone breast implants. FDA has still failed to act on the recommendation by their leading scientists to send Medical Alerts to women with silicone implants warning them of their cancer risks."

Based on his report, Dr. Epstein renews the call for a medical alert. He also urges the development of a long-term surveillance program, at industry's expense, with priority for women with polyurethane implants.

October 26, 1997

Chicago Tribune

Awareness Month Keeps Women Perilously Unaware

This October marks the 13th anniversary of the National Breast Cancer Awareness Month (NBCAM), with its flagship Oct. 17 National Mammography Day. Enthusiastically promoted by the "cancer establishment"—the American Cancer Society and the national Cancer Institute—the American College of Radiology and mainstream women's group, NBCAM is dedicated to reducing breast cancer mortality through early detection by mammography screening. With an estimated 180,000 new cases and 44,000 deaths in 1997—breast cancer is second only to lung cancer as the leading cause of cancer death in women—What could be a more worthy objective!

Unfortunately, the primary focus of NBCAM reveals profoundly misguided priorities and a disturbing lack of commitment to prevention. NBCAM is based on the insistence, exemplified by the American Cancer Society's statement in its "Cancer Facts and Figures—1997," that there are no "practical ways to prevent breast cancer . . . . Since women may not be able to alter their personal risk factors, the best opportunity for reducing mortality is through early detection" by mammography. Similarly, The National Cancer Institute's 1995 Special Presidential Commission on Breast Cancer maintained that breast cancer is "simply not a preventable disease" while requesting more funding for research on detection and treatment.

In fact the benefits of annual screening to women age 40 to 50, who are now being aggressively recruited, are at best controversial. In this age group, one in four cancers is missed at each mammography. Over a decade of premenopausal screening, as many as three in 10 women will be mistakenly diagnosed with breast cancer. Moreover, international studies have shown that routine premenopausal mammography is associated with increased breast cancer death rates at older ages. Factors involved include: the high sensitivity of the premenopausal breast to the cumulative carcinogenic effects of mammographic x-radiation; the still higher sensitivity to radiation of women who carry the A-T gene; and the danger that forceful and often painful compression of the breast during mammography may rupture small blood vessels and encourage distant spread of undetected cancers.

Apart from the dangers and questionable value of premenopausal screening is its apparently unrecognized and prohibitive cost of $2.5 billion annually—based on an average of $125 per mammogram for approximately 20 million U.S. women age 40-50—which is more than the budgets of the National Cancer Institute and American Cancer Society combined.

While the benefits of postmenopausal screening are less controversial, there is little evidence that the usual U.S. overkill of taking four or more mammograms per breast annually is any more effective than the more restrained European practice of a single view every two to three years. Furthermore, there is no evidence that screening at any age is more effective than monthly breast self-examination, especially by women trained in this procedure, combined with an annual clinical examination whose costs are minimal,

Underlying this indifference to prevention are interlocking conflicts of interest between the cancer establishment and the cancer drug industry, and between the American Cancer Society and American College of Radiology and the powerful mammography machine and film industries. More significantly, NBCAM was conceived and funded in 1984 by Imperial Chemical Industries, one of the world's largest petrochemical manufacturers, and its U.S. subsidiary and spinoff Zeneca Pharmaceuticals.

Zeneca is the sole manufacturer of tamoxifen, the world's top-selling cancer drug, widely used for treating breast cancer and also for ill-advised trials to see whether it can prevent the disease in healthy women even though it is itself strongly carcinogenic. Of further concern, Zeneca has recently acquired 11 major cancer centers from Salick Health Care, posing disturbing and precedent-setting conflicts of interest between drug manufacture and prescription. Financial sponsorship by Zeneca gives it editorial control over every leaflet, poster, publication and commercial produced by NBCAM. As such, NBCAM is a masterful public relations coup for Zeneca.

With this background, it is hardly surprising that NBCAM fails to inform women how they can reduce their risks of breast cancer. In fact, we know a great deal about its avoidable causes, which include:

- Prolonged use of oral contraceptives and estrogen replacement therapy.
- High-fat animal and dairy product diets that are heavily contaminated with chlorinated pesticides that are estrogenic and carcinogenic to the breast, and meat contaminated with potent sex hormones following their use to fatten cattle in feed lots prior to slaughter.
- Exposure to petrochemical carcinogens in the workplace that put about 1 million U.S. women at increased risk.
- Exposure to carcinogenic chemicals from hazardous waste sites and petrochemical plants that pollute soil, air and water.
- Exposure to indoor air pollutants, including, carcinogenic pesticides and solvents.
- Prolonged use of black and dark brown permanent or semi-permanent hair dyes.
- Heavy smoking and drinking commencing in adolescence,
- Inactivity and obesity.

Making women aware of these avoidable risks rather than fixating just on early detection should be the goal of a truly effective National Breast Cancer Awareness Month.

June 5, 1998

Chicago Tribune

No Safety in These Implant Numbers

The Tribune editorial "seeking shelter from a legal storm" (May 22) on Dow Corning's decision to file for bankruptcy is misleading in the extreme. The Tribune implies that women are lying about health problems they have suffered from silicone-gel breast implants and openly ignores efforts by Dow Corning to suppress its own evidence on the cancer risks of implants.

In a routine, August 1987 inspection, the Food and Drug Administration discovered the previously unreported results of a Dow Corning carcinogenicity test on the silicone gel used in its implants. Injection under the skin of rats induced a high incidence of malignant tumors. While Dow attempted to trivialize these findings by claiming that these cancers were non-specific "solid state tumors," this claim was dismissed by an FDA task force on grounds that these cancers were highly lethal, invaded distant organs and showed no variation in the incidence between male and female rates.

On the basis of these findings, a senior task-force scientist urged that a medical alert be issued to warn the public of the possibility of malignancy developing in humans following long-term implants or silicone breast prostheses. A July 1994 report by a National Cancer Institute investigator subsequently confirmed that silicone gel is also carcinogenic in mice.

At still higher risk of cancer are some 350,000 women with silicone implants wrapped in industrial-grade polyurethane foam. Evidence on the carcinogenicity of polyurethane was clearly demonstrated in the early 1960's. Subsequent studies showed that the foam breaks down in the breast to other carcinogens, toluene diisocyanate (TDI) and toluene diamine (TDA), which also induce breast cancer in rodents. (TDA was removed from hair dyes by the cosmetic industry in 1971 on the grounds of its carcinogenicity.)

Population studies, claimed as proof of safety by Dow and other implant manufacturers, are too short-term and otherwise flawed to negate the risk of cancer in some 2 million implanted women. Indeed, such studies would have exculpated asbestos in addition to most other recognized carcinogens, which have latencies extending over three decades. The study cited most often by industry as evidence of implants' safety was largely funded by plastic surgeons, who clearly have a vested interest in breast implants.

Rather than persisting in its egregious cover-up of the cancer risk of breast implants, apart from recent efforts to file for Chapter 11 to escape liability in breast-implant litigation, Dow Corning should immediately warn all implant women of their cancer risks, offer to remove their implants and develop long-term cancer surveillance at its own expense.

September 1, 1998

FDA Advisory Committee Urged to Reject Zeneca's Application of Tamoxifen for Preventing Breast Cancer in Healthy Women as the Drug Is Ineffective and Dangerous

On September 2, FDA's Advisory Committee on Oncologic Drugs will review Zeneca Pharmaceutical's New Drug Application (NDA) for approval of tamoxifen "for the prevention of breast cancer in (healthy) women at high risk." Claims that tamoxifen can prevent breast cancer are based on an April 6, 1998 National Cancer Institute (NCI) preliminary report, unsupported by a scientific publication, of a short term trial on some 13,000 healthy women at "high risk" of breast cancer, including women over the age of 60, who were randomly given tamoxifen or a placebo; further details of the report are still not available to the scientific community and the public. The trial was terminated prematurely in view of the reduction in the incidence of breast cancer in all tamoxifen treated age groups. However, serious and sometimes fatal complications, including uterine cancer and pulmonary embolism, were seen in postmenopausal women among whom the incidence of breast cancer was reduced by 1.7%, while the incidence of serious complications was increased by 2.2% in non-hysterectomized women.

The brevity of the trial prevented recognition of other delayed serious health risks. Of particular concern is the fact that tamoxifen is a highly potent carcinogen, inducing liver cancer in rats at low doses equivalent, based on blood levels, to those used in the trial. Disturbingly, women in the trial were not informed of the clear evidence of these risks. The absence of reported liver cancer in women treated with tamoxifen for breast cancer is hardly reassuring as relatively few women have been treated for over 5 years and followed up for a further 20 years before which the development of liver cancer would be most unlikely. Additionally, there are serious questions as to whether tamoxifen actually reduced the incidence of breast cancer or merely delayed its onset by treating small undetected tumors. In fact, two articles published on July 11, 1998 in the highly prestigious journal, The Lancet, reported no evidence of breast cancer prevention by tamoxifen in two major European trials.

In an August 17 written statement, which will be read into the record at the September 2 Advisory Committee Hearing, Dr. Epstein concluded:

"NCI's preliminary April 6 report on the prevention of breast cancer by tamoxifen has still not yet been finalized and published in a scientific journal. The Advisory Committee should also consider the propriety of Zeneca's NDA as it is based, in part, on data which have not been made fully available to the public although the underlying (NCI) research was funded by the public. Furthermore, the claimed evidence for chemoprevention has been discredited by two subsequent scientific publications. Of as great concern is the well documented evidence of short term life-threatening complications, and also risks of delayed fatal complications, evidence for which has been trivialized and suppressed by NCI. Based on these scientific and ethical considerations, the Advisory Committee is urged to deny approval of Zeneca's NDA."

Finally, the NDA poses further serious questions in view of Zeneca's control and funding of the heavily promoted annual October National Breast Cancer Awareness Month. This campaign urges women to have mammography, in spite of its highly questionable effectiveness and risks in premenopausal women, while avoiding any reference to a wide range of scientifically documented safe and effective methods for reducing risks of breast cancer. These include avoidance of prolonged and early onset use of oral contraceptives; obesity and inactivity; and high fat and dairy food products contaminated with carcinogenic and estrogenic industrial chemicals. Such critical omissions are favorable to Zeneca's efforts to influence public policy in favor of approval of large scale tamoxifen chemoprevention, targeted for up to 30 million U.S. women at "high risk" of breast cancer.

ENDORSERS:

Barbara Seaman
Co-Founder
National Women's Health Network
Washington, D.C.

Ann Fonfa
Annie Appleseed Project
New York

January 27, 1999

Misleading Claims by an Industry-Sponsored Study on the Safety of the Pill

A January 1999 study, funded by major international pharmaceutical companies, claims that oral contraceptives pose no risks of breast cancer or other ill effects. While the study was alleged to be the largest ever conducted, it was both small scale and insensitive. The study was based on 23,000 healthy women who had "never used" the pill since 1968 and who were subsequently followed up over a 25 year period. The average age of women at termination of the study was only 49, an age when breast cancer is relatively uncommon. Not surprisingly, the authors admitted that the number of breast and other cancers was so small that "further data is needed to confirm our findings."

In contrast, a 1996 large scale international collaborative analysis of some 54 epidemiological studies, based on over 53,000 women with breast cancer and published in The Lancet in1996, demonstrated that use of the pill starting in adolescence increased risks of breast cancer by 60 percent. These risks are clearly underestimates as reflected by the authors 'recognition that "there is little information about use that ceased more than 20 years ago," a latency much too short to preclude further major increases in breast cancer rates. Reliance on studies based on such short latencies would have exculpated the carcinogenicity of asbestos, besides the majority of other recognized human carcinogens. Other better designed and well controlled studies have reported much higher risks of breast cancer for women starting use of the pill in their teens or early twenties, especially with use before a full term pregnancy and subsequent prolonged use, and among women with a family history of breast cancer.

Moreover, the claim that the current low-dose synthetic ethinyl estradiol pill is much safer than the high-dose mestranol pill used in the 1960's and 1970's is misleading as the former is more potent than the latter, besides being some 40-fold more potent than natural estradiol; additionally, ethinyl estradiol, unlike mestranol, binds to estrogen receptors in the breast. Furthermore, the modern pill is used for much longer periods, often from menarche to menopause, than was the case with the earlier high-dose pills. It should further be emphasized that no studies have yet been conducted on the high potency modern pills and none are reportedly in progress. This is in striking contrast to the intensive investigation by Federal regulatory and health agencies on the endocrine-disruptive effects of estrogenic pesticides and other industrial contaminants whose potency is some 1/500,000th that of ethinyl estradiol.

Of related interest, it should be noted that the incidence of estrogen-dependent breast cancers, particularly among post-menopausal women, has increased by 130 percent from the mid 70s in sharp contrast to only a 27 percent increase in non-estrogen dependent cancers. This may well be relevant to the risks of the pill as a major source of incremental estrogen exposure.

Clearly, unqualified claims on the safety of the current pill reflect interests of the pharmaceutical industry rather than scientifically well-based concerns on women's health.

March 14, 2001

Chicago Tribune Opinion Piece

Mammography's Mixed Blessings

Mammography centers nationwide are scaling down or even closing because of inadequate Medicare payments and concerns about possible malpractice suits. While access to mammography is shrinking, the demand is increasing in the wake of aggressive promotion of premenopausal screening by the American Cancer Society.

Women now are waiting weeks or longer for appointments—potentially dangerous delays for those with lumps needing diagnostic mammography. With breast cancer on the increase—and now striking about 192,000 women and killing 41,000 annually—delayed detection promised by mammography surely poses a health care crisis. However, the crisis is more apparent than real, as screening is unreliable, dangerous—and inflationary.

— Mammography is not a technique for early diagnosis as breast cancer is rarely detectable until about eight years old.

— Evidence that screening allows early detection and treatment of breast cancer is tenuous based on analysis of two large trials, Danish researchers writing in the Lancet recently concluded: "There is no reliable evidence that screening decreases breast cancer mortality [and thus that] screening is unjustified."

— The Canadian National Breast Screening Study recently reported on a trial on some 39,000 postmenopausal women. Half of the women performed monthly breast self-examination, following instruction by trained nurses, had annual clinical breast examinations by trained nurses and also annual mammograms. The others practiced self-exams and had annual clinical exams but no mammograms. The authors of the study concluded that the mammographic detection of non-palpable cancers did not improve survival rates.

— False-negative mammograms are particularly common in premenopausal women because of their denser breast structure, and also in postmenopausal women on estrogen replacement therapy as some develop breast densities, making mammograms difficult to read.

— About one-third of all breast cancers and more still of the aggressive premenopausal cancers are discovered in the interval between successive annual mammograms. Premenopausal women particularly can thus be lulled into a false sense of security and fail to seek medical advice.

— False-positive mammograms, common in premenopausal and postmenopausal women on estrogen replacement therapy, result in needless anxiety, additional mammograms or unnecessary biopsies—even mastectomies. For some, the cumulative risk of false positives can reach as high as 100 percent over a decade of screening.

— Over diagnosis is another risk. As screening becomes more common, pre-invasive breast ducts cancer, or ductal carcinoma-in-situ, is now diagnosed annually in some 40,000 women and often unnecessarily treated as invasive cancer by lumpectomy, plus radiation or even mastectomy. However, most of these pre-invasive cancers never become invasive, even if left untreated, and mortality is very low (1 percent)—the same for those diagnosed and treated early or late.

— Screening poses cumulative cancer risks. The routine of taking four films for each breast results in 1 rad (radiation absorbed dose) exposure, about 1,000 times more than a chest x-ray. The premenopausal breast is sensitive to radiation, each rad exposure increasing risk by 1 percent with a cumulative 10 percent increased risk over 10 years of screening; risks are greater for "baseline" screening at younger ages. Less well recognized dangers are posed by forceful breast compression during premenopausal mammography, which may rupture blood vessels in or around small undetected cancers and result in the spread of malignant cells.

— Finally, screening is inflationary; average Medicare and insurance costs are $70 and $125, respectively. If all 20 million premenopausal women had annual mammograms, minimum aggregate costs would be $2.5 billion; costs would reach $10 billion if the industry succeeds in replacing film machines, costing about $100,000, with digital machines, costing about $400,000, for which there is no evidence of improved effectiveness.

The combination of clinical exams and self-exams is effective, safe and low cost, unlike mammography. In 1985, ACS admitted: "At least 90 percent of the women who develop breast carcinoma discover the tumor themselves."

Nevertheless, the National Cancer Institute and the ACS, with ties to the American College of Radiology, and the mammography industry remain dismissive of breast examination as an alternative to mammography. National networks of clinical exam and self-exam clinics staffed by trained nurses should be established. These clinics would further empower women by providing scientific information on breast cancer prevention, of which women remain largely unaware.

ENDORSER:

Barbara Seaman
Co-Founder
National Women's Health Network
Washington, D.C.

May 3, 2001

The National Breast Cancer Coalition (NBCC) Is Urged by Dr. Samuel Epstein to Consider Breast Examination as a Practical Alternative to Mammography

The NBCC's recommendations against premenopausal mammography will be confirmed and extended by leading epidemiologists at its tenth anniversary May 5-9 Washington, D.C. meeting. However, consideration should also be given to promoting the role of breast examination as an effective and safe alternative to screening.

Dr. Anthony Miller, co-investigator of the recent Canadian National Breast Cancer Screening Study, will report on a unique trial of some 39,000 postmenopausal women. Half performed monthly breast self examination (BSE) following instruction by trained nurses, had annual clinical breast examinations (CBE) by trained professionals, and also had annual mammograms. The other half practiced BSE and had annual CBE's but no mammograms; it may be noted that CBE performance by trained nurses was as good, if not better, than the study surgeons. Dr. Miller concluded: "The addition of annual mammography to physical examination has no impact on breast cancer mortality." Thus, mammographic detection of non-palpable cancers failed to improve survival rates.

Dr. Peter Gotzsche will further challenge claims that screening reduces breast cancer mortality by enabling early detection and treatment. Based on recent analysis of two large Swedish trials, he concluded: "There is no reliable evidence that screening decreases breast cancer mortality—(and thus that) screening is unjustified."

As detailed in a review, in press in the International Journal of Health Services, by Dr. Samuel Epstein, Dr. Rosalie Bertell, and Barbara Seaman, reservations on the efficacy, besides hazards, of screening are further stressed by the following considerations:

- Mammography is not a technique for early diagnosis of breast cancer which is rarely detectable until about eight years old. Screening should thus be recognized as damage control rather than, misleadingly, as "secondary prevention."

- Missed cancers are common in premenopausal women due to their dense breast structure, and also in postmenopausal women on estrogen replacement therapy who often develop breast densities, making their mammograms difficult to read. Also, about one third of all cancers, and more of the aggressive premenopausal cancers, are diagnosed between annual screenings. Women can thus be lulled into a false sense of security by an apparently negative mammogram.

- Misdiagnosed cancers are common in premenopausal women, postmenopausal women on estrogen replacement therapy, and women with a strong family history, and can reach 100% over a decade's screening. Misdiagnoses thus result in anxiety, more mammograms, unnecessary biopsies and even mastectomies.

- Over-diagnosis with subsequent overtreatment is among the major risks of mammography. With increased screening, pre-invasive breast duct cancer or ductal carcinoma-in-situ (DCIS), is now diagnosed in some 40,000 women annually and unnecessarily treated as invasive cancer by lumpectomy plus radiation or even mastectomy. However, most DCIS never becomes invasive even if untreated, and mortality is low, 1%, whether diagnosed and treated early or late.

- Screening poses cumulative cancer risks. Contrary to assurances that radiation exposure is trivial, the routine of taking four breast films results in 1 rad (radiation absorbed dose) exposure, in contrast to about one thousandth less for a chest x-ray. The premenopausal breast is highly sensitive to radiation, each rad exposure increasing cancer risk by 1%, resulting in a cumulative 10% increased risk over 10 years screening; risks are greater for "baseline" screening at younger ages. Risks are even higher for silent carriers of the A-T gene, accounting for up to 20% of all cancers. Less recognized dangers are due to the often painful breast compression during premenopausal mammography. This may rupture blood vessels in or around small undetected cancers with resulting lethal spread of malignant cells.

- Concerns on the unreliability, besides dangers, of premenopausal screening are so pervasive that this practice remains unique to the U.S.

- Screening poses an inflationary threat; average Medicare and insurance costs are $70 and $125, respectively. If all 20 million premenopausal women had annual mammograms, minimal costs would be $2.5 billion. These costs would be quadrupled if the industry succeeds in replacing film machines, costing about $100,000, by digital machines, costing about $400,000, for which there is no evidence of improved effectiveness.

Breast examination, CBE combined with BSE, is effective, safe and low in cost in striking contrast with mammography. The American Cancer Society (ACS) admitted in 1985 that "at least 90% of the women who develop breast carcinoma discover the tumor themselves." Nevertheless, the ACS, National Cancer Institute, American College of Radiology, and the mammography industry, all remain dismissive of breast examination. Claims for the benefits of mammography screening at all ages, in a non-peer reviewed ACS publication in the May issue of Cancer, are highly flawed including by "before-after" comparisons of women unstratified by menopausal status.

National networks of CBE and BSE clinics staffed by trained nurses should be established. These clinics could further empower women by them with scientific information on breast cancer prevention of which women still remain largely unaware.

February 6, 2002

Mammography Is Dangerous besides Ineffective

Recent confirmation by Danish researchers of longstanding evidence on the ineffectiveness of screening mammography has been greeted by extensive nationwide headlines. Entirely missing from this coverage, however, has been any reference to the well-documented dangers of mammography.

Screening mammography poses significant and cumulative risks of breast cancer for premenopausal women. The routine practice of taking four films of each breast annually results in approximately 1 rad (radiation absorbed dose) exposure, about 1,000 times greater than that from a chest x-ray. The premenopausal breast is highly sensitive to radiation, each 1 rad exposure increasing breast cancer risk by about 1 percent, with a cumulative 10 percent increased risk for each breast over a decade's screening. These risks are even greater for younger women subject to "baseline screening."

Radiation risks are some four-fold greater for the 1 to 2 percent of women who are silent carriers of the A-T (ataxia-telangiectasia) gene; by some estimates this accounts for up to 20 percent of all breast cancers diagnosed annually.

Since 1928, physicians have been warned to handle "cancerous breasts with care—for fear of accidentally disseminating cells" and spreading the cancer. Nevertheless, mammography entails tight and often painful breast compression, particularly in premenopausal women, which could lead to distant and lethal spread of malignant cells by rupturing small blood vessels in or around small undetected breast cancers.

Missed cancers are common in premenopausal women owing to their dense breasts, and also in postmenopausal women on estrogen replacement therapy.

Mistakenly diagnosed cancers are common. For women with multiple risk factors including a strong family history and early menarche—just those strongly urged to have annual mammograms—the cumulative risks of false positives can reach as high as 100 percent over a decade's screening.

The widespread acceptance of screening has lead to over diagnosis of pre-invasive cancer (ductal carcinoma in situ), sometimes treated radically by mastectomy and radiation, and even chemotherapy.

As increasing numbers of premenopausal women are responding to aggressively promoted screening, imaging centers are becoming flooded. Resultantly, patients referred for diagnostic mammography are now experiencing potentially dangerous delays, up to several months, before they can be examined.

The dangers and unreliability of screening are compounded by its growing and inflationary costs. Screening all premenopausal women would cost $2.5 billion annually, about 14 percent of estimated Medicare spending on prescription drugs. These costs would be increased some fourfold if the highly profitable industry, enthusiastically supported by radiologists, succeeds in replacing film machines, costing about $100,000 each, with the latest high-tech digital machines recently approved by the FDA, costing about $400,000 each, for which there is no evidence of improved effectiveness.

The ineffectiveness and dangers of mammography pose an agonizing dilemma for the millions of women anxious for reassurance of early detection of breast cancer. However, the dilemma is more apparent than real. As proven by a September 2000 publication, based on a unique large-scale screening study by University of Toronto epidemiologists, monthly breast self-examination (BSE) following brief training, coupled with annual clinical breast examination (CBE) by a trained health care professional, is at least as effective as mammography in detecting early tumors, and also safe. National networks of BSE and CBE clinics staffed by trained nurses should be established to replace screening mammography. Apart from their minimal costs, such clinics would empower women and free them from increasing dependence on industrialized medicine and its complicit medical institutions.

October 9, 2002

Breast Exams Are Just as Effective as Screening Mammography

Contrary to extensive recent media coverage, the Chinese trial on monthly breast self-examination (BSE), published in the October 2 issue of the Journal of the National Cancer Institute, does not disprove its effectiveness in preventing breast cancer deaths. Furthermore, the study is irrelevant to the well-documented effectiveness of BSE, especially when combined with annual clinical breast examination (CBE) by a trained professional.

Contrary to media reports that the Chinese self-exams were done regularly, the researchers admit that BSE was practiced "roughly every 4-5 months" during the first 4-5 years of the 10-year trial, and with unknown frequency subsequently. The researchers also admit evidence, from numerous studies over the last two decades, that: breast cancers detected by BSE "tend to be diagnosed at an earlier stage and to be smaller than cancers diagnosed in the absence of any screening"; that women "practicing BSE tend to have their tumors diagnosed at an earlier stage than women who do not report practicing BSE;" that "women who regularly and competently practice BSE are more likely to find their tumors themselves than women who practice BSE less diligently"; and that tumor size is "inversely associated with the frequency of practicing BSE."

Surprisingly, in their listing of 44 references, the researchers omit reference to the landmark 2000 Canadian National Breast Cancer Screening Study which demonstrates the effectiveness of breast exams in reducing breast cancer mortality. This evidence is confirmed in an editorial commenting on the Chinese study publication: "There is evidence that excellent physical examination practice, whether CBE or BSE, may indeed be effective. Not only is there case-control evidence that excellent BSE may reduce mortality, there is also randomized, controlled trial evidence that excellent CBE done by trained nurse-examiners may be as effective as mammography in reducing breast cancer mortality. The addition of annual mammography screening to physical examination has no impact on breast cancer mortality."

Over the 10-year period of the Chinese trial, the incidence of benign tumors, or false positives, was approximately twice as high in the BSE group as in the controls. This contrasts with a three-fold higher incidence noted in the Canadian mammography group. Such false positives, or over diagnosis, usually lead to unnecessary biopsies and even surgery.

It should be further stressed that, apart from the importance of self-empowering women, the costs of BSE and CBE are trivial compared to the inflationary impact of film mammography. The estimated annual costs for screening pre—and post-menopausal women is about $10 billion, about 5 percent of the $200 billion Medicare budget or about 14 percent of Medicare spending on prescription drugs. Costs for digital mammography, enthusiastically supported by radiologists in the absence for evidence in improved effectiveness, would be approximately four-fold greater.

May 16, 2007

Avoidable Causes of Breast Cancer

The Silent Spring Institute must be warmly commended for compiling very important and well-documented reports on environmental causes of breast cancer, termed "mammary gland carcinogens."

These reports clearly incriminate a wide range of industrial chemicals which have been shown over recent decades to induce breast cancer in standard carcinogenicity tests in rats and mice.

Surprisingly, however, the reports make no reference to unarguable epidemiological evidence on other "mammary gland carcinogens," particularly FDA approved drugs; oral contraceptives; estrogen replacement therapy; and rBGH, a genetically engineered drug, injected in cows to increase milk production.

A long-standing series of studies over the last three decades have clearly incriminated hormonal contraceptives as major risks of breast cancer. These include:

- A 1981 study in the British Journal of Cancer reported a nearly four-fold increased risk in young women who had used oral contraceptives for eight years before their first pregnancy.
- In 1982, the American Journal of Epidemiology announced that women aged 35 to 54 who used oral contraceptives before their first childbirth tripled their risks of breast cancer.
- A 1987 study in the British Journal of Cancer reported that women under the age of 45 who had used the Pill for over four years before their first full-term pregnancy more than doubled their risk.
- A 1988 study published in Neoplasia reported that the risk of breast cancer increased with duration of use of the Pill, particularly for seven or more years. This risk increased to more than seven fold in women with a family history.
- In 1988, the Cancer and Steroid Hormone Study, published in Contraception, revealed that women who had used oral contraceptives for eight years or more, who had never given birth, and who had begun menstruating before the age of 13 were at increased risk for developing breast cancer before the age of 45.

The risk was nearly three-fold for eight to eleven years of use, and twelve fold for twelve or more years of use.

- In 1995, a National Cancer Institute study found a strong link between the length of time oral contraceptives are used and breast cancer risk. A few months of use could increase a woman's risk by 30 percent. An over two-fold risk was found with ten years of use.

The evidence incriminating estrogen replacement therapy (ERT) as a major risk of breast cancer is also long standing and extensive.

- In 1991, an American Journal of Epidemiology article cited eight major studies demonstrating up to 80 percent increased risk of breast cancer among women using ERT for extended periods.
- In 1991, pooled results from sixteen previous studies, published in the Journal of the American Medical Association, found that women who used ERT for fifteen years increased their risk of breast cancer by 30 percent. Ten fold higher risks were reported among women with a family history of breast cancer.
- In 1995, the Harvard Nurses' Health Study confirmed an increased risk of 30 to 70 percent for women on ERT.
- A large-scale study, based on 60,000 postmenopausal women, published in the 1997 New England Journal of Medicine, showed that the use of ERT for over 10 years increased breast cancer deaths by 43 percent.

Also surprising is the failure of the report to make any reference to over 20 publications demonstrating up to a seven fold increased risk of breast cancer from consumption of milk from cows injected with the genetically engineered bovine growth hormone rBGH drug, as approved by the FDA. This evidence is detailed by the author and four colleagues in a May 11, 2007 Citizen Petition to the FDA (www.preventcancer.com).

Evidence of these avoidable causes of breast cancer also lends urgent support for current Senate proposals calling for radical reform of the U.S. Food and Drug Administration to ensure that drugs are safe as advertised.

October 16, 2007

The Breast Cancer Awareness Month Misleads Women

In 1984, the American Cancer Society (ACS) inaugurated the National Breast Cancer Awareness Month (NBCAM), with its October 17 flagship National Mammography Day. The NBCAM was conceived and funded by the Imperial Chemical Industries, a leading international manufacturer of petrochemicals, and its U.S. subsidiary Zeneca Pharmaceuticals. Zeneca is the sole manufacturer of Tamoxifen, claimed to reduce risks of breast cancer, even though it is toxic and carcinogenic.

The NBCAM assured women that "early (mammography) detection results in a cure nearly 100% of the time." More specifically, the NBCAM is primarily directed to claims for reducing the incidence and mortality of breast cancer through early detection by annual mammography starting at age 40.

Still unrecognized by the ACS, and also the National Cancer Institute (NCI), is strong evidence that mammography poses significant risks of breast cancer. The routine practice of taking four films annually for each breast results in approximately 1 rad (radiation absorbed dose) exposure, which is approximately 1,000 times the dose from a single chest x-ray. Each rad exposure increases risks of breast cancer by about one percent, with a cumulative 10 percent increased risk for each breast over a decade's screening.

Moreover, the premenopausal breast is highly sensitive to radiation. Not surprisingly, premenopausal mammography screening is practiced by no nation other than the U.S.

Risks of premenopausal mammography are some four-fold greater for the one to two percent of women who are carriers of the A-T gene (ataxia telangiectasia), and highly sensitive to the carcinogenic effects of radiation. By some estimates, this accounts for up to 20 percent of all breast cancers diagnosed annually.

Compounding these problems, missed cancers are common in premenopausal women due to the density of their breasts.

That most breast cancers are first recognized by women was admitted in 1985 by the ACS. "We must keep in mind that at least 90% of the women who develop breast cancer discover the tumors themselves." Furthermore, an analysis of several 1993 studies showed that women who regularly performed breast self-examination (BSE) detected their cancers much earlier than women failing to examine themselves. The effectiveness of BSE however depends on training by skilled professionals, enhanced by annual clinical breast examination by a professional. In spite of such evidence, the ACS and radiologists dismiss BSE, and claim that "no studies have clearly shown the benefit of using BSE."

A leading Massachusetts newspaper featured a photograph of two women in their twenties in an ACS advertisement that promised early detection by mammography results in a cure "nearly 100 percent of the time." An ACS communications director, questioned by journalist Kate Dempsey, responded in an article published in the Massachusetts Women's Community's journal Cancer "The ad isn't based on a study. When you make an advertisement, you just say what you can to get women in the door. You exaggerate a point . . . Mammography today is a lucrative [and] highly competitive business." She just couldn't be any more correct.

With this background, it is not surprising that the NBCAM neglects to inform women how they can reduce their risks of breast cancer. In fact, we know a great deal about its avoidable causes which are trivialized or ignored by the ACS. These include:

- Prolonged use of the Pill or estrogen replacement therapy.
- High consumption of meat which is heavily contaminated with potent natural or synthetic estrogens, or other sex hormones, implanted in cattle in feedlots prior to slaughter to increase muscle mass.
- Prolonged consumption of milk from cows injected with a genetically engineered growth hormone to increase milk production. This milk is contaminated with high levels of a natural growth factor, which increases breast cancer risks by up to seven-fold.
- Prolonged exposure to a wide range of unlabeled hormonal ingredients in cosmetics and personal care products.
- Living near hazardous waste sites, petrochemical plants, power lines, and nuclear plants.

- Occupational exposures of over one million women to carcinogens. These include benzene, ethylene oxide, methylene chloride, phenylenediamine hair dyes, and agricultural pesticides, including DDT residues.

ENDORSER:

Rosalie Bertell, PhD

Former President of the International Institute of Concern for Public Health, Toronto, Canada

Regent of the International Physicians for Humanitarian Medicine, Geneva, Switzerland

July 22, 2009

Safe Breast Self-Examination by Young Women Vs. Risky Mammography

Critics of a Bill promoting training secondary school students to do breast self examinations to detect cancer are ignoring the risks of premenopausal mammography.

On March 26 this year, Representatives Debbie Wasserman-Schultz (D-FL) and Amy Klobuchar (D-MN), supported by other leading Representatives introduced the Breast Cancer Education and Awareness Requires Learning Young, <u>EARLY</u>, Act of 2009. The object of this Act is "to increase awareness of the risks of breast cancer in young women, and to provide support for those diagnosed with breast cancer." The bill has 260 co-sponsors, enough to guarantee passage by the House. However, the measure has stalled in the Senate.

The Bill met with a storm of protests by "experts in breast cancer prevention." These included Dr. Donald Berry, chairman of the Department of Biostatistics at the M.D. Anderson Cancer Center, who warned that the bill is misguided. "I leave politics to the politicians, why can't they leave science to the scientists? Except for family history, there are no important risks . . . for women younger than 40."

Dr. Leslie Bernstein, director of the City of Hope Comprehensive Cancer Center, also claimed that "We have no known environmental causes of breast cancer other than radiation . . . except when you are having a mammogram," a surprising and damaging admission.

However, these and other critics of EARLY are unaware of the scientific evidence on a wide range of avoidable causes of breast cancer. These include the Pill, estrogen replacement therapy, and living close to hazardous waste sites and nuclear plants.

Not surprisingly, the American Cancer Society (ACS), a strong proponent of routine premenopausal mammography, failed to comment on EARLY. In 1984, with its October flagship National Mammography Day, the ACS inaugurated the National Breast Cancer Awareness Month. This assured women that annual mammography starting at the age of 40 "results in a cure nearly 100 percent of the time." However, and still denied by the ACS, screening mammography poses significant dangers of radiation.

The routine practice of taking two films of each breast annually over 10 years, results in approximately 0.5 rad (radiation absorbed dose) exposure. This is about 500 times greater than exposure from a single chest x-ray, broadly focused on the entire chest rather than narrowly on the breast. Moreover, the premenopausal breast is highly sensitive to radiation. Each rad exposure increases risks of breast cancer by about 1%, with a cumulative 5% increased risk for each breast over a decade's screening. So, a premenopausal woman having annual mammograms over 10 years is exposed to roughly 5 rads. This is the approximate level of radiation received by a Japanese woman a mile or so away from where the Hiroshima or Nagasaki atom bombs were exploded.

Radiation risks are increased by fourfold for the 1% to 2% of women who may be unknowing and silent carriers of the A-T (ataxia-telangiectasia) gene, and thus highly sensitive to the carcinogenic effects of radiation. By some estimates, this accounts for up to 20% of all breast cancers diagnosed annually.

Of additional concern, missed cancers are common in premenopausal women due to the density of their breasts. Mammography also entails tight and often painful breast compression, particularly in premenopausal women. This may lead to the rupture of small blood vessels in or around small undetected breast cancers, and the lethal distant spread of malignant cells.

That most breast cancers are first recognized by women themselves was even admitted as early as 1985 by the American Cancer Society (ACS), the world's largest "non-profit" organization. At least 90 percent of women who develop breast cancer discover the tumors themselves."

As detailed in my 1999 publication in the prestigious *International Journal of Health Services*, the ACS is knee deep in conflicts of interest with the mammography industry. Five radiologists have served as ACS presidents and, in its every move, the ACS promotes the interests of the major manufacturers of mammogram machines and films, including Siemens, DuPont, General Electric, Eastman Kodak, and Piker. The mammography industry also conducts "research" for the ACS, to which it donates considerable funds. This blatant conflict of interest is hardly surprising. *The Chronicle of Philanthropy*, the world's leading charity watchdog, warned in 1993 that the ACS is "more interested in accumulating wealth than saving lives."

Not surprisingly, ACS promotion continues to lure women of all ages into mammography centers, leading them to believe that mammography is their best hope against breast cancer. An ACS communications director, questioned by journalist Kate Dempsey, admitted in an article published by the Massachusetts Women's Community's journal *Cancer*, "The ad isn't based on a study. When you make an advertisement, you just say what you can to get women in the door. You exaggerate a point . . . Mammography today is a lucrative [and] highly competitive business."

Furthermore, an analysis of several 1993 studies showed that women who regularly performed monthly breast self-examination (BSE) detected their cancers much earlier than those who failed to do so. However, the ACS and radiologists still claim that "no studies have clearly shown any benefit of BSE."

Apart from the importance of self-empowering women, the costs of BSE are trivial compared to the inflationary impact of mammography. The estimated annual costs for screening pre—and post-menopausal women are in excess of $10 billion, equivalent to about 14 percent of Medicare spending on prescription drugs. Costs of digital mammography, enthusiastically supported by radiologists and the radiology industry, are approximately four-fold greater, even in the absence of any evidence for its improved effectiveness.

Finally, and not surprisingly, premenopausal mammography is practiced by no nation other than the United States. As recently reported by the British journalist Liz Savage, "Earlier this year, *The Times of London* published a letter, signed by two dozen physicians and patient advocates, reprimanding the UK's National Health Service for not providing women with adequate information about the risks of screening mammography." The letter described "the harms associated with early detection of breast cancer by screening that are not widely acknowledged. The most important of these harms are over-diagnosis—and its frequent consequence, over-treatment."

ENDORSER:

Rosalie Bertell, PhD

Former President of the International Institute of Concern for Public Health, Toronto, Canada

Regent of the International Physicians for Humanitarian Medicine, Geneva, Switzerland

November 24, 2009

Risks of Mammography: Hidden Role of the American Cancer Society

The series of recent articles on mammography which report the harm done by overscreening, written by New York Times columnist Gina Kolata, as well as in other newspapers, have made no reference to the critical role of the American Cancer Society, warns Samuel S. Epstein, M.D., chairman of the Cancer Prevention Coalition.

Five radiologists have served as presidents of the American Cancer Society (ACS). In its every move, the ACS promotes the interests of the major manufacturers of mammogram machines and films, including Siemens, DuPont, General Electric, Eastman Kodak, and Piker.

This bias hypes mammography, which Dr. Epstein and Rosalie Bertell, PhD of the International Physicians for Humanitarian Medicine emphasize is an avoidable cause of breast cancer.

"The mammography industry conducts research for the ACS and its grantees, serves on its advisory boards, and donates considerable funds," they warn. "DuPont also is a substantial backer of the ACS Breast Health Awareness Program; sponsors television shows and other media productions touting ACS literature for hospitals, clinics, medical organization, and doctors; produces educational films; and aggressively lobbies Congress for legislation promoting the nationwide availability of mammography services."

In virtually all its actions, the ACS has been and remains strongly linked with the mammography industry. Meanwhile, it ignores or attacks breast self examination (BSE), following training by expert nurses or clinicians, which is the safe and effective alternative, say Drs. Epstein and Bertell.

ACS promotion continues to lure women of all ages into mammography centers, leading them to believe that mammography is their best hope against breast cancer. A leading Massachusetts newspaper featured a photograph of two women in their twenties in an ACS advertisement that promised early detection results in a cure "nearly 100 percent of the time."

An ACS communications director, questioned by journalist Kate Dempsey, admitted in an article published by the Massachusetts Women's Community's journal Cancer, "The ad isn't based on a study. When you make an advertisement, you just say what you can to get women in the door. You exaggerate a point . . . Mammography today is a lucrative [and] highly competitive business."

Not surprisingly, the prestigious Chronicle of Philanthropy, the leading charity watch dog, has warned that the ACS "is more interested in accumulating wealth than saving lives."

This evidence on the complicity of the ACS was made available to Gina Kolata at her request on October 20th, Dr. Epstein says. However, in her subsequent series of articles, she made no reference to the role of the ACS in concealing the dangers of mammography from the nation's women.

Routine mammography delivers an unrecognized high dose of radiation, warn Drs. Epstein and Bertell. If a woman follows the current guidelines for premenopausal screening, over a 10 year period she would receive a total dosage of about 5 rads. This approximates the level of exposure to radiation of a Japanese woman one mile from the epicenter of atom bombs dropped on Hiroshima or Nagasaki.

"Mammography is a striking paradigm of the capture of unsuspecting women by run-away powerful technological and global pharmaceutical industries, with the complicity of the cancer establishment, particularly the ACS, and the rollover mainstream media," they warn.

Drs. Epstein and Bertell emphasize, "Promotion of the multibillion dollar mammography screening industry has also become a diversionary flag around which legislators and women's product corporations can rally, protesting how much they care about women, while studiously avoiding any reference to avoidable risks of breast cancer.

Screening mammography should be phased out in favor of annual clinical breast examination, (CBE), by a trained nurse and monthly breast self examination (BSE), also following training by a trained nurse. This is an effective, safe, and low-cost alternative, to diagnostic mammography, the two experts advice.

"Such action is all the more critical and overdue in view of the still poorly recognized evidence that mammography does not lead to decreased breast cancer mortality," they say.

Drs. Epstein and Bertell envision nationwide networks of BSE and CBE clinics, staffed by trained nurses, saying, "These low-cost clinics would also empower women by providing them with scientific evidence on the risks of breast cancer, and also on its prevention."

This information is of particular importance, they say, in view of the high incidence of breast cancer, which has increased by 18% from 1975, in spite of the multi-billion dollar U.S. insurance and Medicare costs of mammography. Such funds should be diverted to establishing BSE clinics nationwide and providing public information on the wide range of avoidable causes of breast cancer.

This information was detailed in 2001 in a scientific article on "The Dangers and Unreliability of Mammography: Breast Examination As A Safe Effective and Practical Alternative," published in the prestigious International Journal of Health Services as long ago as 2001. This was co-authored by Dr. Epstein, Dr. Bertell, a leading international expert on radiation hazards, and the late Barbara Seaman, the leader and founder of the women's breast cancer movement.

ENDORSER:

Rosalie Bertell, PhD
Former President of the International Institute of Concern for Public
    Health, Toronto, Canada
Regent of the International Physicians for Humanitarian Medicine,
    Geneva, Switzerland

February 16, 2010

Food and Drug Administration Admits Medical Radiation Risks, Ignores Mammography Dangers

The Cancer Prevention Coalition notes with approval that on February 9, the Food and Drug Administration announced that it would take stringent action to regulate "the most potent forms of medical radiation," particularly those from increasingly popular CT scans.

Cancer Prevention Coalition Chairman Samuel S. Epstein, M.D. commends the FDA for warning that such radiation is unsafe and equivalent to that of about 400 chest x-rays, 0.4 rads (radiation absorbed dose), and "can increase a person's lifetime cancer risk."

However, says Dr. Epstein, "the FDA remains strangely unaware that radiation from routine premenopausal mammography poses significant and cumulative risks of breast cancer."

This warning is contrary to conventional assurances that radiation exposure from mammography is trivial, about 1/1,000 of a rad, and similar to just that from a chest x-ray. However, Dr. Epstein explains, the routine practice of taking two films of each breast results in exposure of about 0.4 rads, focused on the breast rather than on the entire chest.

"Thus, premenopausal women undergoing annual screening over a ten-year period are exposed to a total of at least 4 rads for each breast, at least 8 times greater radiation than FDA's "cancer risk" level," Dr. Epstein calculates, warning, "Such high radiation exposure approximates to that of Japanese women living approximately 1 mile away from the site of the Hiroshima atom bomb explosion."

This alarming information is not new, explains Dr. Epstein. In 1972, the prestigious National Academy of Sciences warned that the overall risks of breast cancer increase by 1% for every single rad exposure. This totals a 10% risk from 10 years annual premenopausal mammography.

This warning was emphasized in Dr. Epstein's 1978 book, The Politics of Cancer, which states, "Whatever you may be told, refuse routine mammograms, especially if you are pre-menopausal. The x-rays may increase your chances of getting cancer."

A 1993 Swedish study involving 42,000 women showed that those under the age of 55 who received regular premenopausal mammography experienced a 29 percent greater risk of dying from breast cancer.

Based on a detailed review of these and a wide range of other such studies, the late Dr. John Gofman, the leading international authority on medical radiation, published an analysis in his classic 1995 book, Preventing Breast Cancer. He stressed that medical radiation is probably the single most important cause of the modern breast cancer epidemic.

These warnings were further detailed in a 2001 article, with some 50 scientific references, "The Dangers and Unreliability of Mammography: Breast Self Examination As A Safe Effective and Practical Alternative," published in the prestigious International Journal of Health Services. This was co-authored by Dr. Epstein, by Dr. Rosalie Bertell, a leading international expert on the dangers of radiation, and by the late Barbara Seaman, founder and leader of the women's breast cancer movement.

An analysis of several 1993 studies showed that women who regularly performed monthly breast self-examination (BSE), particularly following training by qualified nurses, detected their cancers much earlier than those who failed to do so. That most breast cancers are first recognized by women themselves was even admitted by the American Cancer Society (ACS) as early as 1985, when the organization stated, "We must keep in mind that at least 90 percent of women who develop breast cancer discover the tumors themselves."

The International Journal of Health Services article further stressed that cancer risks from mammography are up to fourfold higher for the 2 percent of women who are silent carriers of a gene known as the A-T (ataxia-telangiectasia), and highly sensitive to the carcinogenic effects of radiation. This accounts for up to about 20 percent of all breast cancers diagnosed annually.

"This wide range of concerns on the still unrecognized dangers of routine premenopausal mammography are critical, especially in view of the current high incidence of breast cancer," Dr. Epstein warns. "Disturbingly, this has increased by about twenty percent since 1975 in spite of routine

Imperial Chemical Industries is one of the largest manufacturers of petrochemical industrial chemicals, and Zeneca is the sole manufacturer of Tamoxifen, the world's top selling cancer drug widely used for breast cancer.

"The ICI/Zeneca financial sponsorship gives them control over every leaflet, poster, publication, and commercial produced by NBCAM," warns Dr. Epstein.

"The ICI also supports the ACS blame-the-victim claim, which attributes escalating rates of breast, besides cancers to heredity and faulty lifestyle," he says. "This false and self-interested claim diverts attention away from avoidable exposures to carcinogenic industrial contaminants of air, water, food, consumer products, and the workplace."

Dangers of Screening Mammography

"Radiation from routine premenopausal mammography poses significant cumulative risks of promoting breast cancer," Dr. Epstein warns.

"Contrary to conventional assurances that radiation exposure from mammography is trivial and similar to that of a chest x-ray, about 1/1000 of a rad (radiation absorbed dose), the routine practice of taking four films for each breast results in some 1,000-fold greater exposure, 1 rad, focused on each breast rather than on the entire chest," he explains. "Thus, premenopausal women undergoing annual screening over a 10-year period are exposed to a total of about 10 rads for each breast."

As emphasized some three decades ago, the premenopausal breast is highly sensitive to radiation, each rad exposure increasing breast cancer risk by 1 percent, resulting in a cumulative 10 percent increased risk over 10 years.

In striking contrast, annual clinical breast examination (CBE) by a trained health professional, in addition to monthly breast self-examination, is safe, at least as effective as mammography, and low, if any, in cost.

A national program for training nurses how to perform clinical breast examination, and also teach breast self examination, is critical and decades overdue, Dr. Epstein advises.

Mammography is not a technique for early diagnosis, contrary to popular belief and assurances by the ACS, and also the media. Dr. Epstein says that in fact, a breast cancer has usually been present for about eight years before it can be belatedly detected by mammography

The Mammography Industry

The ACS has close connections to the mammography industry, as Dr. Epstein detailed in his 1998 book, "The Politics of Cancer Revisited." "In fact, if every woman followed ACS and NCI mammography guidelines, the annual revenue to health care facilities would be a staggering $5 billion," he says today.

"The ACS promotion continues to lure women of all ages into mammography centers, leading them to believe that mammography is their best hope against breast cancer," said Dr. Epstein.

He cites a leading Massachusetts newspaper that featured a photograph of two women in their twenties in an ACS advertisement that promised early detection results in a cure "nearly 100 percent of the time."

An ACS communications director, questioned by journalist Kate Dempsey, responded in an article published by the Massachusetts Women's Community's journal Cancer, saying, "The ad isn't based on a study. When you make an advertisement, you just say what you can to get women in the door. You exaggerate a point. Mammography today is a lucrative [and] highly competitive business."

Dr. Epstein warns that the ACS exposes premenopausal women to radiation hazards from mammography with little or no evidence of benefits. The ACS also fails to tell them that their breasts will change so much over time that the "baseline" images have little or no future relevance. This is truly an American Cancer Society crusade. But against whom, or rather, for whom?

The American Cancer Society's Conflicts of Interest

About half of the ACS board members are clinicians, oncologists, surgeons, radiologists, and basic molecular scientists, mostly with close ties to the NCI. Many board members and their colleagues apply for and obtain funding from both the ACS and the NCI. Substantial NCI funds also go to ACS directors who sit on key NCI committees. Although the ACS asks board members to leave the room when the rest of the board discusses their funding proposals, this is just a token formality. In this private club, easy access to funding is one of the perks as the board routinely rubber-stamps approvals. A significant amount of ACS research funding goes to this extended membership.

Frank conflicts of interest are evident in many ACS priorities. These include their advocating mammography and the National Breast Cancer Awareness campaign and supporting the pesticide and cancer drug industries. These conflicts even extend to the privatization of national cancer policy.

Public Relations

- 1998-2000: PR for the ACS was handled by Shandwick International, whose major clients included RJ Reynolds Tobacco Holdings.
- 2000-2002: PR for the ACS was handled by the Edelman Public Relations, whose major clients included Brown & Williamson Tobacco Company, and the Altria Group, the parent company of Philip Morris, and Kraft.

Industry Funding

ACS has received contributions in excess of $100,000 from a wide range of "Excalibur donors." Some of these companies were responsible for environmental pollution with carcinogens while others manufactured and sold products containing toxic and carcinogenic ingredients.

These donors include:

- Petrochemical companies (DuPont, BP, and Pennzoil)
- Industrial waste companies (BFI Waste Systems)
- Big Pharma (AstraZeneca, Bristol-Myers Squibb, GlaxoSmithKline, Merck & Company, and Novartis)
- Auto companies (Nissan and General Motors)
- Cosmetic companies (Christian Dior, Avon, Revlon, and Elizabeth Arden)
- Junk food companies (Wendy's International, McDonalds's, Unilever/Best Foods, and Coca-Cola.
- Biotech companies (Amgen and Genentech)

B.
Hormonal Milk

Hormonal Milk

Citizen Petition "Imminent Health Hazard" Seeking the Withdrawal of the New Animal Drug Application Approval for Posilac®-Recombinant Bovine Growth Hormone (rBGH) Milk*

January 12, 2010

Kathleen Sebelius
Secretary of Health and Human Services
U.S. Department of Health and Human Services

Margaret Hamburg, M.D.
Commissioner of Food and Drugs

This petition is based on scientific evidence of increased risks of cancer, particularly breast, colon, and prostate, from the consumption of milk from cows injected with Posilac®, the genetically modified (recombinant) Bovine Growth Hormone (also known as rBGH, sometribove, recombinant bovine somatotropin, or rBST). Posilac® is the trademark for Monsanto's rBGH product, registered with the U.S. Patent and Trademark Office, and is approved for marketing by the Food and Drug Administration (FDA). This petition is also based on abnormalities in the composition of rBGH milk, resulting from the recognized veterinary toxicity of rBGH, particularly increased levels of insulin like growth factor (IGF-1).

A. AGENCY ACTION REQUESTED

This petition requests the Secretary and the Commissioner to take the following action:

Suspend approval of Posilac®, and/or require milk and other dairy products produced with the use of Posilac® to be labeled with warnings such as, "Produced with the use of Posilac®, and contains elevated levels of IGF-1, a major risk factor for breast, prostate, and colon cancers."

---

*   This Petition is based on 61 scientific references and endorsed by 5 leading national experts, is a re-submission of the May 11, 2007 Petition, which the FDA ignored.

B. STATEMENT OF GROUNDS

1. The Veterinary Toxicity of Posilac®

Evidence of these toxic effects was first detailed in confidential Monsanto reports, based on records of secret nationwide rBGH veterinary trials, submitted to the FDA prior to October 1989 when they were leaked to one of the petitioners, Dr. Epstein. He then made these reports available to Congressman John Conyers, Chairman of the House Committee on Government Operations. On May 8, 1990, Congressman Conyers issued the following statement. "I find it reprehensible that Monsanto and the FDA have chosen to suppress and manipulate animal health test data." Details of these toxic effects were subsequently admitted by Monsanto and the FDA, and disclosed on the drug's veterinary label (Posilac®) in November, 1993. These include injection site lesions, a wide range of other toxic effects, and an increased incidence of mastitis, requiring the use of medication and antibiotics, and resulting in their contamination of milk.

2. Abnormalities in rBGH Milk

In a Monsanto Executive Summary, Posilac, January 1994, it was claimed that "natural milk is indistinguishable" from rBGH milk and that "There is no legal basis requiring its labeling." However, there are a wide range of well-documented abnormalities in rBGH milk, apart from increased IGF-1 levels. These include: reduction in casein; reduction in short-chain fatty acid and increase in long-chain fatty acid levels; increase in levels of the thyroid hormone triiodothyronine enzyme; contamination with unapproved drugs from treating mastitis; and frequency of pus cells due to mastitis.

3. Increased Levels of IGF-1 in rBGH Milk

A wide range of publications have documented excess levels of IGF-1 in rBGH milk, with increases ranging from four—to 20-fold. Based on six unpublished industry studies, FDA admitted that IGF-1 levels in rBGH milk were consistently and statistically increased, and that these were further increased by pasteurization; these increases were also admitted by others. Included among these is one by Lilly Industries, in its application for marketing authorization to the European Community Committee for Veterinary Products, admitting that rBGH milk may contain more than 10-fold increase in IGF-1 levels. It should also be noted that pasteurization increases IGF-1 levels by a further 70%, presumably by disrupting protein binding, and since standard analytic techniques for IGF-1 in rBGH milk may underestimate its levels by up to 40-fold.

4. IGF-1 Is Readily Absorbed from the Intestine into the Blood

Contrary to Section 2 of FDA's 6/8/2000 response to the December 5, 1998 Citizen Petition of the Center for Food Safety, IGF-1 is a peptide and not a protein, and as such is readily absorbed into the blood. Even more compelling is evidence of marked growth promoting effects following short-term feeding tests in rats. FDA's Section 2 thus reflects a misunderstanding relating to "the possibility of IGF-1 surviving digestion."

5. Increased IGF-1 Levels Increase Risks of Breast, Colon and Prostate Cancers

Thus, increased levels of IGF-1 have been shown to increase risks of breast cancer by up to seven-fold in 19 publication, risks of colon cancer in 10 publication, and prostate cancer in 7 publications.

6. Increased IGF-1 Levels Inhibit "Apoptosis"

Of generally unrecognized, critical importance is the fact that increased IGF-1 levels block natural defense mechanisms against the growth and development of early submicroscopic cancers, known as apoptosis or programmed self destruction.

7. Bovine Growth Hormone Increases Twinning Rates

As increased rate of twinning in cows injected with rBGH was admitted by Monsanto on its November 1993 Posilac label. rBGH increases ovulation and embryo survival, and increases the incidence of fraternal twins. "Because multiple gestations are more prone to complications such as premature delivery, congenital defects and pregnancy-induced hypertension in the mother than singleton pregnancies, the finding s of this study suggest that women contemplating pregnancy might consider substituting meat and dairy products with other protein sources, especially in countries that allow growth hormone administration to cattle."

8. The International Ban on the Use and Imports of rBGH Dairy Products

Based on the veterinary and public health concerns detailed in this Petition, the use and import of rBGH dairy products has been banned by Canada, 29 European nations, Norway, Switzerland, Japan, New Zealand, and Australia.

It should further be noted that on June 30, 1999, the Codex Alimentarius Commission, the United Nations Food Safety Agency representing 101 nations worldwide, ruled unanimously not to endorse or set a safety standard for rBGH milk.

9. The FDA Policy on Labeling rBGH Milk

The FDA has misled dairy producers and consumers with regard to its requirement for labeling of rBGH milk, to the effect that "No significant difference has been shown between milk derived from rBST-treated and non-rBST treated cows." This, however, is misleading in extreme as the "FDA has determined it lacks the basis for requiring such labeling in its statute." This was admitted in a 7/27/94 letter by Jerold R. Mande, Executive Director to the FDA Commissioner, to Harold Rudnick, State of New York Department of Agriculture and Markets.

This petition, based on 61 scientific references, was submitted by:

Samuel S. Epstein, M.D.
Chairman, Cancer Prevention Coalition
Professor emeritus Occupational and Environmental Medicine
University of Illinois at Chicago

Ronnie Cummins, Executive Director, Organic Consumers Association

John Kinsman, President, Family Farm Defenders

Arpad Pusztai, PhD, FRSE

Jeffrey Smith, Executive Director, Institute for Responsible Technology

July 27, 1989

Los Angeles Times

Growth Hormones Would Endanger Milk

With the Food and Drug Administration ready to approve the use of genetically engineered growth hormones in cows to boost milk production, concerns are mounting among dairy farmers, state legislatures, animal-rights activists and consumer and public-interest groups.

These hormones, known as BGH, are manufactured by giant chemical companies—Monsanto, American Cyanamid, Upjohn and Eli Lilly together with Dow-who anticipate $500-million annual worldwide sales.

Their promotional hype claims that the hormones are natural," that they are not found in milk, that they increase milk yields up to 25%, that they do not harm cows, that they do not alter milk quality and that they are safe for humans. The FDA also agrees that bovine growth hormones are safe and have allowed the sale of unlabeled milk and meat from BGH cows for about five years. These claims, which are based on industry-contracted research at more than 20 U.S. university dairy science departments, are misleading in the extreme.

Apart from the national surplus of milk and anticipated foreclosure of thousands of small dairy farms if milk production is increased and milk prices reduced, the effectiveness of bovine growth hormones is exaggerated. Furthermore, the nutritional quality of milk and cheese is altered; fat is increased and casein decreased. Stress effects have been noted in cows hyper-stimulated by BGH. These include increased susceptibility to infection, infertility, loss of fat, heat intolerance and "burnout" or lactational failure; severe stress diseases including gastric ulcers, arthritis and kidney and heart abnormalities have also been induced in pigs. Additionally, bovine growth hormones are likely to be misused as a growth promoter in calves, pigs and sheep, particularly as there are no practical methods for detecting the hormone in meat, and in view of the abusive track record of the meat industry regarding hormonal and other feed additives.

Apart from economic and veterinary concerns, bovine growth hormones pose grave consumer health risks that have not been investigated by the industry or FDA.

Bovine growth hormones are not "natural." The FDA now admits that they are up to "3% different in molecular structure" from the normal hormone. Increased BGH levels in milk and blood have been found in injected cows. BGH and its digested products could be absorbed from milk into blood, particularly in infants, and produce hormonal and allergic effects.

Increased levels of cell-stimulating growth factors, apparently identical to those in humans, have been reported in BGH milk. These could induce premature growth and breast stimulation in infants, and possibly promote breast cancer in adults.

Increased bacterial infections in BGH cows will require treatment with antibiotics that will pass into milk. This is likely to result in antibiotic-resistant infections in the general population. Also, the stress effects of bovine growth hormones in cows could suppress immunity and activate latent viruses, such as bovine leukemia (Leukosis) and bovine immunodeficiency viruses, which are related to the AIDS complex and may be infectious to humans.

Steroids and adrenaline-type stressor chemicals induced in cows by these hormones are likely to contaminate milk and may be harmful, particularly to infants and young children.

The fat and milk of cows are already contaminated with a wide range of carcinogenic contaminants, including dioxins and pesticides. Bovine growth hormones reduce body fat and are likely to mobilize these carcinogens into milk, with cancer risks to consumers.

What is to be done? State legislatures should be pressured to ban BGH. The FDA should be petitioned to ban the manufacture, domestic sale and export of the hormones until all safety questions can be resolved. Congressional oversight should focus on industry's misleading and self-interested claims on BGH, and the FDA's regulatory abdication. Finally, consumers should recognize these hormones as industry's latest unsafe contribution to the brave new world of chemicalized food and mechanized farming.

August 1989

Madison Capital Times, **Editorial**

We Must Ban Growth Hormones until All Questions Are Answered

With the Food and Drug Administration ready to approve the use of genetically engineered growth hormones in cows to boost milk production, concerns are mounting among dairy farmers, state legislatures, animal rights activists, and consumer and public interest groups.

These hormones, known as BGH, are manufactured by giant chemical companies—Monsanto, American Cyanamid, Upjohn, and Eli Lilly together with Dow—who anticipate $500 million in annual worldwide sales.

Their promotional hype claims that the hormones are "natural," that they are not found in milk, that they increase milk yields up to 25 percent, that they do not harm cows, that they do not alter milk quality and that they are safe for humans.

The FDA also agrees that BGH is safe and has allowed the sale of unlabeled milk and meat from BGH cows for about five years. These claims, which are based on industry-contracted research at more than 20 U.S. university dairy science departments, are misleading in the extreme.

Apart from the national surplus of milk and anticipated foreclosure of thousands of small dairy farms if milk production is increased and milk prices reduced, the effectiveness of BGH is exaggerated.

Furthermore, the nutritional quality of milk and cheese is altered; fat is increased and casein decreased. Stress effects have been noted in cows hyper-stimulated by BGH. They include increased susceptibility to infection, infertility, loss of fat, heat intolerance and "burnout," or lactational failure; and severe stress diseases including gastric ulcer and arthritis. Also, kidney and heart abnormalities have been found in pigs.

Additionally, BGH is likely to be misused as a growth promoter in calves, pigs and sheep, particularly as there are no practical methods for detecting the hormone in meat, and in view of the abusive track record of the meat industry regarding hormonal and other feed additives.

Apart from economic and veterinary concerns, BGH poses grave consumer health risks that have not been investigated by the industry or the FDA.

BGH is not "natural." The FDA now admits that it is up to "3 percent different in molecular structure" from the normal hormone. Increased BGH levels in milk and blood have been found in injected cows. BGH and its digested products could be absorbed from milk into blood, particularly in infants, and produce hormonal and allergenic effects.

Increased levels of cell-stimulating growth factors, apparently identical to those in humans, have been reported in BGH milk. These could induce premature growth and breast stimulation in infants, and possibly promote breast cancer in adults.

Increased bacterial infection in BGH cows would require treatment with antibiotics that would pass into milk. That is likely to result in antibiotic-resistant infections in the general population. Also, the stress effects of BGH in cows could suppress immunity and activate latent viruses, such as bovine leukemia (Leukosis) and bovine immunodeficiency viruses, which are related to the AIDS complex and may be infectious to humans.

Steroids and adrenaline-type stressor chemicals induced in cows by these hormones are likely to contaminate milk and may be harmful, particularly to infants and young children.

The fat and milk of cows are already contaminated with a wide range of carcinogenic contaminants, including dioxins and pesticides. BGH reduces body fat and is likely to mobilize the carcinogens into milk, with cancer risks to consumers.

What can be done? State legislatures should be pressured to ban BGH. The FDA should be petitioned to ban the manufacture, domestic sale and export of the hormones until all safety questions can be resolved.

Congressional oversight should focus on industry's misleading and self-interested claims on BGH, and the FDA's regulatory abdication.

Finally, consumers should recognize the hormones as industry's latest unsafe contribution to the brave new world of chemicalized food and mechanized farming.

June 2, 1990

Austin American Statesman

FDA Is Ignoring Dangers of Bovine Growth Hormone

On May 8, 1990, Rep John Conyers, D–Md., chairman of the House Committee on Government Operations, requested Inspector General Richard Kusserow of the Department of Health and Human Services to immediately investigate the Food and Drug Administration for "abdication of regulatory responsibility" with regard to its review of biosynthetic bovine growth hormones used to artificially boost milk production.

On the basis of recently available confidential industry files, Conyers charged that "Monsanto and the FDA have chosen to suppress and manipulate animal health test data—in efforts to approve commercial use of BGH." In prompt response to these revelations, Sen. Patrick Leahy, D–Vt., pressured the FDA into accepting an independent review by the National Institutes of Health to evaluate consumer hazards from BGH milk. European reactions and concerns are not lagging far behind.

In flagrant contradiction of repeated industry and FDA assurances, on the basis of which unlabeled milk and dairy products from secret nationwide trials on BGH have been sold to the public for the past six years, the confidential files reveal unarguable evidence of serious disease in BGH-injected cows and of contamination of their milk.

The toxic effects of BGH are evidenced at autopsy by increased organ weights, a high incidence of widespread "multifocal adhesions"—and chronic inflammation of internal organs, including the heart and lungs.

Nearly half the injected cows became infertile.

An increased incidence of chronic mastitis and anemia is documented.

Photographs reveal ulcerating injection site reactions and deep carcass damage.

Unapproved antibiotics and drugs were used to treat BGH-induced infections; one cow received 120 drug treatments during a single lactation.

In practice, such treatment would result in heavy contamination of milk with antibiotics, posing serious consumer hazards.

High levels of BGH were found in milk and still higher levels, in blood of injected cows. Such contamination poses potential hazards to consumers, particularly infants, from the absorption of partially digested products of BGH proteins, especially as these products are known to be metabolically active. These concerns prompted the FDA in 1982 to require withdrawal of BGH administration for at least five days before human consumption of milk was permitted. These concerns were further emphasized in a 1987 FDA memorandum that again warned of the activity of digested BGH products.

These revelations have climaxed growing consumer concerns on the dangers of BGH. They have also vindicated recent national and international regulatory actions including the April 1990 ban on the sale of BGH dairy products in Wisconsin and Minnesota, the moratorium on BGH until December 1990 by the European Economic Community and the proposed ban by the European Parliament. Nevertheless, the FDA has made no secret of its continuing intent to ignore these concerns and to approve the commercial use of BGH by the spring of 1991. In this, the FDA is fully supported by the administration. Agriculture Secretary Clayton Yeutter in a recent letter to the EEC, warned that a European ban on BGH "would certainly contravene our mutual objective of achieving international harmonization in the sensitive area of food safety." Ambassador Thomas Niles, in a confidential April 6, 1990, letter to the EEC, urged approval of BGH and reiterated FDA claims "that milk and meat from treated cows are safe and wholesome for human consumption."

BGH is a product for which there is no demand by consumers or the overwhelming majority of dairy farmers. Increased milk production due to BGH will be more than offset by costs of the hormone and extra cattle feed, by currently unrecognized costs due to infertility, mastitis, other cattle diseases and their treatment and by decreased milk consumption reflecting well-based consumer concerns. These broadly based society costs are no balanced by profits to the BGH manufacturing industries, Monsanto, American Cyanamid, Upjohn Co., and Elanco in conjunction with Dow Chemical Co., form anticipated sales of $500 million in 1991.

January 23, 1996

New Study Warns Of Breast and Colon Cancer Risks from rBGH Milk: Advocacy Groups Escalate Efforts against rBGH

The Cancer Prevention Coalition and Food & Water released a new study today which concludes that milk from cows injected with recombinant Bovine Growth Hormone (rBGH) increases risks of breast and colon cancers in humans. This study is published in the January issue of the International Journal of Health Services, a peer-reviewed, leading international public health journal.

The study summarizes evidence that rBGH increases levels of insulin-like growth factor (IGF-1) in milk. IGF-1 is a powerful stimulator and regulator of cell-growth and division in humans and cows. The study concludes that increased IGF-1 levels are risk factors for breast and colon cancer.

rBGH poses an even greater risk to human health than ever considered," warned Samuel Epstein M.D., Professor of Environmental Medicine at the University of Illinois School of Public Health and Chairman of the Cancer Prevention Coalition, author of the new report. "The FDA and Monsanto have a lot to answer for. Given the cancer risks, and other health concerns, why is rBGH milk still on the market?"

Since 1986, independent scientists have expressed concern about the lack of research on the potential health effects of IGF-1 in rBGH milk. More recently, the Council of Scientific Affairs of the American Medical Association admitted that: "Further studies will be required to determine whether the ingestion of higher than normal concentrations of bovine IGF-1 is safe."

Increased IGF-1 levels in rBGH milk exert their cancer promoting effects directly on cells lining the colon, and on breast cells, following absorption into the blood.

"Monsanto's claims that rBGH is perfectly safe have been proven dead wrong today. This study further validates the health concerns of millions of consumers about this controversial product," said Michael Colby,

Executive Director of Food and Water. "Only Monsanto is benefiting from this drug. It's time for dairy companies to side with consumers by adopting a policy that they will not allow rBGH, under any circumstances, to be used by their farmers."

Epstein concluded, "The entire nation is currently being subjected to a large-scale adulteration of an age-old dietary staple by a poorly characterized and unlabeled biotechnology product which is very different than natural milk."

Statement by the Cancer Prevention Coalition on Igf-1 and Breast and Colon Cancer*

The FDA has ignored the wide range of converging evidence that associates increased consumption of insulin growth factor-i (IGF-1), which increases in milk from rBGH treated cows, with a potential risk of breast and other types of cancer.

Published research shows that rBGH use on dairy cows induces a marked and sustained increase in levels of insulin-like growth factor-1, or IGF-1, in cow's milk. This is admitted by FDA (Juskevich & Guyer, 1990), and more explicitly by others (Prosser 1988; Prosser 1989; Mepham, 1992). A recent admission by another manufacturer of rBGH (Eli Lilly & Co.) reports a tenfold increase in IGF-1 levels. Furthermore, there is suggestive evidence that IGF-1 in rBGH milk is more bioactive than in non-hormonal milk (Mepham, 1992).

IGF-1 regulates cell growth, division and differentiation, particularly in children. Human and normal bovine IGF-1 are identical, they are largely bound in protein and thus probably less biologically active than unbound IGF1 in rBGH derived milk.

IGF-1 is not destroyed by pasteurization. In fact this process substantially increases IGF-1 levels in milk. (Juskevich and Guyer, 1990). Nor is IGF-1 destroyed by digestion. Moreover, FDA admits that IGF-1 is readily absorbed across the intestinal wall (Juskevich & Guyer, 1990); this was also previously admitted by Monsanto in 1987. Further confirmation is also provided by other authorities (e.g. Mepham, 1992). Additionally, recent research indicates that IGF-1 can be absorbed into the bloodstream where it can affect other hormones. (Donovan and Odle, 1994)

FDA and other industry sources have not published any detailed studies on the oral toxicity of IGF-1 Rather, they have consistently refused to make available their findings and raw data. A highly condensed summary of an IGF-1 Monsanto short term test in mature rats was released by FDA (Juskevich & Guyer, 1990). The agency alleges that this study confirms IGF-1's "lack of oral activity." At the outset it should be noted that the Monsanto test was contracted out to Hazelton Laboratories, which has a two decade history of misrepresentation of scientific data. (Epstein, 1978). However, even the cited Monsanto/Hazelton data explicitly reveal statistically significant evidence of growth promoting effects. Feeding relatively low doses of IGF-1 to mature rats for only two weeks resulted in statistically significant and biologically highly significant systemic effects: increased body weight; increased liver weight; increased bone length; and decreased epiphyseal width. These results are confirmatory of prior theoretical predictions.

The FDA has completely failed to investigate the effects of long-term feeding of IGF-1 and treated milk on growth, or on more sensitive sub-cellular effects, in infant rats or infants of any other species.

Significantly, cows injected with rBGH show heavy localization of IGF-1 in breast (udder) epithelial cells; this does not occur in untreated cows. (Furlanetto, et al, 1984; Gregor, et al, 1985; Campbell, et al, 1986.) IGF-1 induces rapid division and multiplication of normal human breast epithelial cells in tissue cultures. It is highly likely that IGF-1 promotes transformation of normal breast epithelium to breast cancers. (Furlanetto, et al, 1984; Harris, et al, 1992, growth factors such as IGF-1 "are responsible at least in part for the evolution of normal breast epithelia to breast cancer . . . '). Moreover, IGF-1 maintains the malignancy of human breast cancer cells, including their invasiveness and ability to spread to distant organs. (Lippman, 1991, 1993). IGF-1 has been similarly associated with colon cancer (Tricolo, et al, 1986).

The undifferentiated pre-natal and infant breast is particularly susceptible to hormonal influences (Ekbom, et al. 1992). Such imprinting by IGF-1 may increase future breast cancer risks, and may also increase the sensitivity of the breast to subsequent unrelated risks such as mammography and the carcinogenic and estrogen-like effects of pesticide residues in food, particularly in pre-menopausal women (Elwood, et al, 1993).

Concerns about increased levels of IGF-1 in milk from cows treated with rBGH are not new. In 1990, the National Institutes of Health (NIH) Consensus panel on rBGH expressed concerns on adverse health effects of IGF-1 in rBGH milk, calling for further study on the treated milk's impacts, especially on infants (NIH, 1991). In a 1989 letter to the FDA, I warned that the effects of IGF-1 "could include premature growth stimulation in infants, [breast enlargement] in young children and breast cancer in adult females." More recently, the Council on Scientific Affairs of the American Medical Association stated: "Further studies will be required to determine whether the ingestion of higher than normal concentrations of bovine insulin-like growth factor is safe for children, adolescents and adults" (AMA, 1991). Instead of further study, the FDA allowed for uncontrolled, unlabeled sales of treated milk to unwitting consumers.

Given the potential health impacts of consumption of milk and other dairy products derived from rBGH treated cows, all such products at a minimum be labeled so that consumers are aware of what they are purchasing and consuming. More prudently the FDA approval of rBGH should be withdrawn until the agency performs adequate long term testing on the impacts of increased levels of IGF-1 in milk and other dairy products derived from rBGH treated cows.

March 30, 1998

Gene Therapy Weekly

Risk Factors: Hormonal Milk Poses Prostate Cancer and Other Cancers Risks

As reported in a January 23, 1998, article in Science, men with high blood levels of the naturally occurring hormone insulin-like growth factor (IGF-1) are over four times more likely to develop [advanced] prostate cancer than are men with lower levels. The report emphasized that high IGF-1 blood levels are the strongest known risk factor for prostate cancer, only exceeding that of a family history, and that reducing IGF-1 levels is likely to prevent this cancer. It was further noted that IGF-1 markedly stimulates the division and proliferation of normal and cancerous prostate cells and that it blocks the programmed self-destruction of cancer cells thus enhancing the growth and invasiveness of latent prostate cancer. These findings are highly relevant to any efforts to prevent prostate cancer, whose rates have escalated by 180 percent since 1950, which is now the most common cancer in non-smoking men with an estimated 185,000 new cases and 39,000 deaths in 1998.

While warning that increasing IGF-1 blood levels by treating the elderly with growth hormone (GH) to slow aging may increase risks of prostate cancer, the 1998 report appears unaware of the fact that the entire U.S. population is now exposed to high levels of IGF-1 in dairy products. In February 1995, the Food and Drug Administration approved the sale of unlabeled milk from cows injected with Monsanto's genetically engineered bovine growth hormone, rBGH, to increase milk production. As detailed in a January 1996 report in the International Journal of Health Services, rBGH milk differs from natural milk chemically, nutritionally, pharmacologically and immunologically, besides being contaminated with pus and antibiotics resulting from mastitis induced by the biotech hormone. Most critically, rBGH milk is supercharged with high levels of abnormally potent IGF-1, up to 10 times more potent. IGF-1 resists pasteurization and digestion by stomach enzymes and is well absorbed across the intestinal wall. Still unpublished Monsanto tests, disclosed by FDA in summary form in 1990, showed that statistically significant growth stimulating effects were induced in organs of adult rats by feeding IGF-1 levels and to increase risks of developing prostate cancer and promoting its invasiveness. Apart from prostate cancer, multiple lines of evidence have also incriminated the role of IGF-1 as risk factors for breast, colon, and childhood cancers.

Faced with escalating rates of prostate and other avoidable cancers, FDA should withdraw its approval of rBGH milk, whose sale benefits only Monsanto while posing major public health risks form the entire U.S. population. Failing early FDA action, consumers should demand explicit labeling and only buy rBGH-free milk.

July 21, 1998

Monsanto's Hormonal Milk Poses Serious Risks of Breast Cancer, Besides Other Cancers

As reported in a May 9 article in The Lancet, women with a relatively small increase in blood levels of the naturally occurring growth hormone Insulin-like Growth Factor I (IGF-1) are up to seven times more likely to develop premenopausal breast cancer than women with lower levels. Based on those results, the report concluded that the risks of elevated IGF-1 blood levels are among the leading known risk factors for breast cancer, and are exceeded only by a strong family history or unusual mammographic abnormalities. Apart from breast cancer, an accompanying editorial warned that elevated IGF-1 levels are also associated with greater than any known risk factors for other major cancers, particularly colon and prostate.

This latest evidence is not unexpected. Higher rates of breast, besides colon, cancer have been reported in patients with gigantism (acromegaly) who have high IGF-1 blood levels. Other studies have also shown that administration of IGF-1 to elderly female primates causes marked breast enlargement and proliferation of breast tissue, that IGF-1 is a potent stimulator of human breast cells in tissue culture, that it blocks the programmed self-destruction of breast cancer cells, and enhances their growth and invasiveness.

These various reports, however, appear surprisingly unaware of the fact that the entire U.S. population is now exposed to high levels of IGF-1 in dairy products. In February 1995, the Food and Drug Administration approved the sale of unlabelled milk from cows injected with Monsanto's genetically engineered bovine growth hormone, rBGH, to increase milk production. As detailed in a January 1996 report in the prestigious *International Journal of Health Services*, rBGH milk differs from natural milk chemically, nutritionally, pharmacologically and immunologically, besides being contaminated with pus and antibiotics resulting from mastitis induced by the biotech hormone. More critically, rBGH milk is supercharged with high levels of abnormally potent IGF-1, up 10 times the levels in natural milk and over 10 times more potent. IGF-1 resists pasteurization, digestion by stomach enzymes, and is well absorbed across the intestinal wall. Still unpublished

1987 Monsanto tests, disclosed by FDA in summary form in 1990, revealed that statistically significant growth stimulating effects were induced in organs of adult rats by feeding IGF-1 at low dose levels for only two weeks. Drinking rBGH milk would thus be expected to significantly increase IGF-1 blood levels and consequently to increase risks of developing breast cancer and promoting its invasiveness.

Faced with escalating rates of breast, besides colon, prostate and other avoidable cancers, FDA should withdraw its approval of rBGH milk, whose sale benefits only Monsanto while posing major public health risks for the entire U.S. population. A Congressional investigation of FDA's abdication of responsibility is well overdue.

March 21, 1999

International Scientific Committee Warns of Serious Risks of Breast and Prostate Cancer from Monsanto's Hormonal Milk

The European Commission (EC) has just released a report by its authoritative international 16-member scientific committee, based on meticulous scientific documentation, confirming excess levels of the naturally occurring Insulin-like Growth Factor-1 (IGF-1) in milk of cows injected with Monsanto's biotech hormone (rBGH). The report concludes that the excess levels of IGF-1 pose serious risks of breast and prostate cancer. "Experimental evidence for an association between IGF-1 and breast and prostate cancer is supported by epidemiological—evidence arising from recently published cohort studies—." The report also warns that excess levels of IGF-1 may promote the growth and invasiveness of any cancer by inhibiting programmed self-destruction of cancer cells (apoptosis), and that contamination of milk with residues of antibiotics used to treat mastitis in rBGH cows is likely to spread antibiotic resistant infections in the general population. The EC human health report finally emphasized the need for additional investigation of several other potential risks of rBGH milk. A parallel EC report also warns of serious veterinary risks of rBGH. It may be noted that FDA has ignored such evidence reported in detail by the author in peer reviewed scientific publications over the last decade. The EC warnings are in sharp conflict with the policies of the Food and Drug Administration, largely based on unpublished and confidential Monsanto claims, that hormonal milk is safe. As seriously, the report raises serious questions on the competence and conflicts of interest of Codex, the WHO organization responsible for setting international food safety standards, which has given an unqualified clean bill of health to rBGH milk. It should further be emphasized that senior FDA officials and industry consultants are members of Codex, which meets in secrecy and relies on unpublished industry assurances of safety. Interlocking relationships between U.S. and Canadian regulatory officials and Codex are matters of critical concern to U.S. consumers and global food safety.

Faced with escalating rates of breast and prostate cancers, besides other avoidable public health hazards, FDA should immediately withdraw its approval of rBGH milk whose sale benefits only Monsanto while posing major public health risks for the entire U.S. population. A Congressional investigation of FDA's abdication of responsibility and of its reliance on Codex authority for food safety, analogous to that recently conducted on rBGH milk by the Canadian Parliament, is well overdue.

August 18, 1999

Monsanto's Genetically Modified Milk Ruled Unsafe by the United Nations

The Codex Alimentarius Commission, the U.N. Food Safety Agency representing 101 nations worldwide, has ruled unanimously in favor of the 1993 European moratorium on Monsanto's genetically engineered hormonal milk (rBGH). This unexpected ruling, revealingly greeted by the U.S. press with deafening silence, is a powerful blow against U.S. global trade policies which are strongly influenced by powerful multinational corporations, such as Monsanto. The Codex Commission ruling has also forced the U.S. to abandon its threats to challenge the European moratorium before the World Trade Organization later this year. As importantly, the ruling represents the first large scale defeat of genetically modified foods on unarguable scientific grounds, apart from ethical and ideological concerns.

Since the Food and Drug Administration approved the sale of unlabeled rBGH milk in February 1994, the U.S. has exerted considerable pressure on Mexico and other trading partners to approve rBGH in efforts to increase pressure on Europe through the World Trade Organization. In this, they have been strongly supported by reports from the Food and Agriculture/World Health Organization's (FAO/WHO) Joint Expert Committees on Food Additives (JECFA), including its latest September 1998 report, which unequivocally absolved rBGH from any adverse veterinary and public health effects. However, these JECFA committees, besides others such as those claiming the safety of meat from cattle treated with sex hormones, operate under conditions of non-transparency and conflicts of interest, and are predominantly staffed by unelected and unaccountable U.S. and Canadian regulatory officials and industry consultants with no expertise in public health, preventive medicine and carcinogenesis. The 1998 JECFA report on rBGH was then submitted to the Codex Committee on Residues of Veterinary Drugs in Foods, chaired by FDA's Director for Veterinary Medicine Dr. Stephen Sundloff, who also played a prominent role in the 1998 JECFA Committee. The Codex Committee promptly rubber stamped JECFA's seal of approval for rBGH with the confident expectation that this would be subsequently endorsed by the parent Codex Commission. However, the best laid plans of Monsanto and the FDA were aborted by an unexpected turn of events.

Bowing to growing pressure in 1998 by Canadian advocacy groups, "dissident" government scientists and the Senate Agriculture Committee. Health Canada convened expert committees on veterinary and human safety under the auspices of the Canadian Veterinary Medical Association and the Royal College of Physicians and Surgeons, respectively. Based on conclusions on the adverse veterinary effects of rBGH, particularly an increased incidence of mastitis, lameness and reproductive problems, Health Canada reluctantly broke ranks with the U.S. in January 1999, and issued a formal "notice of non-compliance," disapproving future sales of rBGH.

Meanwhile, the European Commission had commissioned two independent committees of internationally recognized experts to undertake a comprehensive review of the scientific literature on both the veterinary and public health effects of rBGH. The veterinary committee fully confirmed and extended the Canadian warnings and conclusions. The public health committee confirmed earlier reports of excess levels of the naturally occurring Insulin-like-Growth Factor One (IGF-1), including its highly potent variants, in rBGH milk and concluded that these posed major risks of cancer, particularly of the breast and prostate, besides promoting the growth and invasiveness of cancer cells by inhibiting their programmed self-destruction (apoptosis). Faced with this latest well documented scientific evidence from both Canada and Europe, the U.S. bowed to the inevitable and failed to challenge the Codex ruling in support of the European moratorium.

It is now 15 years since Monsanto embarked on a series of large scale veterinary trials on rBGH all over the U.S., and sold milk from these trials to an uninformed and unsuspecting public with the full approval of the FDA. Since then, Monsanto and the FDA, strongly supported by a network of indentured university academics, aggressive lobbying by the National Dairy Council and its well organized "hit squads" targeting rBGH opponents, and an overwhelmingly uncritical media, have ignored or trivialized substantial scientific evidence on the hazards of rBGH milk, including a series of publications over the last decade in the International Journal of Health Services, the most prestigious international public health publication. Also ignored by the media have been charges in 1981 by Congressman John Conyers (then Chairman of the House Committee on Government Operations), on the basis of a leaked confidential Monsanto study revealing serious pathology in cows injected with rBGH, that

"Monsanto and the FDA have chosen to suppress and manipulate animal health test data in efforts to approve commercial use of rBGH."

These considerations reinforce growing concerns on the extreme unreliability of Monsanto and other biotech industry claims of the safety of genetically modified soy and other foods, especially in the absence of comprehensive testing by independent scientific experts, who should be funded by industry and not consumers.

August 23, 1999

Postscript to PR Newswire, August 18 Press Release on "Monsanto's Genetically Modified Milk"

In response to the strong interest and supportive calls, apart from some narrow legalistic questions, on this press release, I would like to further clarify the Codex ruling.

Since 1995, the U.S. has pressured the Codex Commission to adopt a standard, based on tolerances or Maximum Residue Limits, for residues of rBGH in milk in attempts to prove its safety and promote its international export. At its June 30 meeting, the Commission unanimously rejected further consideration of this U.S. proposal, particularly in light of the recent Canadian ban or "notice of non-compliance," and of recent reports to the European Commission by two committees of independent international experts on the cancer and other risks of Monsanto's milk. By such action, the Commission explicitly ruled that national governments have absolute rights to decide whether or not to permit imports of rBGH milk in view of well based public health concerns. My August 18 press release is clearly consistent with these events, notwithstanding the self-interested protestations by spokesmen for the FDA, the highly flawed and unaccountable Joint Expert Committee on Food Additives and Monsanto.

It may be further noted that the premier health and science U.K. journalist George Monbiot in his July 22 article in The Guardian, reported that "three weeks ago the European Union routed an American attempt to force—(Europe) to accept (rBGH milk) since safety concerns about rBGH milk could not be ignored." Monbiot also commented on the "deluge of absolutely no coverage at all" with which this unprecedented and momentous ruling against genetically modified food has been greeted.

January 18, 2000

Austria Urged to Take Initiatives to Protect the Public against Cancer and Other Risks of Monsanto's Genetically Modified rBST Dairy Products

Austrian concerns on animal welfare, food safety, and genetically modified (GM) foods are among the highest in the world. However, these concerns are complicated by the fact that the GM milk hormone, rBST, is exclusively manufactured in Austria by Biochemie Kundl, a Novartis plant under license to Monsanto; in 1998, over 100 million doses of the GM hormone were exported to the U.S. and also to 16 other Third World Countries. While the administration of rBST to cows in Europe was banned this month on unarguable animal health and welfare grounds, there are no restrictions yet on the import of GM dairy products, nor any requirements for their GM labeling.

Austria could resolve this dilemma with two initiatives. First, a grass roots campaign and/or government ruling requiring the labeling of imported GM dairy products; the labeling of such GM foods is now under consideration by the EC. Second, representation to the European Parliament and European Council by the Austrian government to ban imports of GM dairy products from the U.S. and other Third World Countries on human health grounds on the basis of the well-recognized "Precautionary Principle."

GM milk, produced by injecting cows with the hormone rBST, is qualitatively and quantitatively different from natural milk. These differences include: contamination of milk by the GM hormone rBST; contamination by pus and antibiotics resulting from the high incidence of mastitis in rBST injected cows; contamination with illegal antibiotics and drugs used to treat mastitis and other rBST induced disease; increased concentration of the thyroid hormone enzyme thyroxin-5'-monodeiodinase; increased concentration of long chain and decreased concentration of short chain fatty acids; reduction in casein levels; and major excess levels of the naturally occurring Insulin-like Growth Factor, IGF-1, including its highly potent variant.

There are very persuasive grounds for invoking the "Precautionary Principle" with regard to the public health hazards of GM milk. Evidence for these hazards, published in peer-reviewed scientific literature, is over a decade old. This evidence has recently been fully endorsed in the March 15-16, 1999, EC risk assessment report, by a team of 16 internationally recognized experts, on "Public Health Aspects of the Use of Bovine Somatotropin."

These hazards include: allergic reactions, antibiotic resistance, and cancer risks from residues in milk of antibiotics used to treat mastitis in GM-hormone injected cows; unresolved concerns relating to elevated thyroid hormones; cardiovascular disease from elevated levels of long chain fatty acids; immunological effects of rBST absorbed from the gastrointestinal tract; and growth promoting and cancer risks from elevated IGF-1 levels.

Multiple lines of converging evidence have strongly incriminated elevated IGF-1 milk levels with major excess risks of breast, prostate, and colon, besides possibly other cancers. Furthermore, IGF-1 is known to inhibit the programmed self-destruction (apoptosis) of cancer cells, thus promoting their growth and invasiveness, and also decreasing their responsiveness to chemotherapy. In spite of such fully-documented evidence, in July 1999 the London-based Committee for Veterinary Medicinal Products of the European Agency for the Evaluation of Medicinal Products Veterinary Medicines Evaluation Unit (EMEA), rejected the proposed ban on the GM hormone on public health grounds. It should, however, be stressed that a minority Committee report expressed strongly divergent views, stressing their recognition of the cancer risks of GM milk. Furthermore, the EMEA agency has no track record of competence and scientific authority in the relevant area of cancer prevention.

Even accepting that there possibly may be scientific uncertainty with regards to the public health hazards of GM milk, there is more than a sufficient weight of preponderant evidence to unreservedly invoke the "Precautionary Principle," whose validity has achieved substantial support internationally and in the European Parliament. The "Precautionary Principle" could also be used in support of labeling requirements for GM dairy products and/or for a ban of all such imports. Finally, the "Precautionary Principle" mandates the categorical responsibility of industry to unequivocally establish the safety of new candidate products, as opposed to imposing a heavy burden on regulatory agencies and citizens to prove risks. Monsanto has completely failed to comply with this requirement with regards to the cancer, and other, risks of its GM hormone and GM milk.

May 19, 2003

Genetically-Engineered Anti-Aging Medication, Monsanto Milk Are Major, Unrecognized Risks of Breast Cancer

Anti-aging medication with genetically-engineered human growth hormone (HGH) poses major risks of breast cancer. Equally unrecognized are risks of drinking unlabeled milk from cows injected with Monsanto's genetically-engineered bovine growth hormone (BGH), marketed since 1994 to increase milk production. These risks are especially critical in view of the escalating incidence of breast cancer, particularly in post-menopausal women, over recent decades. As critical is the fact that women have still not been warned of both these avoidable risks.

The anti-aging effects of HGH are due to its stimulating the liver to increase production of the natural Insulin-like Growth Factor-1 (IGF-1), whose blood levels normally decline with increasing age. BGH milk also has high levels of IGF-1, which is readily absorbed through the gut.

There are numerous publications, in prestigious scientific journals since the early 1990's, showing that elevated IGF-1 levels are strongly associated with major excesses of breast, besides colon and prostate, cancer. By 1992, a leading authority on IGF-1 warned that it was strongly incriminated in the transformation of normal breast cells to cancer cells. Even minor elevations of IGF-1 are associated with up to a 7-fold increased risk of breast cancer. This is almost as high as that in women carrying genes (BRCA1 and BRCA2) with the strongest hereditary predisposition. Additionally, IGF-1 inhibits the naturally programmed ability of cancer cells to self-destruct. This results in stimulating the growth and invasiveness of small, undiagnosed cancers, and increasing their resistance to chemotherapy. These concerns on risks of high levels of IGF-1 in BGH milk are particularly strong in view of evidence that prenatal and infant breasts are highly susceptible to stimulatory and hormonal influences. This early life "imprinting" is thus likely to result in progressive increases in risks of breast cancer over future decades.

Use of HGH for anti-aging medication has become a major growth industry. Suppliers of HGH, including those offering mail order prescriptions, are proliferating on Internet web sites. The Chicago-based ten-year old American Academy of Anti-Aging Medicine, with over

8,000 members, promotes injectable HGH in programs claiming to stop or even reverse aging, including decreasing body fat, and increasing muscle mass and bone density. However, practitioners of this burgeoning "health" industry are either ignorant of or fail to warn of well-documented information on the grave cancer risks of HGH medication.

HGH medication should only be used by qualified endocrinologists for highly restricted medical disorders, such as dwarfism due to pituitary gland deficiency, as approved by the FDA in 1985. It should be further stressed that anti-aging medication has never received any such approval.

The public should also boycott unlabeled dairy products in favor of those labeled as rBGH-free, which are becoming increasingly available.

February 4, 2005

The "Milk Is Milk" Industry Campaign Threatens Public Health

Last month, the Hudson Institute's agribusiness-funded Center for Global Food Issues launched an aggressive "Milk is Milk" campaign to assure consumers that there is no difference between natural milk and that from cows injected with Monsanto's genetically-engineered or recombinant Bovine Growth Hormone (rBGH) to increase milk production and profitability. This campaign is also aimed at preventing organic dairy farmers and retailers from making "false or misleading claims to be hormone-free, (and) nutritional and animal welfare perceptions, such as happier cows." Responding to Hudson's complaints, the Food and Drug Administration (FDA) announced that it will take action against such misleading marketing practices.

However, contrary to Hudson, there is a wealth of scientific information on the toxic veterinary effects of rBGH, major differences between rBGH and natural milk, and cancer risks posed by rBGH milk. Revealingly, Hudson uses the term rBST, recombinant Bovine Somatotropin, avoiding any reference to the word "Hormone" in Monsanto's original acronym rBGH.

Cows hyper-stimulated by repeated rBGH injections are seriously stressed. Such evidence, detailed in confidential Monsanto files submitted to the FDA in 1987, was anonymously leaked to one of us (Epstein) in November 1989. These files revealed widespread pathological lesions, infertility, and chronic mastitis, treated with illegal antibiotics. Acting on this information, in 1990 the House Committee on Government Operations charged "that Monsanto and the FDA have chosen to suppress and manipulate animal health test data—in efforts to approve commercial use" of rBGH. This charge is also consistent with the Committee's 1986 report, "Human Food Safety and the Regulation of Animal Drugs." This concluded that the "FDA has consistently disregarded its responsibility—has repeatedly put what it perceives are interests of veterinarians and the livestock industry ahead of its legal obligation to protect consumers—jeopardizing the health and safety of consumers of meat, milk and poultry."

By 1994, when FDA approved the use of rBGH under Monsanto's trade name Posilac, the label insert, seen only by dairy farmers, admitted that "its use is associated with increased frequency of use of medication in cows for mastitis, "and some 20 other toxic effects. Such information on the Posilac label is clearly inconsistent with Hudson's criticism of "happier cow" claims by organic dairy farmers.

Also contrary to Hudson, rBGH milk differs qualitatively and quantitatively from natural milk. Fat levels, particularly long chain saturated fatty acids incriminated in heart disease, are increased, while levels of a thyroid hormone enzyme are increased. Furthermore, the high incidence of chronic mastitis in rBGH injected cows results in contamination of their milk with pus, and with antibiotics used to treat the infection, with risks of allergic reactions and nationwide antibiotic resistance. Less well recognized is contamination of rBGH milk with the hormone itself, and immunological evidence of absorption of the hormone from the intestine.

Even more seriously, rBGH milk is contaminated with high levels of the natural Insulin-like Growth Factor-1 (IGF-1), which regulates cell growth, division and multiplication throughout life, particularly in infants and young children; Eli Lilly, in its application for registration of rBGH, admitted that IGF-1 blood levels of injected cows are increased up to ten-fold. IGF-1 is resistant to pasteurization and digestion, and is readily absorbed from the small intestine. Monsanto's own data revealed that feeding IGF-1 to adult rats for only two weeks significantly increased body and liver weights, and bone length.

More critically, increased IGF-1 blood levels have been incriminated as a major cause of cancer. IGF-1 induces uncontrolled growth of normal human breast cells in tissue culture, and has been incriminated in their transformation to cancer cells. Some 30 publications, dating back to 1985, have reported strong associations between increased IGF-1 blood levels with increased risks of colon, and breast cancers. A 1998 study, based on 300 healthy nurses, showed that elevated IGF-1 blood levels are strongly associated with up to a seven-fold increased risk of developing premenopausal breast cancer. This is the highest known risk, approximating to that of a strong family history. More recent studies have also shown strong associations between increased IGF-1 blood levels and prostate cancer.

Of related concern is evidence that elevated IGF-1 levels inhibit the body's normal ability to protect itself from microscopic cancers by the natural process of programmed cell destruction, known as "apoptosis." This promotes the growth and invasiveness of early cancers, and also decreases their responsiveness to chemotherapy.

Acting on this cumulative evidence, a 1999 European Commission report by a team of internationally recognized experts concluded: "Avoidance of rBGH dairy products in favor of natural products would appear to be the most practical and immediate dietary intervention to . . . (achieve) the goal of preventing cancer." Furthermore, this warning has been endorsed (in our 2002 publication in a leading scientific journal) by over 100 leading independent experts in cancer prevention and public health, besides citizen activist groups. This endorsement was coupled with insistence that the public has an absolute right-to-know of information on avoidable causes of cancer, a democratic right which the agribusiness and FDA continue to subvert.

ENDORSERS:

Ronnie Cummins
National Director
Organic Consumers Association

June 27, 2006

Hormonal Milk Poses Greater Risks than Just Twinning

As widely covered in the national media, a recent article by Dr. Gary Steinman in The Journal of Reproductive Medicine reported that women drinking milk and eating dairy products from cows injected with Monsanto's genetically engineered growth hormone drug are up to five times more likely to risk giving birth to fraternal twins than non-dairy product vegans.

This news is hardly surprising. Hormonal milk contains up to ten-fold increased levels of the natural Insulin-like Growth Factor, known as IGF, long known to increase ovulation and twinning rates in cows. The hormone also makes cows sick. Monsanto has been forced to admit to 20 toxic veterinary effects on its drug label.

Monsanto has also recently admitted that about one third of dairy cows in the nation are now in herds where the hormone is used.

Hormonal milk is very different than natural milk. Hormonal milk is often contaminated with pus cells, resulting from mastitis in cows due to hyperstimulation of milk production, and also with antibiotics used to treat the mastitis. Other abnormalities include increased fatty acids, which are incriminated in heart disease.

More serious are major risks of breast, colon, and prostate cancers due to increased IGF levels in hormonal milk. Evidence for this has been documented in about 50 scientific publications over the past three decades. Among them is the 1998 Harvard Nurses' Health Study, based on a follow-up of 300 healthy nurses. Those with elevated IGF blood levels were shown to have up to a seven-fold increased risk of breast cancer.

A less well-recognized risk is evidence that IGF blocks natural, self-destructive, defense mechanisms against early submicroscopic cancers, technically known as apoptosis.

Acting on these lines of evidence, a 1999 European Commission Report, by internationally recognized experts, concluded that avoidance of hormonal dairy products in favor of natural organic products "would appear to be the most practical and immediate dietary intervention to . . . achieve the goal of preventing cancer." Warning of these risks were confirmed in my 2002 publication in the International Journal of Health Services, endorsed by over 50 leading independent experts in cancer prevention and public health.

Of particular concern are risks to infants and children in view of their high susceptibility to cancer-causing products and chemicals. Nevertheless, few schools make organic milk available, nor do most state governments, under low-income food programs, particularly the Special Supplemental Nutrition Program for Women, Infants, and Children.

Nevertheless, the Food and Drug Administration remains indifferent to these risks, in spite of Congressional concerns. Illustrative is the 1986 report, "Human Food Safety and Regulation of Animal Drugs," by the House Committee on Government Operations. This concluded that the "FDA has consistently disregarded its responsibility—has repeatedly put what it perceives are interests of veterinarians and the livestock industry ahead of its legal obligations to protect consumers—jeopardizing the health and safety of consumers of meat, milk, and poultry."

However, these risks are avoidable. According to The Hartman Group, a prominent Seattle consulting firm, organic milk is now among the first organic product that consumers buy. Organic milk is also becoming increasingly available, with an annual growth rate of about 20 percent, while overall milk consumption is dropping by about 10 percent.

Wal-Mart is now the biggest seller of certified organic milk, followed by Horizon Organic, owned by Dean Foods, the nation's largest dairy producer, and by Groupe Danone, the leading French dairy company. While growth in this market is still held back by the higher price of organic milk, this problem is likely to be resolved by Wal-Mart's competitive pricing.

In sharp contrast to the U.S., 24 European nations, Norway, Switzerland, New Zealand, Japan, and Canada have banned the use and imports of hormonal milk and dairy products. However, in spite of the ban, Canada imports over 20 percent of its total dairy products from the U.S., without any restrictions.

Our government has failed to warn its citizens of the dangers of hormonal milk. The media could now play a critical role in alerting the nation to these avoidable dangers.

September 22, 2006

The Organic Milk Wars: It's Not Just the Price

Shoppers' appetite for organic food is steadily growing. Leading the way is USDA certified organic milk, with this year's growth rate of 25 percent, while overall consumption decreased by 10 percent. Organic milk is now among the first organic product that consumers buy.

What's more, the price of organic milk, besides other organic food, is dropping sharply to a narrow margin above conventional products. Leading the way, and far ahead of the field, is Wal-Mart, the nation's largest grocer and retailer.

Price apart, this is very good news for consumers. Organic milk is very different, and safer than milk from cows injected with rBGH, a highly potent genetically engineered version of BGH, the natural bovine growth hormone.

Manufactured by Monsanto, rBGH is sold to dairy farmers under the trade name Posilac. Injection of this hormone forces cows to increase their milk production by about 10%. However, this is of little or no benefit in view of the current national surplus. Monsanto has stated that about one third of dairy cows in the nation are in large herds where the hormone is now used. rBGH factory farms now pose a major threat to the viability of small organic dairy farms, and enriches Monsanto without any benefits to consumers.

Monsanto, strongly supported by the Food and Drug Administration (FDA), still insists that hormonal milk is indistinguishable from natural milk, and that it is safe. This is blatantly false:

- rBGH makes cows sick. Monsanto has been forced to admit to about 20 toxic effects, including mastitis, on its Posilac drug label.
- rBGH milk is often contaminated with pus, due to mastitis commonly induced by rBGH, and also with antibiotics used to treat the mastitis. This poses risks of nationwide antibiotic resistance to life threatening infections.

- rBGH milk is chemically, and nutritionally different than natural milk. These differences include increased levels of milk fat, posing cardiovascular risks.
- Milk from cows injected with rBGH is contaminated with the hormone, traces of which are absorbed through the gut into the blood, and provoke foreign antibodies.
- rBGH milk is supercharged with high levels of a natural growth factor (IGF-1), which is readily absorbed through the gut. These levels are further increased following pasteurization.
- In numerous published scientific studies over the last two decades, excess levels of IGF-1 have been incriminated as causes of breast, colon, and prostate cancers.
- IGF-1 blocks natural defense mechanisms, technically known as apoptosis, against the growth of early submicroscopic cancers.

Based on such well-documented scientific evidence, a 1999 European Commission Report, by a group of well recognized international experts, concluded that avoidance of rBGH dairy products in favor of natural organic products "would appear to be the most practical and immediate dietary intervention to . . . achieve the goal of preventing cancer." Warnings of these risks were detailed in my 1996 publication in the prestigious *International Journal of Health Services*, endorsed by over 50 leading national and international independent experts in cancer prevention and public health, besides by activist consumer groups, and in my 2006 book *What's In Your Milk?*

Based on such scientific evidence, Canada, 28 European Member States, Norway, Switzerland, New Zealand, and Japan have all banned the use and import of U.S. rBGH milk and dairy products.

In sharp contrast, the FDA continues to turn a blind eye to the dangers of Monsanto's hormonal milk. This indifference has been supported by longstanding conflicts of interest between Monsanto and the White House, the American Medical Association, and the American Cancer Society, which still remain unrecognized by the media. Also unrecognized have been Congressional expressions of concern. These include a 1990 charge by Congressman John Conyers, then Chair of the House Committee on Government Operations. "I find it reprehensible that Monsanto and the FDA have chosen to suppress and manipulate animal health test data in efforts to approve commercial use of rBGH . . . without regard to the adverse effects on humans."

As recently warned by Ben Cohen, Cofounder of Ben & Jerry's Ice Cream, "rBGH is a bad and dangerous . . . bio-technological solution to a problem that does not exist."

April 10, 2006

National School Lunches: Unsafe at Any Eating

On April 6, a bipartisan Congressional group, with strong support in both Houses, announced plans to introduce legislation amending the National School Lunch Act. This would prohibit the sale in schools of sugary or fatty junk foods, notably soft drinks and French fries.

This initiative officially endorses longstanding efforts by many school districts to provide only healthy foods, and hopefully reduce the growing incidence of childhood obesity and related diseases.

Enforcement of this initiative would be the responsibility of the U.S. Department of Agriculture (USDA), which is in charge of the current Public School Lunch Program. This extended authority was applauded by the Center for Science in the Public Interest, a national food safety activist group, stating that "The Agency has done a good job with the official school lunch and could do a good job with all other foods." This endorsement may well be warranted nutritionally. However, it certainly is not warranted by the USDA's failure to disclose well-documented scientific evidence on the risks to health of the two school lunch staples, milk and meat.

Much of the nations milk supply comes from cows injected with a genetically engineered variant of their natural growth hormone, technically known as rBGH (recombinant Bovine Growth Hormone). Manufactured by Monsanto, and sold to dairy farmers under the trade name POSILAC. Injection of the hormone forces cows to increase their milk yield by about 10 percent, while making them sick in the process.

Monsanto and the USDA insist that rBGH milk is indistinguishable from natural milk, and that it is safe for children and other consumers. This is scientifically and medically untrue. rBGH milk makes cows sick. Monsanto has been forced to admit to some 20 toxic veterinary effects on its POSILAC label. These include mastitis, resulting in pus cells in milk, and antibiotics used to treat the mastitis. rBGH milk is also chemically, and nutritionally different than natural milk, and is supercharged with excess levels of a natural growth factor (IGF-1), which is readily absorbed through the intestines into the blood. Of major concern is a wealth of longstanding scientific evidence incriminating these excess levels as delayed causes of breast, colon, and prostate cancers.

Reacting to the fully documented scientific evidence on the dangers of rBGH milk, a wide range of nations including all of Europe, Canada, Australia, New Zealand and Japan have banned rBGH milk.

U.S. beef is heavily contaminated with sex hormones. When U.S. beef cattle enter feedlots, sex hormone pellets are implanted under the ear skin, a process that is repeated at the midpoint of their 100-day pre-slaughter fattening period. These hormones increase the weight of the cattle, adding to profits by about $80 per animal.

The hormones in past and current use include the natural estradiol, progesterone, and testosterone, and their more potent synthetic counterparts, zeranol, trenbolone, and melengesterol. The U.S. Food and Drug Administration (FDA) and the USDA have both maintained and still claim that residues of these hormones in meat are safe and within normal limits.

However, confidential industry reports to the FDA, obtained under the Freedom of Information Act, have revealed high residues of the hormones in meat products. Following a single ear implant in steers of Synovex-S, a combination of estradiol and progesterone, their residues in meat were found to be up to 20-fold higher than normal. The amount of estradiol in two hamburgers eaten in one day by an 8-year-old boy could increase his total hormone levels by as much as 10 percent, particularly as young children have very low natural hormone levels.

Increased levels of sex hormones are linked ever more closely to the escalating increase of reproductive cancers in the U.S., 36 percent for post-menopausal breast cancer, 51 percent for testicular cancer, and 88 percent for prostate cancer, since 1975. These concerns have been strongly reinforced by recent evidence, from researchers at Ohio State University, that meat and blood from cattle implanted with zeranol have powerful hormonal effects, which resist cooking.

Europe has viewed longstanding U.S. claims with considerable skepticism. Since 1989, all 25 European nations have banned the sale of beef from hormone-treated cattle.

The national School Lunch Program is a major focus of the current Midwest BioETHICS 2006 (www.bioethics2006.org) conference in Chicago. This culminates in a Tuesday evening session on the critical need for certified organic milk and meat to replace the current dangerous staples. The conference coincides with the national Biotechnology Industry Organization, which aggressively promotes the industrialization of the nation's food supply.

November 9, 2006

Chicago Tribune

Got Hormone-Free Milk?

Recent campaigns by consumer groups have attacked Starbucks for not offering rBGH-free milk, or milk from cows that have not been treated with Monsanto's synthetic growth hormone, Posilac.

But should Starbucks cave to the pressure—and so far, it hasn't—it wouldn't necessarily have to use pricey organic milk, which consumers are screaming for these days.

A new category of milk known as "organic light" is creeping onto store shelves around the country in response to consumer demand for products free of added Posilac. The genetically engineered bovine growth hormone, used in about one-third of the nation's dairy cows, is also known as recombinant bovine somatratropin (rBST) in Canada and Europe.

Consumers don't seem to care that the Food and Drug Administration and the dairy industry both say the use of Monsanto's patented Posilac is safe or that proponents argue it's an economical way to hike milk production by 10 percent a year.

Many, like me, prefer not to take their chances, especially if an alternative to conventional milk is available.

Hormone-free milk isn't officially organic because it doesn't meet all the requirements and doesn't cost as much to produce. So it can enjoy the marketing cachet of natural foods and be priced higher than conventional milk but still cost less than organic.

The movement, which is entirely consumer-driven and began in the Northeast and on the West Coast, is now rippling across the United States. This week, Dean Foods Co. announced it's expanding the marketing of rBST-free milk and recently began rolling out its hormone-free Schepps brand in Dallas.

Next year, the trend is expected to converge in the Midwest, including Illinois, according to a recent article in the St. Louis Post Dispatch.

And unbelievably, it could mean we're in the early days of the end of the unnecessary use of bovine growth hormone.

The consumer rejection of Posilac has been something of a shock to Monsanto, which has set up a Web site with a handy profit calculator showing dairy farmers how the use of Posilac can increase profits.

But to most consumers, the issue is one of health and unknown consequences of added growth hormone, not economics.

Though the FDA says rBGH milk is safe and indistinguishable from natural organic milk, Samuel Epstein, professor emeritus of environmental medicine at the University of Illinois at Chicago School of Public Health, finds the notion ludicrous.

In his new book *What's in Your Milk* (Trafford Publishing, $24.95), he charges that rBGH milk can increase the risk of breast, colon and prostate cancer and is profitable to Monsanto while posing dangers with no benefits to consumers.

Then there is the question of whether rBGH milk is a biotech solution to a problem that doesn't exist. In the introduction of Epstein's book, Ben Cohen, co-founder of Ben & Jerry's Ice Cream and president for Business Leaders with Sensible Priorities argues that:

- rBGH is not needed to increase America's supply of dairy products. Oversupply by factory farms is a problem, not an answer.
- rBGH is not needed to improve the health of dairy cows. The manufacturer's own label warns that the growth hormone can trigger a wide range of harmful effects.
- rBGH is not needed to help family farmers. Their costs already are too high, without another artificial chemical to buy. And the artificial hormone makes cows sick, leading to higher costs for veterinary care and antibiotics.
- rBGH is very different than natural milk and poses cancer and other risks to consumers.

While we wait for more evidence on the health effects of added growth hormone, there are other issues to consider. If Posilac really can't be detected in milk, how will consumers know whether the products they're paying more money for are really hormone-free or not?

And more than 60 percent of the milk produced in the U.S. is used in the production of cheese, yogurt and other products. So even if you buy hormone-free fluid milk, you might be getting a dose of Posilac in your cheese pizza or your coffee frappuccino.

January 3, 2007

What's in Your Milk?

rBGH (recombinant Bovine Growth Hormone) is a genetically engineered, potent variant of the natural growth hormone produced by cows. Manufactured by Monsanto, it is sold to dairy farmers under the trade name POSILAC. Injection of this hormone forces cows to increase their milk production by about 10%. Monsanto has stated that about one third of dairy cows are in herds where the hormone is used.

Monsanto, supported by the Food and Drug Administration (FDA), insist that rBGH milk is indistinguishable from natural milk, and that it is safe for consumers. This is blatantly false:

- rBGH makes cows sick. Monsanto has been forced to admit to about 20 toxic effects, including mastitis, on its Posilac label.
- rBGH milk is contaminated by pus, due to the mastitis commonly induced by rBGH, and antibiotics used to treat the mastitis.
- rBGH milk is chemically, and nutritionally different than natural milk.
- Milk from cows injected with rBGH is contaminated with the hormone, traces of which are absorbed through the gut into the blood.
- rBGH milk is supercharged with high levels of a natural growth factor (IGF-1), which is readily absorbed through the gut.
- Excess levels of IGF-1 have been incriminated as a cause of breast, colon, and prostate cancers.
- IGF-1 blocks natural defense mechanisms against early submicroscopic cancers.
- rBGH factory farms pose a major threat to the viability of small dairy farms.
- rBGH enriches Monsanto, while posing dangers, without any benefits, to consumers, especially in view of the current national surplus of milk.

Of still greater concern, based on 37 published scientific studies as detailed in the book, excess levels of IGF-1 in rBGH milk pose major risks of breast, colon and prostate cancers.

The introduction to *What's in Your Milk?* by Ben Cohen, cofounder of Ben & Jerry's Ice Cream, with a Foreword by Jeffrey M. Smith, author of the bestseller Seeds of Deception

Many prominent experts in the environmental field have endorsed the new book including Congressman John Conyers, Jr., Ranking Democrat, House Judiciary Committee, Mark Achbar, Executive Producer of the multiple prize-winning documentary The Corporation, Ronnie Cummins, National Director, Organic Consumers Association, and Dr. Joseph Mercola, founder of the world's most visited natural health website.

The book is a unique resource on rBGH milk. It presents Dr. Epstein's trailblazing scientific publications since 1989, which have played a major role in influencing other nations, including Canada, 24 European nations, Norway, Switzerland, Australia, New Zealand, and Japan to ban rBGH milk. The book also presents: the author's editorials and letters to major newspapers, and correspondence with the FDA, Congressman John Conyers, and other key members of Congress and the Senate. Epstein also details evidence of interlocking conflicts of interest between Monsanto and the White House, the American Medical Association and American Cancer Society. He also details evidence of Monsanto's white collar crime; the suppression and manipulation of information on the veterinary and public health dangers of rBGH milk; and evidence of Monsanto's "Hit Squad," which attempted to stifle and discredit him.

Of compelling interest is the story behind Fox Television's firing of Jane Akre, a veteran journalist, following her in-depth interview on rBGH with Dr. Epstein, his subsequent day-long deposition by Monsanto on her behalf, her subsequent litigation against Fox, and Fox's successful counter suit.

Monsanto's corporate recklessness, compounded by FDA's complicity and refusal to require labeling of rBGH milk, more than justify the rejection of any assurances of its safety. Of further interest is the critical relevance of this information to the ongoing growing concerns and debate on genetically engineered foods, including irrefutable evidence discrediting the "trust us" safety assurances of Monsanto, and other industries.

The book also presents resource materials, including listings of national and international anti-biotech, public health, veterinary and animal rights activist groups. Also listed are rBGH-free U.S. dairy producers, such as Horizon Organic, and Swiss Valley Farms.

What's in Your Milk's critical message to consumers is BOYCOTT rBGH HORMONAL MILK IN FAVOR OF CERTIFIED ORGANIC MILK.

February 22, 2007

CPC Submits Petition Calling for a Ban on Genetically Engineered Milk

On February 20, three major activist organizations representing dairy farmers, consumers, and public health experts filed a Citizen Petition to the U.S. Department of Health and Human Services. This requested immediate disapproval of Monsanto's veterinary drug Posilac on the grounds of "imminent hazards."

The petition also requested the FDA Commissioner to suspend approval of Posilac, and require milk and other dairy products to be labeled "with a cancer warning."

It should further be recognized that the FDA has willfully misled dairy producers and consumers with regard to its requirement for labeling of rBGH milk, to the effect that "No significant difference has been shown between milk derived from rBGH-treated and non-BST treated cows."

Apart from being willfully false, it is misleading in extreme as the "FDA has determined it lacks the basis for requiring such labeling in its statute." This was admitted in a July 1994 letter from Jerold R. Mande, Executive Director to the FDA Commissioner, to Harold Rudnick, New York State Department of Agriculture and Markets.

Posilac is a genetically engineered hormone also known as rBGH. About 25 percent of the nation's cattle are injected with Posilac to increase their milk production.

Since 1994, a wide range of toxic veterinary effects have been belatedly admitted by Monsanto and the FDA, and detailed on Posilac's veterinary label.

Milk containing Posilac is very different from natural milk. It may be contaminated with antibiotics and drugs used to treat injection site reactions and mastitis, and milk fat is increased, particularly levels of fatty acids incriminated in heart disease.

Most importantly, there are increased levels of a natural insulin-like growth factor known as IGF-1, ranging up to 20-fold.

IGF-1 is a small molecule, known as a peptide, and is readily absorbed from the small intestine into the blood. It is responsible for normal growth and development.

However, elevated levels of IGF-1 have been shown, in over 50 publications in leading scientific journals, to increase risks of breast, colon and prostate cancer, in some instances, by up to seven fold. Elevated levels have also been shown to block natural defense mechanisms against early submicroscopic cancers, known as apoptosis.

Based on the veterinary and public health concerns detailed in this Petition, the use and import of rBGH dairy products has been banned by Canada, 20 European nations, Norway, Switzerland, Japan, New Zealand, and Australia.

It should further be noted that on June 30, 1999, the Codex Alimentarius Commission, the United Nations Food Safety Agency representing 101 nations worldwide, ruled unanimously not to endorse or set a safety standard for rBGH milk.

The reckless conduct of the FDA detailed in the petition is consistent with its long track record of brazen denials and cover-up. A January 1986 report, "Human Food Safety and Regulation of Animal Drugs," unanimously approved by the House Committee on Government Operations concluded that the "FDA has consistently disregarded its responsibility . . . has repeatedly put what it perceives are interests of veterinarians and the livestock industry ahead of its legal obligation to protect consumers . . . jeopardizing the health and safety of consumers of meat, milk, and poultry."

This petition was submitted on behalf of the Cancer Prevention Coalition, Samuel S. Epstein, M.D., Chair; the Organic Consumers Association, Ronnie Cummins, Executive Director; and Family Farm Defenders, John Kinsman, President.

August 12, 2009

FDA Needs to Dismiss Former Monsanto Counsel

The Cancer Prevention Coalition is cautioning Americans that the recent appointment of Michael Taylor as the Senior Food Safety Advisor of the U.S. Food and Drug Administration (FDA) is of major public health concern.

In 1984, then FDA Deputy Commissioner Taylor, former counsel for Monsanto and the leading national biotech umbrella organization, warned dairy producers and retailers against "hormone-free" labels on milk from cows that had not been injected with Monsanto's biotech milk stimulant, known as recombinant bovine growth hormone, rBGH, to increase milk production.

On the basis of Taylor's explicit assurances, FDA claimed that such labeling could be "false or misleading," as there was "no significant difference between milk from treated and untreated cows."

However, "Taylor's assurance was blatantly false," according to Samuel S. Epstein, M.D., who chairs the Cancer Prevention Coalition.

"The hormone rBGH induced toxic effects in cows including mastitis," Dr. Epstein says. "Also, rBGH milk is significantly different from natural milk chemically, nutritionally, pharmacologically and immunologically."

Further, says Dr. Epstein, "rBGH milk also is contaminated with pus and antibiotics resulting from mastitis induced by the biotech hormone."

"However, in spite of such well-documented scientific evidence, the FDA authorized the sale and marketing of GE milk in 1984, while blocking any labeling," Dr. Epstein says.

He warns that drinking rBGH milk increases consumers' risk of breast, colon and prostate cancer.

"Of further and major concern, as detailed in my 2006 book What's In Your Milk?" (Trafford Publishing), drinking rBGH milk had been shown to increase risks of breast cancer in 1984. This evidence was later confirmed by over a dozen other scientific publications," Dr. Epstein says.

"rBGH milk was also subsequently shown to increase risks of prostate and colon cancers."

Meanwhile, he says, the FDA's permissive policies on rBGH milk have remained unchanged for over two succeeding decades.

Based on these considerations, it is anticipated that the FDA Commissioner Margaret Hamburg, M.D. will request the resignation of Michael Taylor.

October 14, 2009

Cancer Expert Counters Reckless Claims That Hormonal Milk Is Safe

The Cancer Prevention Coalition is criticizing a widely publicized recent report, "Recombinant Bovine Somatotropin" (rBST) which claims that milk from cows injected with this genetically engineered hormone is safe.

The report was authored by eight paid consultants to rBST companies, including Elanco and Monsanto, points out Dr. Samuel S. Epstein, Chairman of the Cancer Prevention Coalition. "All of these consultants were paid for their so-called 'safety assessments,'" he says.

The hormone rBST is injected in about 20% of U.S. dairy cows to increase milk production. While the industry claims that the hormone is safe for cows, and that the milk is safe for consumers, this is "blatantly false," says Dr Epstein, who authored the 2006 book, *What's In Your Milk?* (Trafford Publishing).

Dr. Epstein warns:

rBST makes cows sick. Monsanto has been forced to admit to about 20 toxic effects, including mastitis, on the label of Posilac, the rBST product that when administered to cows makes them produce more milk. Monsanto's Posilac product was acquired by Eli Lilly in 2008.

rBST milk is contaminated by pus, due to mastitis, an infection of the udder commonly induced by the hormone, and also by antibiotics used to treat the mastitis.

rBST milk is chemically and nutritionally different than natural milk.

Milk from cows injected with rBST is contaminated with the hormone, traces of which are absorbed through the gut into the blood of people who consume this milk or products made from it.

rBST milk is supercharged with high levels of the natural growth factor (IGF-1), which is readily absorbed through the gut.

Excess levels of IGF-1 have been incriminated in well-documented scientific publications as causes of breast, colon, and prostate cancers. Additionally, IGF-1 blocks natural defense mechanisms against early submicroscopic cancers.

Cancer Prevention Coalition warnings of these risks in 1990 were endorsed by the National Family Farm Coalition, representing 30 organizations, and also by the Campaign Against rBST, representing 10 organizations.

A 2007 Cancer Prevention Coalition petition to the U.S. Food and Drug Administration (FDA), "Seeking Withdrawal of the New Animal Drug application for rBST," was endorsed by the Organic Consumers Association, Farm Defenders, and the Institute for Responsible Technology.

Nevertheless, the FDA has remained indifferent to these risks, in spite of longstanding Congressional concerns.

Illustrative is the 1986 Congressional report, "Human Food Safety and Regulation of Animal Drugs," by the House Committee on Government Operations. This report concluded that the "FDA has consistently disregarded its responsibility . . . has repeatedly put what it perceives are interests of veterinarians and the livestock industry ahead of its legal obligations to protect consumers—jeopardizing the health and safety of consumers of meat and milk."

Of particular concern are risks to infants and children in view of their high susceptibility to cancer-causing ingredients in consumer products, warns Dr. Epstein.

Dr. Epstein says these risks are readily avoidable by consuming organic milk. According to The Hartman Group, a prominent Seattle consulting firm, organic milk is now among the first organic product that consumers buy. Organic milk is also becoming increasingly available, with an annual growth rate of about 20%, while overall milk consumption is dropping by 10%.

"Nevertheless," Dr. Epstein emphasizes, "only a few schools make organic milk available, nor do most state governments, under low-income food programs, particularly by the Special Supplemental Nutrition Program for Women, Infants and Children."

Wal-Mart is now the biggest seller of certified organic milk, followed by Horizon Organic, owned by Dean Foods, the nation's largest dairy producer, and by Groupe Danone, the leading French dairy company.

While growth in this market is still held back by the higher price of organic milk, this problem is likely to be resolved by Wal-Mart's competitive pricing.

In sharp contrast to the United States, the European Union nations as well as Norway, Switzerland, New Zealand, Japan, and Canada all have banned the use and imports of hormonal milk and dairy products.

This news release has been sent to state governors and senior officials in all 50 state health departments as well as to senior federal officials in all relevant agencies, and also staff members of relevant Congressional committees.

It was anticipated that Dr. Margaret Hamburg, the new FDA Commissioner, would take prompt action to protect the unsuspecting public from the dangers of rBST milk. However, she has failed to do so.

October 28, 2009

Dr. Samuel Epstein's 20-Year Fight against Biotech, Cancer-Causing Milk

Twenty years ago, back when Frank Young, M.D. was Commissioner of the U.S. Food and Drug Administration, he received a report from Samuel S. Epstein, M.D. entitled "Potential Public Health Hazards of Biosynthetic Milk Hormones," warning of the public health dangers of consuming milk from hormone-treated cows.

Injection of cows with recombinant Bovine Growth Hormone (rBGH), the genetically engineered, potent variant of the natural growth hormone produced by cows, sharply elevates levels of insulin-like growth factor (IGF-1) in milk, Dr. Epstein warned the commissioner.

IGF-1, which is readily absorbed through the small intestine, increases the risk of cancer in people who drink milk from cows treated with rBGH, he warned. In 1989, Dr. Epstein had found evidence of breast cancer resulting from IGF-1 ingestion; a few years later colon and prostate data began to emerge.

In his role as professor of environmental and occupational medicine with the School of Public Health, University of Illinois Medical Center in Chicago, Dr. Epstein urged the FDA Commissioner to ban the manufacture and sale of rBGH, as well as milk from treated cows, until all public and veterinary health and safety concerns were resolved.

Manufactured by Monsanto, rBGH is sold to dairy farmers under the trade name Posilac. Injection of this hormone forces cows to increase their milk production by about 10%. Monsanto has stated that about one third of dairy cows are in herds where the hormone is used.

Dr. Epstein warns that rBGH milk is often contaminated with pus, due to mastitis, an udder infection commonly induced by rBGH, and also with antibiotics used to treat the mastitis. This poses risks of nationwide antibiotic resistance to life threatening infections, he warns.

His 1989 report criticized Monsanto for failing to disclose their unpublished data and for the company's refusal to label milk from rBGH treated cows, which denies consumers the right to know when they consume hormonal milk.

"These concerns are further exacerbated by the abdication of regulatory responsibility by the FDA and USDA," Dr. Epstein wrote.

Dr. Epstein did not wait for government action.

In the September/October 1989 issue of the journal The Ecologist, of which he was associate editor, Dr. Epstein published the first major warning to reach the public about the risks of consuming rBGH milk.

In addition to increased risk of breast cancer, consuming hormonal milk increased stress, increased susceptibility to allergens, and suppressed the body's immune system, making the consumer more vulnerable to infectious diseases, the Ecologist article stated.

In Britain, the article explained, field trials of the hormone were being conducted secretly.

In the United States, the FDA granted the industry immunity from measuring hormone concentrations in milk from cows treated with rBGH.

Dr. Epstein objected that this exemption violated the 1938 Federal Food Drug and Cosmetic Act, which requires the FDA to have a "prescribed and approved test method" for determining whether a drug is being improperly used with resulting illegal residues in food. But no test was available for rBGH milk.

In September 1989, Dr. Epstein testified on these matters to the Wisconsin State Assembly Committee on Agriculture, and the following year, published an article based on his testimony in the International Journal of Health Services.

He has repeatedly called on government to require the industry to "fund research in accordance with independently approved protocols" supervised by a "neutral, independent intermediary" such as the National Institutes of Health or the National Science Foundation.

In December 1990, Dr. Epstein presented these views at a conference hosted by the National Institutes of Health, warning that high IGF-1 levels could increase the risk of breast cancer in people who drink rBGH milk.

Nevertheless, in 1993, the FDA approved the commercial sale of milk from rBGH treated cows and issued regulations banning the labeling of rBGH milk.

In 1994, FDA Commissioner David Kessler, M.D. received a letter from Dr. Epstein expressing his "grave concerns" about the risks of breast and colon cancer from consumption of hormonal milk.

Now chairman of his new nonprofit organization, the Cancer Prevention Coalition," Dr. Epstein wrote, "IGF-1 induces malignant transformation of normal human breast epithelial cells. IGF-1 is a growth factor for human breast cancer cells, maintaining their malignancy, progression and invasiveness. IGF-1 has similarly been associated with colon cancer."

The letter urged Kessler to revoke the agency's approval of rBGH registration.

Given these concerns, dairy farmers began assuring the public by putting "hormone-free" labels on milk from cows that had not been injected with rBGH. A month later, the Los Angeles Times published an article by Dr. Epstein blasting the FDA for the labeling ban.

The labeling ban was challenged by nationwide grassroots consumers groups, and by two milk suppliers, both of whom were sued by Monsanto.

In a range of public arenas, from 1996 Chicago hearings on the labeling of genetically modified foods to a 1998 article in the "International Journal of Health Services," Dr. Epstein continued to warn that rBGH milk poses increased risks for breast and colon cancer.

"In short," he wrote in the 1998 article, "with the active complicity of the FDA, the entire nation is currently being subjected to an experiment involving large-scale adulteration of an age-old dietary staple by a poorly characterized and unlabeled biotechnology product. Disturbingly, this experiment benefits only a very small segment of the agri-chemical industry while providing no matching benefits to consumers. Even more disturbingly, it poses major public health risks for the entire U.S. population."

In March 1998, Dr. Epstein added a new warning about consumption of rBGH milk—prostate cancer.

In the journal Gene Therapy Weekly, he wrote that rBGH milk is "supercharged with high levels of abnormally potent IGF-1, up to 10 times the levels in natural milk and over 10 times more potent."

"Apart from prostate cancer," he warned, "multiple lines of evidence have also incriminated the role of IGF-1 as risk factors for breast, colon and childhood cancers."

After 10 years of warnings based on in-depth scientific documentation, Dr. Epstein began to get support in his fight against hormonal milk.

In March 1999, the Scientific Committee of the European Commission released a report finding excess levels of IGF-1 in milk of cows injected with rBGH. The report concluded that the excess IGF-1 poses serious risks of breast and prostate cancer.

Commenting on the Scientific Committee's report, Dr. Epstein criticized Codex, the World Health Organization responsible for setting international food safety standards, which had approved hormonal milk. "FDA officials and industry consultants are members of Codex, which meets in secrecy and relies on unpublished industry assurances of safety," he wrote.

Just five months later, in August 1999, Codex unexpectedly ruled in favor of the 1993 European Union moratorium on rBGH milk. The ruling forced the United States to abandon its threat to challenge the moratorium at the World Trade Organization.

Cancer Prevention Coalition warnings were endorsed by the National Family Farm Coalition, representing 30 organizations, and also by the Campaign Against rBGH, representing 10 organizations.

The Organic Consumers Association and Director Ronnie Cummins endorsed the campaign to educate the public about the dangers of rBGH milk. In a joint 2005 editorial in the journal Medical Veritas Epstein and Cummins wrote, ". . . increased IGF-1 blood levels have been incriminated as a major cause of cancer."

Over 100 leading independent experts in cancer prevention and public health, plus citizen activist groups endorsed this warning, wrote Epstein and Cummins.

This endorsement was coupled with insistence that the public has "an absolute right-to-know" of information on avoidable causes of cancer, "a democratic right which the agribusiness and FDA continue to subvert," they wrote.

In 2006, Dr. Epstein published the book, *What's in Your Milk? An Exposé of Industry and Government Cover-Up on the Dangers of the Genetically Engineered (rBGH) Milk You're Drinking*, (Trafford Publishing).

Monsanto, supported by the FDA, insists that rBGH milk is indistinguishable from natural milk, and that it is safe for consumers. "This is blatantly false," wrote Dr. Epstein, listing the dangers of milk from cows treated with the hormone.

rBGH makes cows sick. Monsanto has been forced to admit to about 20 toxic effects, including mastitis, on its Posilac label.

rBGH milk is contaminated by pus, due to the mastitis commonly induced by rBGH, and antibiotics used to treat the mastitis.

rBGH milk is chemically, and nutritionally different than natural milk.

Milk from cows injected with rBGH is contaminated with the hormone, traces of which are absorbed through the gut into the blood.

rBGH milk is supercharged with high levels of the natural growth factor, IGF-1, which is readily absorbed through the gut.

Excess levels of IGF-1 have been incriminated as a cause of breast, colon, and prostate cancers.

IGF-1 blocks natural defense mechanisms against early submicroscopic cancers.

rBGH factory farms pose a major threat to the viability of small dairy farms.

rBGH enriches Monsanto, while posing dangers, without any benefits, to consumers, especially in view of the current national surplus of milk.

Of still greater concern, based on 37 published scientific studies as detailed in the book, excess levels of IGF-1 in rBGH milk pose major risks of breast, colon and prostate cancers.

Not surprisingly rBGH milk is banned in Canada, the EU and internationally.

The book features an Introduction by Ben Cohen, cofounder of Ben and Jerry's Ice Cream and president of the group Business Leaders for Sensible Priorities. The Foreword was written by Jeffrey M. Smith, author of the bestseller Seeds of Deception.

The book attracted endorsements from Congressman John Conyers, chairman of the House Judiciary Committee; Mark Achbar, executive producer of the multiple prize-winning documentary The Corporation; Dr. Joseph Mercola, founder of the world's most visited natural health website; Quentin Young, M.D., chairman of the Health and Medicine Policy Research Group and past president of the American Public Health Association; and Peter I. Hardin, editor and publisher of "The Milkweed," an influential monthly publication covering the dairy industry.

Other endorsers included Ken Ausubel, author of "Seeds of Change" and director of the Bioneers conferences; and Anna Lappe, author of "Diet for a Small Planet."

The book is a unique resource on rBGH milk. It presents Dr. Epstein's trailblazing scientific publications since 1989, which have played a major role in influencing other nations, including Canada, 24 European nations, Norway, Switzerland, Australia, New Zealand, and Japan to ban rBGH milk.

The book also presents: the author's editorials and letters to major newspapers, and correspondence with the FDA, Congressman Conyers, and other key members of Congress.

In the book, Epstein also details evidence of interlocking conflicts of interest between Monsanto and the White House, the American Medical Association and American Cancer Society. He presents evidence of

Monsanto's white collar crime; the suppression and manipulation of information on the veterinary and public health dangers of rBGH milk; and evidence of Monsanto's "Hit Squad," which attempted to stifle and discredit him.

Monsanto's corporate recklessness, compounded by FDA's complicity and insistence that there is no significant difference between rBGH and rBGH-free milk, more than justify the rejection of any assurances of its safety. Of further interest is the critical relevance of this information to the ongoing growing concerns and debate on genetically engineered foods, including irrefutable evidence discrediting the "trust us" safety assurances of Monsanto, and other industries.

The book also presents resource materials, including listings of national and international anti-biotech, public health, veterinary and animal rights activist groups. Also listed are rBGH—free U.S. dairy producers, such as Horizon Organic, and Swiss Valley Farms.

What's In Your Milk's critical message to consumers is, BOYCOTT rBGH HORMONAL MILK IN FAVOR OF CERTIFIED ORGANIC MILK. The book is available from Trafford Publishing, www.trafford.com/06-0676

In 2007, Andrew C. von Eschenbach, M.D. was the FDA Commissioner. The Cancer Prevention Coalition petitioned the FDA, "Seeking Withdrawal of the New Animal Drug application for rBST." This petition was endorsed by the Organic Consumers Association, Farm Defenders, the Institute for Responsible Technology and by Hungarian biologist Arpad Pusztai.

The petition asks that the FDA suspend approval of the rBGH product Posilac and/or require that milk and other dairy products produced by injecting Posilac carry warning labels stating, "Produced with the use of Posilac, and contains elevated levels of IGF-1, a major risk factor for breast, prostate and colon cancers."

It is currently estimated that about 20% of U.S. milk is produced with the use of rBGH.

Still considered the leading international scientific expert on hormonal milk, Dr. Epstein is not waiting for government action on rBGH milk, although all the concerns he has expressed over the past 20 years are still outstanding.

On October 14, 2009, he criticized a widely publicized report, "Recombinant Bovine Somatotropin," which repeats claims that milk from cows injected with rBGH is safe, pointing out that the report was authored by eight paid consultants to rBST companies, including Elanco and Monsanto.

November 13, 2009

American Public Health Association Supports Ban on Hormonal Milk and Meat

The Cancer Prevention Coalition is pleased to announce that the Governing Council of the American Public Health Association has voted to oppose the continued sale and use of genetically engineered hormonal rBGH milk, and also meat adulterated with sex hormones. This decision is based on long-standing scientific and public policy information developed and published by the Cancer Prevention Coalition over the last two decades, as summarized below.

rBGH MILK

This hormone is injected in about 20% of U.S. dairy cows to increase milk production. While the industry claims that the hormone is safe for cows, and that the milk is safe for consumers, this is blatantly false.

rBGH makes cows sick. Monsanto has been forced to admit to about 20 toxic veterinary effects, including mastitis, on the label of Posilac (rBGH,) which is injected in cows to increase milk production. Monsanto's Posilac product was acquired by Eli Lilly in 2008.

rBGH milk is contaminated by pus, due to mastitis, an udder infection commonly induced by the hormone, and also by antibiotics used to treat the mastitis.

rBGH milk is chemically and nutritionally different than natural milk.

Milk from cows injected with rBGH is contaminated with the hormone, traces of which are absorbed through the gut into the blood of people who consume this milk or its products.

rBGH milk is supercharged with high levels of the natural growth factor (IGF-1), which is readily absorbed through the gut.

Excess levels of IGF-1 have been incriminated in well-documented scientific publications by the Chairman of the Cancer Prevention Coalition as causes of breast, colon, and prostate cancers. Additionally,

IGF-1 blocks natural defense mechanisms against early submicroscopic cancers.

Cancer Prevention Coalition Chairman Samuel S. Epstein, M.D. says, "These warnings, and related information were updated in my 2006 book, *What's in Your Milk* (Trafford Publishing) supported by over 320 references, and endorsed by Jeffrey Smith, Executive Director, Institute for Responsible Technology, and by Dr. Quentin Young, Past President American Public Health Association."

Warnings by the Cancer Prevention Coalition of these risks in 1990 have been endorsed by the National Family Farm Coalition, representing 30 organizations, and also by the Campaign Against rBST, representing 10 organizations.

A 2007 Cancer Prevention Coalition petition to the U.S. Food and Drug Administration (FDA), "Seeking Withdrawal of the New Animal Drug application for rBST," was endorsed by the Organic Consumers Association, Farm Defenders, and the Institute for Responsible Technology. However, the FDA failed to responded to or act on this petition. This petition was endorsed by the Organic Consumers Association, the Family Farm Defenders, and the Institute for Responsible Technology.

Furthermore, the FDA has remained indifferent to these risks, in spite of longstanding Congressional concerns. Illustrative is the 1986 Congressional report, "Human Food Safety and Regulation of Animal Drugs," by the House Committee on Government Operations. This report concluded that the "FDA has consistently disregarded its responsibility . . . has repeatedly put what it perceives are interests of veterinarians and the livestock industry ahead of its legal obligations to protect consumers—jeopardizing the health and safety of consumers of meat and milk."

Of particular concern are risks to infants and children in view of their high susceptibility to cancer-causing ingredients in consumer products.

These risks are readily avoidable by consuming organic milk. According to The Hartman Group, a prominent Seattle consulting firm, organic milk is now among the first organic product that consumers buy. Organic milk is becoming increasingly available, with an annual growth rate of about 20%, while overall milk consumption is dropping by 10%.

Nevertheless, only a few schools make organic milk available, nor do most state governments, under low-income food programs, particularly by the Special Supplemental Nutrition Program for Women, Infants and Children."

Wal-Mart is now the biggest seller of certified organic milk, followed by Horizon Organic, owned by Dean Foods, the nation's largest dairy producer, and by Groupe Danone, the leading French dairy company. While growth in this market is still held back by the higher price of organic milk, this problem is likely to be resolved by Wal-Mart's competitive pricing.

In sharp contrast to the United States, the European Union nations, as well as Norway, Switzerland, New Zealand, Japan, and Canada, all have banned the use and imports of hormonal milk and dairy products.

This information was recently sent by the Cancer Prevention Coalition to state governors, besides senior officials in all 50 state health departments as well as to senior federal officials in all relevant agencies, and also staff members of relevant Congressional committees.

It is anticipated that Dr. Margaret Hamburg, the highly respected new Commissioner of the FDA, will take prompt action to protect the unsuspecting public from the dangers of rBST milk.

HORMONAL BEEF

Beef produced in the United States is heavily contaminated with natural or synthetic sex hormones, which are associated with an increased risk of reproductive and childhood cancers.

Increased levels of sex hormones are linked to the escalating incidence of reproductive cancers in the United States since 1975-60% for prostate, 59% for testis, and 10% for breast, warns the Cancer Prevention Coalition.

The hormones in past and current use include the natural estrogen, progesterone and testosterone, and the synthetic zeranol, trenbolone, and melengesterol.

When beef cattle enter feedlots, pellets of these hormones are implanted under the ear skin, a process that is repeated at the midpoint of their

100-day pre-slaughter fattening period. These hormones increase carcass weight, adding over $80 in extra profit per animal.

The Cancer Prevention Coalition warned that, "Not surprisingly, but contrary to longstanding claims by the U.S. Food and Drug Administration (FDA) and the U.S. Department of Agriculture (USDA), residues of these hormones in meat are up to 20-fold higher than normal. Still higher residues result from the not uncommon illegal practice of implantation directly into muscle. Furthermore, contrary to misleading assurances, meat is still not monitored for hormone residues." Nevertheless, the FDA and USDA still maintain that hormone residues in meat are within "normal levels," while waiving any requirements for residue testing.

Following a single ear implant in steers of Synovex-S, a combination of estrogen and progesterone, residues of these hormones in meat were found to be up to 20-fold higher than normal.

The amount of estradiol in two hamburgers eaten in one day by an 8-year-old boy could increase his total hormone levels by as much as 10%, particularly as young children have very low natural hormone levels. Not surprisingly, the coalition warns, the incidence of childhood cancer has increased by 38% since 1975.

These concerns are not new. As evidenced in a series of General Accountability Office investigations and Congressional hearings, FDA residue-tolerance programs and USDA inspections are in near total disarray, aggravated by brazen denials and cover-ups.

A January 1986 report, "Human Food Safety and the Regulation of Animal Drugs," unanimously approved by the House Committee on Government Operations, concluded that "the FDA has consistently disregarded its responsibility—has repeatedly put what is perceives are interests of veterinarians and the livestock industry ahead of its legal obligation to protect consumers, thus jeopardizing the health and safety of consumers of meat, milk and poultry."

On January 1, 1989, the European Community placed a ban on meat imports from animals treated with growth inducing hormones. This had a direct impact on the U.S. beef industry, which used the hormones in more than half of the cattle sent to market each year.

Twenty-years later, on May 6, 2009, the European Union and the United States settled their long—running dispute over hormone-treated beef. Under terms of the four-year deal the EU will be permitted to maintain its ban on hormone-fed beef. In return, the EU has agreed to increase the amount of hormone-free beef that can be imported from the U.S. without duty.

It is well recognized that American women have a greater risk of breast cancer than women in countries that do not permit the sale of hormonal beef.

THE WHITE HOUSE

On November 4, 2009, the Cancer Prevention Coalition submitted a 10/21/09 press release on "Hormones in U.S. Beef Linked to Increased Cancer Risks," and a 10/28/09 release on "Dr. Epstein's 20 Year Fight Against Biotech Cancer Causing Milk" to Katie McCormick, Press Secretary to First Lady of the United States Michelle Obama; to Jocelyn Frey, Deputy Assistant to the President and Director of Policy; and to Sam Kass, White House Food Initiative Coordinator and the Obama family's personal chef at the White House. Replies are pending.

January 15, 2010

An FDA Ban on Genetically-Engineered Milk Is Twenty Years Overdue

In May 2007, Samuel S. Epstein, M.D., Chairman of the Cancer Prevention Coalition, and four other leading national experts on genetically-engineered, recombinant bovine growth hormone (rBGH) milk filed a Petition to the Food and Drug Administration (FDA), "Petition Seeking the Withdrawal of the New Animal Drug Application Approval for Posilac®-Recombinant Bovine Growth Hormone (rBGH)."

In the absence of any response, on January 12, 2010, Dr. Epstein resubmitted this Petition to Michael Taylor, Deputy Commissioner of the Food and Drug Administration.

As detailed in this Petition, Posilac® poses major public health hazards. Dr. Epstein requested his review and support of an early ban of Posilac®.

This Petition requests the Secretary of Health and Human Services, and the Commissioner of Food and Drugs to suspend the approval of rBGH, a genetically engineered bovine growth hormone, and require milk and other dairy products produced with its use to be labeled with a warning such as, "Produced with the use of rBGH, and contains elevated levels of insulin-like growth factor, IGF-1, which poses major risks of breast, prostate, and colon cancers."

STATEMENT OF GROUNDS

THE VETERINARY TOXICITY OF rBGH

Evidence of these toxic effects was first detailed in confidential Monsanto reports, based on records of secret nationwide rBGH veterinary trials, submitted to the FDA prior to October 1989 when they were leaked to one of the petitioners, Dr. Epstein. He then made these reports available to Congressman John Conyers, Chairman of the House Committee on Government Operations. On May 8, 1990, Congressman Conyers issued the following statement, "I find it reprehensible that Monsanto and the FDA have chosen to suppress and manipulate animal health test data."

Details of these toxic effects were subsequently admitted by Monsanto, and by the FDA, and were disclosed on the drug's veterinary label (Posilac®) in November, 1993. These toxic effects include injection site lesions, a wide range of other toxic effects, and an increased incidence of mastitis requiring the use and antibiotics, with resulting contamination of milk.

ABNORMALITIES IN rBGH MILK

A January 1994 Monsanto Executive Summary on rBGH, claimed that "natural milk is indistinguishable" from rBGH milk, and that "there is no legal basis requiring its labeling." However, there are a wide range of well-documented abnormalities in rBGH milk. These include: reduction in short-chain fatty acid and increase in long-chain fatty acid levels; increase in levels of a thyroid hormone enzyme; contamination with unapproved drugs for treating mastitis; and frequency of pus cells due to mastitis.

INCREASED LEVELS OF INSULIN-LIKE GROWTH FACTOR 1 (IGF-1) IN rBGH MILK

A wide range of publications have documented excess levels of IGF-1 in rBGH milk, with increases ranging from four—to 20-fold. Based on six unpublished industry studies, FDA admitted that IGF-1 levels in rBGH milk were consistently and statistically increased, and that these were further increased by pasteurization. These increases were also admitted by the pharmaceutical company Eli Lilly, in application for marketing authorization in the European Community. It should also be noted that pasteurization of milk increases IGF-1 levels.

IGF-1 IS READILY ABSORBED FROM THE INTESTINE INTO THE BLOOD

IGF-1 is a small protein component known as a peptide. As such it is readily absorbed into the blood. It survives digestion, and has marked growth promoting effects following short-term feeding tests in rats.

INCREASED IGF-1 LEVELS IN MILK INCREASE RISKS OF BREAST, COLON AND PROSTATE CANCERS

Increased levels of IGF-1 have been shown to increase risks of breast cancer in 19 scientific publications, risks of colon cancer in 10 publications, and prostate cancer in 7 publications.

INCREASED IGF-1 LEVELS INHIBIT "APOPTOSIS"

Of critical importance is the fact that increased IGF-1 levels block natural defense mechanisms, known as apoptosis, against early submicroscopic cancers.

rBGH INCREASES TWINNING RATES

An increased rate of twinning in cows injected with rBGH was admitted by Monsanto on its November 1993 Posilac® label, and the incidence of fraternal twins. Monsanto also admitted that it increases "and complications such as premature delivery, congenital defects and pregnancy-induced hypertension."

THE INTERNATIONAL BAN ON THE USE AND IMPORTS OF U.S. rBGH DAIRY PRODUCTS

Based on well-documented veterinary and public health concerns, in June 30, 1999, the United Nations Food Safety Agency, representing 101 nations worldwide, ruled unanimously not to endorse or set a safety standard for rBGH milk. Effectively, this has resulted in an international ban on U.S. milk, approximately 20% of which is rBGH.

FDA POLICY ON LABELING rBGH MILK

The FDA continues to mislead dairy producers and consumers with regard to its requirement for labeling of rBGH milk, with its deliberately false claim that "No significant difference has been shown between milk derived from rBST-treated and non-rBST treated cows."

"In fact," warns Dr. Epstein, "rBGH milk continues to pose major cancer and other risks to the entire U.S. population."

The 2007 Petition has been endorsed by four other leading experts on genetically-engineered, recombinant bovine growth hormone (rBGH) milk. We look forward to a response.

ENDORSERS:

Ronnie Cummins
National Director
Organic Consumers Association

John Kinsman
President
Family Farm Defenders

Arpad Pusztai, PhD, FRSE
Consultant Biologist
Scotland

Jeffrey Smith
Executive Director
Institute for Responsible Technology

April 2, 2010

Cancer Prevention Coalition Challenges "Honest Food Labels" Article

March 18, New York Times editorial, "Honest Food Labels," FDA Commissioner, Margaret Hamburg, M.D., publicized letters to 17 food companies accusing them of—"masking undesirable ingredients"—in their products. She also emphasized the importance of "providing nutrition information that consumers can rely on." Unfortunately, she has failed to take any such action with regard to the two major dietary staples, milk and meat.

About 20% of our milk is genetically engineered, technically known as rBGH (recombinant Bovine Growth Hormone), which contains high levels of a natural growth factor known as IGF-1 (Insulin-like Growth Factor one). This survives digestion and is readily absorbed from the small intestine into the blood. Increased levels of IGF-1 have been shown to increase risks of breast cancer in 19 scientific publications, risks of colon cancer in 10 publications, and prostate cancer in 7 publications. Of further concern, increased IGF-1 levels block natural defense mechanisms against early microscopic cancers, known as apoptosis.

Based on these concerns, on June 3, 1999, the United Nations Food Safety Agency, representing 101 nations worldwide, ruled unanimously not to endorse or set safety standards for rBGH milk. Effectively, this has resulted in an international ban on U.S. milk.

Also based on these concerns, the Cancer Prevention Coalition, endorsed by five leading national experts, petitioned the FDA in May 2007 to label rBGH milk with an explicit cancer warnings. In the absence of any response, we resubmitted this petition in January 2010 to Dr. Hamburg, and are waiting for a response.

U.S. cattle are implanted with natural or synthetic sex hormones prior to entering feed lots 100 days prior to slaughter in order to increase their meat yield. Not surprisingly, our meat is contaminated with high levels of sex hormones. Based on these concerns, and as warned by the Cancer Prevention Coalition and five leading national experts, our meat poses increased risks of hormonal cancers, which have escalated since 1975:

breast by 23%, prostate by 60%, and testis by 60%. Not surprisingly, U.S. meat is banned worldwide.

Furthermore, as clearly evidenced in a series of General Accounting Office investigations and Congressional hearings, the FDA, besides the U.S. Department of Agriculture (USDA), have failed to take any regulatory action to protect the public from the dangers of hormonal meat. A 1986 report, "Human Food Safety and Regulation of Animal Drugs," unanimously approved by the House Committee on Government Operations, concluded that the "FDA has consistently disregarded its responsibility—has repeatedly put what it perceives are interests of veterinarians and the livestock industry ahead of its legal obligation to protect consumers—jeopardizing the health and safety of consumers meat, milk, and poultry."

In response to questions on the dangers of hormonal meat raised by the European Commission in February 1996, the USDA responded with unsubstantiated claims that less than 0.25% of animals tested annually proved positive for "residue violations." In fact, meat has not been and is still not monitored for sex hormone levels by the USDA or FDA.

Together with other leading scientific experts, on January 29, 2010, the Cancer Prevention Coalition submitted a Citizens Petition to the FDA on the "Imminent health Hazard" from hormonal meat, supported by 59 scientific references. We are waiting for a response.

Not surprisingly, U.S. milk and meat are banned virtually worldwide.

C.
Hormonal Meat

Hormonal Meat

Citizen Petition Seeking Labeling of Nitrite-Preserved Hot Dogs for Childhood Cancer Risk[*]

April 25, 1995

David A. Kessler, M.D.
Commissioner, Food and Drug Administration

This Petition is based on accumulating scientific information on excess risks of childhood brain tumors and leukemia from the consumption of hot dogs containing nitrite preservatives.

A. AGENCY ACTION REQUESTED

This petition requests the FDA to take the following action:

Immediately require nitrite-containing hot dogs to be labeled with warnings such as hot dogs containing nitrites have been shown to pose risks of childhood cancer.

B. STATEMENT OF GROUNDS

Nitrites are widely used as preservatives in hot dogs, besides other meat products. Nitrites combine with amines naturally present in meat to form carcinogenic N-nitroso compounds. N-nitrosodimethylamine has been identified in nitrite-preserved meat products. There is overwhelming evidence on the carcinogenicity of N-nitrosodimethylamine in animal experiments. Furthermore, epidemiologic evidence has associated N-nitroso carcinogens with cancer of the oral cavity, urinary bladder, esophagus, stomach and brain.

There is substantial evidence on the risks of childhood cancer from the consumption of meats containing nitrites. In 1982, Preston-Martin, et al. found that consumption during pregnancy of meats cured with sodium nitrite has been associated with development of brain tumors in the offspring.

---

[*]   This Petition is based on twenty-four scientific references.

Recent case-control studies have confirmed the risks of cancer from consumption of hot dogs. Eating many hot dogs by children, as well maternal hot dog consumption during pregnancy, has been shown to be associated with brain cancer and leukemia in children.

Bunin, et al. studied children who were diagnosed with brain cancer before age six, between 1986 and 1989. Of 53 foods and beverages and three alcoholic beverages consumed by mothers during pregnancy, only hot dogs were associated with an excess risk of childhood brain tumor.

Sarusua and Savitz studied 234 childhood cancer cases in Denver and found a strong association between the consumption of hot dogs and brain cancer. Children born to mothers who consumed hot dogs one or more times per week during pregnancy had approximately doubled the risk of developing brain tumors. Children who ate hot dogs one or more times per week were also at higher risk of brain cancer. In addition, children who ate hot dogs and took no vitamins, which retard the formation of N-nitroso carcinogens, were more strongly associated with both acute lymphocytic leukemia (ALL) and brain cancer. Sarusua and Savitz concluded:

"The results linking hot dogs and brain tumors (replicating an earlier study) and the apparent synergism between no vitamins and meat consumption suggest a possible adverse effect of dietary nitrites and nitrosamines."

Peters, et al., studied the relationship between the intake of certain foods and the risk of leukemia in children from birth to age 10 in Los Angeles County between 1980 and 1987. The researchers found that children who ate 12 or more hot dogs per month had approximately nine times the normal risk for developing childhood leukemia. A strong risk for childhood leukemia also existed for those children whose fathers' intake of hot dogs was 12 or more per month. Peters, et al. concluded:

"Our results provide evidence for an association between consumption of hot dogs and risk of childhood leukemia. Adjustments for all factors thought to be potential confounders did not affect these associations. Independent risks were associated with both children's and fathers' consumption . . . The findings, if correct, suggest that reduced consumption of hot dogs could reduce leukemia risks, especially in those consuming the most.

These findings are of particular significance considering a 38 percent increase in the incidence of brain and nervous system cancers in children from 1973-1991. Brain tumors account for about one in five childhood cancers.

This petition, based on twenty-four scientific references, was submitted by:

Samuel S. Epstein, M.D.
Chairman, Cancer Prevention Coalition
Professor Occupational and Environmental Medicine
University of Illinois at Chicago

Michael Deutsch, Esq., Legal Director, Center for Constitutional Rights, New York

Citizen Petition "Imminent Health Hazard" From Hormonal Beef

January 29, 2010

Kathleen Sebelius
Secretary of Health and Human Services
U.S. Department of Health and Human Services

Margaret Hamburg, M.D.
Commissioner of Food and Drugs

CC: Congressman John Conyers
CC: Congressman Dennis Kucinich

Citizen Petition "IMMINENT HEALTH HAZARD" FROM HORMONAL BEEF

The undersigned submits this petition on behalf of the Cancer Prevention Coalition, Samuel S. Epstein, M.D., Chairman; Massachusetts Institute of Technology, Nicholas Ashford, PhD, JD, Professor of Technology and Policies; Organic Consumers Association, Ronnie Cummins, Executive Director; and Health and Medicine Policy Research Group, Quentin D. Young, M.D., Chairman.

Based on a review of the scientific literature, Food and Drug Administration (FDA) Freedom of Information Summaries, other U.S. Government reports, and World Health Organization (WHO) reports, we conclude that the use of natural and synthetic anabolics in meat production poses serious carcinogenic and other hazards to consumers, with particular reference to breast and other reproductive cancers. For these reasons, we petition the federal government to:

- Recognize these hazards as "imminent hazards" for the purpose of future regulatory action, and
- Take appropriate action to eliminate their use and likely human exposure.

---

* This Petition is based on fifty-nine scientific references.

170

This Petition is based on the following evidence:

1. The Carcinogenicity of Natural Anabolics

    a. Estradiol-17B

Based on an exhaustive review of the scientific literature, the International Agency for Research on Cancer (IARC) confirmed the carcinogenicity of estradiol in experimental animals, inducing mammary, testicular, other reproductive tumors, and tumors at other sites, and concluded that it was of comparable potency to diethylstilbestrol, an illegal synthetic anabolic. IARC subsequently concluded that the evidence of estradiol's carcinogenicity to animals was "sufficient," and that it was "causally associated" with reproductive cancers in women.

    b. Testosterone

On the basis of a review of the scientific literature, testosterone was classified by IARC as a Group 2A carcinogen. IARC concluded that the evidence of its carcinogenicity in rodents was "sufficient," and that it "may be involved in the genesis of (prostatis) tumors in humans." These carcinogenic effects have also been recognized by WHO. Following administration of testosterone to rodents, "the incidence of prostatic tumors was higher than in control animals (and the incidence of uterine tumors was surprisingly high."

    c. Progesterone

On the basis of a review of the scientific literature, IARC concluded that the evidence for its carcinogenicity, based on the induction of mammary, ovarian and uterine cancers in rodents, was "sufficient."

    d. Enhanced infant sensitivity

There is substantial literature on the enhanced carcinogenic sensitivity of neonatal rodents to natural anabolics, both individually and in combination, and to synthetic anabolics, such as diethylstilbestrol. Illustratively, "neonatal exposure of mice to progesterone plus estradiol-17B resulted in an increased incidence of mammary tumors. Furthermore, there is a substantial literature on the increased susceptibility of infant and young rodents and humans to a wide range of carcinogens, including natural anabolics and diethylstilbestrol (DES).

2.   The Carcinogenicity of Synthetic Anabolics

   a.   Trenbolone Acetate

There are no published data on the carcinogenicity of Trenbolone, a synthetic steroid resembling testosterone. However, unpublished and inadequately documented industry data have demonstrated its carcinogenicity to mice and rates. These findings include: "Significant increases in hepatic proliferative lesions (neoplasia and hyperplasia) in male and female (mice)—and in increased incidence of pancreatic islet tumors" in rats. These carcinogenic effects have also been recognized by WHO. However, these conclusions were dismissed by FDA "on the basis of direct and ancillary evidence."

   b.   Zeranol

There are no published data on the carcinogenicity of Zeranol, a non-steroidal synthetic estrogen. However, unpublished and inadequately documented industry data have demonstrated the "induction of anterior lobe pituitary adenomas" in male rates. These carcinogenic effects have also been recognized by WHO.

   c.   Melengesterol Acetate (MGA)

There are no published data on the carcinogenicity of MGA, a synthetic progestin. A 1966 Food Additive Petition to the FDA, summarizing the toxicology of MGA and on the basis of which its use was approved, omitted any reference to carcinogenicity. However, an internal industry report documented the induction of a statistically significant incidence of mammary tumors in female mice; these results were subsequently published.

3.   Residues of Anabolics Following Legal Administration for Meat Production

The legal route for administration of natural anabolics and of synthetic anabolics, other than MGA, is subcutaneous implantation of pellets in the ear. In October 1989, FDA approved the re-implantation of steers with estradiol benzoate and progesterone (Synovex-S) in the mid-point of their feeing period. There has been no requirement for any pre-slaughter withdrawal period for over three decades.

Both USDA and FDA have assured the public that meat products are routinely monitored for residues of animal drugs and other industrial chemicals through offensive statements:

- Since 1987, USDA and FDA have been monitoring volatile levels of residues of animal
drugs, pesticides, and industrial chemicals in food animals.
- The program has expanded greatly since its inception, and because the use of many
pesticides has declined, a greater emphasis is now placed on testing for animal drugs.
- The program is designed to ensure that the compounds most likely to be present in food animals are included in the nationwide monitoring residue plan. The program has the
flexibility to keep up with current usage of animal drugs.
- Samples of meat and poultry products are collected from healthy appearing animals at
domestic slaughter establishments using a statistically based, random sampling plan.
- Surveillance programs are designed to distinguish those areas of the livestock and poultry populations in which residue problems exist, to measure the extent of the problems, and to evaluate the impact of actions initiated to reduce the occurrence of residues.
- FSIS (Food Safety and Inspection Service of USDA) collects samples for testing when a
problem with residues is suspected.
- Most residue monitoring program has been supported by an education program targeted at food animal producers, and its success has assisted in the decline of residue violators.
- The residue monitoring program has been supported by an education program targeted at food animal producers, and its success has assisted in the decline of residue violators.
- In 1993, approximately one-fourth of one percent of animals tested showed positive for residue violation. In other words, almost 99.74 percent of animals tested showed no residue violations.

However, in contrast to these highly misleading published assurances, FSIS 1993 data indicate that none of approximately 120 million head of livestock slaughtered annually have been monitored for any residues of natural or synthetic anabolics.

The only available residue data are provided in "New Animal Drug Application" (NADA) petitions to FDA, by pharmaceutical companies, manufacturing and formulating the anabolic drugs, as detailed in Freedom of Information Summaries obtained from the FDA. Residue levels were determined by specialized techniques, radio-immune assays, which are not practical for routine monitoring. Despite the requirement of Section 512 of The 1968 Animal Drug Amendments to the Federal Food Inspection Act which stipulates that a manufacturer submitting a NADA must provide "a description of practical methods" for analysis and monitoring of carcinogenic residues in food, no such methods were available in 1973; over two decades later, none are still available. FDA, however, has circumvented this legislative mandate by claiming that "a regulatory method is not needed for the assurance of safety of the approved use of (anabolic) implants because the maximum increased exposure, even considering probable misuse of the drug, is demonstrated to be far below those concentrations considered unsafe."

a. Estradiol

Following implantation of steers with Synovex-S (estradiol benzoate and progesterone), estradiol residues in liver, kidney, muscle and fat at 15 days were increased over normal background levels by 6, 9, 12 and 23-fold, respectively; the average residue in fat of untreated controls was 1.8ppt (μg/kg). However, minimizing these data, WHO claimed that estradiol implants "—may produce two-fold to five-fold increases in residue levels and that these fall within the normal range found in untreated bovine animals—," the comparability of which was, however, unspecified.

b. Testosterone

Following implantation of heifers with Synovex-H (estradiol benzoate and testosterone propionate), testosterone residues in kidney, liver, muscle and fat at 30 days were increased over normal background levels by 2, 3, 5 and 30-fold, respectively; the average fat level in untreated animals was 26ppt (μg/kg). Similar increased residues have been reported by WHO.

c. Trenbolone

Following implantation of heifers with Revalor (Trenbolone acetate and estradiol), the total average residues in beef liver were 50 ppb (μg/kg) at 30 days, while "residues in muscle, kidney and fat were much lower." In contrast to these data, WHO, however, claimed that the 50ppb liver residues were the "highest mean concentrations."

d. Zeranol

Following implantation of Ralgro (Zeranol) in steers and heifers, total average residues in muscle, fat, kidney and liver at 15 days were 0.1, 0.3, 1.7, and 8.2ppb. Similar residues have been reported by WHO.

e. Melengesterol Acetate (MGA)

Following feeding heifers with MGA, 139 of 174 fat samples contained residues below 10ppb, while the remainder had residues ranging from 10-19ppb at 12 to 24 hours after the last feeding; the sensitivity level of this assay was only 10ppb. It should be noted that WHO has still failed to evaluate the use of MGA; this is in contrast to the requirement that it evaluates all veterinary drugs regulated in at least one country.

4. Residues of Anabolics Following Illegal Administration

No data are available on the much higher local and distant residue levels anticipated following intramuscular implantation or injection. A 1986 USDA survey revealed that as many as half the cattle in 32 large feedlots had "misplaced implants." FDA's response was limited in extreme: "part of the carcass containing pellets should continue to be condemned." Such action ignores the probability of high residues in distant organs and tissues due to the anticipated increased absorption of anabolics from highly vascular muscle in contrast to relatively avascular subcutaneous ear tissue. Furthermore, visual inspection and random monitoring could not reveal evidence of intramuscular injection, as opposed to implantation.

5. Public Health Hazards from Residues of Natural Anabolics in Meat Products

FDA has consistently dismissed concerns on hazards of natural anabolics in meat:

No harmful effects will occur in individuals chronically ingesting animal tissues that contain an incremental increase of endogenous steroid equal to 1% or less of the amount produced daily by the segment of the population with the lowest daily production rate. In the case of Estradiol, prepubertal boys synthesize the least; in the case of testosterone, prepubertal girls synthesize the least. The calculated incremental increase permitted in beef muscle above the amount naturally present in untreated animals are 120ppt for Estradiol and 0.64ppb for Testosterone. Based upon relative consumption of other tissues versus muscle, safe incremental levels of 480ppt and 2.6ppb for Estradiol and Testosterone, respectively, are established for fat, 360ppt and 1.9ppb for kidney, and 240ppt and 1.3ppb for liver.

When the sponsor can demonstrate with a suitable assay that under the proposed conditions of use the concentration of residue of the endogenous sex steroid in treated food-producing animals is such that the actual increase in exposure of people will not exceed the permitted increase, then the compound is shown to be safe.

These assurances of safety are flawed for reasons including the following:

a. Consumption of meat products with incremental residues of a specific exogenous anabolic not only increases normal body hormonal levels, but also disturbs complex patters of normal hormonal interaction and balances. Such imbalances pose carcinogenic hazards.

b. The amount of endogenous steroids "produced by the segment of the population with the lowest daily production rate" are infants and young, rather than prepubertal children; daily estradiol production for prepubertal boys, 6.5 μg, is over 50-fold in excess of levels for children under 8, based on IARC data. This is of particular significance in view of the enhanced sensitivity of infants to the carcinogenic effects of estrogens (see Section 1d).

c. In the absence of routine monitoring, there is no assurance that "the proposed conditions of use" of the anabolics corresponds to routine feedlot practice. There is in fact evidence to the contrary, resulting in unmonitored residue levels well in excess of those anticipated by FDA (see Section 3).

d. FDA assurances are based on the alleged absence of "harmful effects" of individual anabolics. However, in practice, most implants contain two natural anabolics or one natural and one synthetic anabolic thus invalidating FDA's calculated assumptions. Furthermore, the probability of additive, let alone synergistic hormonal effects has apparently not been considered by FDA (see Section 1d). Of related concern is recent evidence that two xenobiotic pesticides induce synergistic estrogenic effects some 1000-fold greater than those resulting from individual exposures.

e. FDA has failed to consider incremental, additive or synergistic, carcinogenic and estrogenic effects of anabolic steroids together with those of xenoestrogenic pesticides and other industrial chemical contaminants in meat products.

f. FDA has failed to recognize the long standing evidence of the approximately 10,000-fold higher potency of estradiol than xenoestrogenic pesticides whose feminizing hazards are of increasing public health concern; such hazards may also include reduction in human male fertility.

6. Therapeutic Administration of Anabolics

The therapeutic uses of anabolics do not pose public health hazards. Such uses are extremely limited, compared to large-scale routine feedlot use, and are prescribed by qualified veterinarians, in contrast to feedlot operators. Furthermore, determination of therapeutic effectiveness necessitates pre-slaughter withdrawal.

7. Public Health Hazards from Residues of Synthetic Anabolics in Meat Products

The hazards of synthetic anabolics have been trivialized or dismissed by both FDA and WHO:

> "Safe concentrations" or tolerances have been established by FDA for residues of Trenbolone in spite of explicit industry data on its carcinogenicity (see Section 2a); these tolerances range from 50-20ppb for different organs and tissues. Similarly, WHO has established "maximum residue levels" (MRL) based on "Acceptable Daily Intakes" (ADI) for meat and dairy products.

"Safe concentrations" for total Zeranol residues have also been established by FDA, in spite of explicit industry carcinogenicity data, recognized by WHO, and the carcinogenicity of its metabolite Zearalenone (see Section 2b). Similarly, WHO have established ADI-based "Acceptable Residue Levels."

FDA has established a tolerance "in edible tissues" for MGA in spite of explicit industry carcinogenicity data (see Section 2c). WHO has failed to evaluate MGA in spite of its use in the U.S. for nearly three decades.

The public health hazards of synthetic anabolics are in general comparable to those of natural anabolics. Of particular concern, however, are the much higher residues of synthetic (in the ppb range), than the natural anabolics (in the ppt range). The concepts of tolerances, ADI and MRL are inappropriate in extreme for any carcinogen, let alone for high residues of carcinogens deliberately introduced into the food supply.

There is substantial evidence challenging the validity of classifying carcinogens as epigenetic, on the basis of bacterial gene mutation tests, for which thresholds or Acceptable Daily Intake (ADI) levels are claimed, as genotoxic. It should be emphasized that asbestos, benzene, arsenic and non-steroidal and steroidal estrogens, all IARC recognized potent Group 1 carcinogens, are inactive in bacterial tests and hence classified as epigenetic, However, they are all mutagenic and thus genotoxic in mammalian systems. Apart from this, hormonal anabolics are mutagenic in mammalian test systems and are thus genotoxic (Tables 1 and 2). There is also substantial scientific evidence challenging the existence of thresholds for any carcinogen. This evidence is even more persuasive for exposures involving unpredictable synergistic interactions. There is no scientific basis for WHO claims that ADI levels can be set for natural and synthetic anabolic carcinogens, or for claims that ADI levels can be based on "no-hormonal-effect levels" of synthetic anabolic carcinogens.

8. Misleading Assurances of Safety by U.S. Regulatory Agencies and "Expert Committees"

The repeated misleading assurances by USDA and FDA since 1979 on the safety of natural and synthetic anabolics are consistent with a similar prior record with regard to DES, including suppression of residue data. Compounding these concerns is longstanding evidence of conflicts of interest in senior agency personnel and their consultants.

As clearly evidenced in a series of General Accounting Office investigations and Congressional hearings, USDA inspection and FDA registration and residue-tolerance programs are in near total disarray. A 1986 report, "Human Food Safety and Regulation of Animal Drugs," unanimously approved by the House Committee on Government Operations, concluded that the "FDA has consistently disregarded its responsibility—has repeatedly put what it perceives are interests of veterinarians and the livestock industry ahead of its legal obligation to protect consumers—jeopardizing the health and safety of consumers meat, milk, and poultry." These criticisms appear equally appropriate today. Illustratively, in response on questions on hormonal meat raised in February 1996 by the European Commission Washington Delegation, the USDA responded with assurances that less than 0.25% of animals tested annually proved positive for "residue violations." In fact, however, no cattle have been monitored for sex hormones.

Similar concerns relate to exculpatory reports by Joint WHO Expert Committees on Food Additives. The membership of these committees reflects disproportionate representation of U.S. senior regulatory officials and of veterinary and food scientists, with minimal if any involvement of independent experts in preventive medicine, public health and carcinogenesis. The European Commission Scientific Conference of November 29-December 1, 1995 also reflects such imbalanced representation. While Conference participate of "scientists directly employed" by industry was "generally refused," no apparent attempt was made to identify or exclude industry consultants, contractees or grantees. Furthermore, the Conference based its finding and conclusions largely on unpublished industry data. As admitted by Steering Committee member Dr. F. W. Kenny, "all assessment data are provided by companies and this implies a regulatory gap," particularly in view of the confidentially of these data; industry is "capable of giving good results, but they will not necessarily always do so." Similar constraints in data generated and interpreted by industry and their consultants have been well documented.

9. Conclusions

Some three decades ago, Roy Hertz, then director of endocrinology of the National Cancer Institute and world authority on hormonal cancer, warned of the carcinogenic risks of estrogenic feed additives, particularly for hormonally sensitive tissues such as breast tissue, because they could increase normal body hormonal levels and disturb delicately poised hormonal balances. Hertz pointed to evidence from innumerable animal tests and human clinical experience that such imbalance can be carcinogenic. Hertz also warned of the essentially uncontrolled and unregulated use of these extremely potent biological agents, no dietary levels of which can be regarded as safe. These warnings are even more apt today.

Lifelong exposure to hormonal anabolics poses significant carcinogenic risks, particularly for breast and other reproductive cancers, whose rates have sharply escalated over recent decades. Such exposures may also pose serious feminizing risks.

TABLE 1: CARCINOGENICITY AND GENOTOXICITY OF HORMONAL ANABOLICS

ANABOLIC	CARCINOGENICITY	MAMMALIAN GENOTOXICITY
ESTRADIOL-17B	+	+
TESTOSTERONE	+	+
PROGESTERONE	+	+
TRENBOLONE-17B	+	+
ZERANOL	+	-
MELENGESTEROL	+	No Data Available

TABLE 2: GENETIC TOXICITY OF HORMONES

HORMONES	TEST SYSTEM
ESTRADIOL-17B	Aneuploidy, aberrant nucleotides and UDS rodent cells in vitro Micronuclei human cells in vitro Transformation, and DNA adducts by metabolites Chromosome aberrations by metabolites in vitro
TESTOSTERONE	As for estradiol in view of in vivo aromatization Transformation hamster cells in vitro
PROGESTERONE	Chromosome aberrations human cells in vitro Chromosome aberrations dog and hamster meiotic cells in vivo
TRENBOLONE-17B	Micronuclei and transformation hamster cells by metabolites in vitro
ZERANOL	Positive Rec-assay B, subtilis
ZEARALENONE	Positive Rec-assay B. subtilis Chromosome aberrations hamster cells in vitro DNA adducts in mice in vivo

This petition, based on fifty-nine scientific references, was submitted by:

Samuel S. Epstein, M.D.
Chairman, Cancer Prevention Coalition
Professor emeritus Occupational and Environmental Medicine
University of Illinois at Chicago

Nicholas Ashford, PhD, JD, Professor of Technology and Policy, Massachusetts Institute of Technology

Ronnie Cummins, Executive Director, Organic Consumers Association

Quentin D. Young, M.D., Chairman, Health & Medicine Policy Research Group, Past President, American Public Health Association

March 8, 1989

Austin American-Statesman

U.S. Policy Turns Blind Side to Dangers of Meat Additives

The United States is alone among other meat-exporting countries, including Argentina and Australia, in accusing the European Economic Community of unfair trade practices in its Jan. 1 ban of hormone-treated U.S. meat and threatening retaliatory sanctions. These actions ignore questions on the dangers of contaminated meat that concern European consumers who pressured the EEC into banning hormones additives two years ago.

Growth-promoting additives, fed or implanted in ears of U.S. cattle, are synthetic non-steroids, such as Zeranol; natural sex steroids, such as estrogen; or pituitary hormones, such as somatotropins. Although the carcinogenicity of the synthetic DES in test animals was known by 1938, its use was approved in 1947 by the U.S. Department of Agriculture and the Food and Drug Administration. Repeated congressional hearings on DES led to the 1958 Delaney law, banning the deliberate addition to food of any level of carcinogens, reflecting the scientific consensus that there is no way of setting safe levels for carcinogens. Nevertheless, continued use of DES was allowed on the alleged grounds that this did not result in detectable residues in meat products, and that Delaney could not be applied retroactively. In spite of infrequent federal sampling, residues were found at levels higher than those inducing cancer experimentally. Vaginal cancers were reported in daughters of women treated with DES in pregnancy by 1971, when DES-treated meat was banned in 20 foreign countries. However, misleading assurances of safety by the FDA and the USDA, including suppression of residue data, stonewalled an U.S. ban until 1979.

The industry then switched to other carcinogenic additives, particularly natural hormones. Unlike the synthetic DES whose residues can be monitored and whose use was conditional on seven days' pre-slaughter, withdrawal, natural hormone residues are not detectable as they cannot be routinely differentiated form hormones produced in the body. Since 1983, the FDA has allowed unregulated use of these additives right up to slaughter, subject only to the non-enforceable requirement that meat residues must be under 1 percent of children's daily hormonal production.

The dangers of hormone additives were signaled by an epidemic of premature sexual development and ovarian cysts in 3,000 Puerto Rican infants and children from 1979 to 1981. These effects were traced to contamination of meat and were reversed by dietary changes. Using research techniques, meat products were found highly contaminated with estrogens, and Zeranol and excess estrogens were found in the blood of afflicted children. This epidemic also was associated with increased uterine and ovarian cancers in adults.

More than a decade ago, Roy Hertz then director of endocrinology of the National Cancer Institute and a leading authority on hormonal cancer, warned of the carcinogenic risks of estrogenic additives which can increase and imbalance normal hormonal levels. Hetz also warned of uncontrolled use of these potent carcinogens, no dietary levels of which are safe—part per trillion estrogen levels in a dime-size piece of meat contain billions of trillions of molecules.

All Americans from conception till death consume unknown amounts of hormones in meat products without warning or labeling. In 1986, half the cattle sampled had hormones illegally implanted in muscle, resulting in high residues which the FDA admitted could result in "adverse effects." Unanswered is whether such estrogen dosage is involved in increasing cancers now striking one in three Americans, particularly the 50 percent increase in breast cancer since 1965. This is of further concern in view of recent confirmation of the associations between breast cancer and oral contraceptives, whose estrogen dosage over a fraction of a lifetime is known and controlled.

Hormones are part of larger problems of thousands of other feed additives, including antibiotics, tranquilizers, pesticides, drugs, flavors and industrial wastes. The runaway technologies of meat and pharmaceutical industries are supported by academic consultants, contractees, lobbyists and revolving doors between industry and regulatory agencies. This was personified by Reagan agriculture secretaries John Block, a former Illinois hog farmer, and Richard Lyng, former head of the American Meat Institute.

As evidence in Government Accounting Office investigations and congressional hearings, USDA and FDA regulation is in near-total disarray, aggravated by denials and cover-ups. A January 1986 House Committee on Government Operations report, "Human Food Safety and the Regulation of animal Drugs," concluded AFDA has consistently disregarded its responsibility—repeatedly put what it perceives are interests of veterinarians and the livestock industry ahead of its legal obligation to protect consumers—jeopardizing the health and safety of consumers of meat milk and poultry. "Most additives are used without evidence of efficacy, monitoring methods and minimal safety of consumers of meat, milk and poultry." Most additives are used without evidence of efficacy; monitoring methods and minimal safety data. The hazards of U.S. meat have retrogressed from random fecal and bacterial contamination of Upton Sinclair's The Jungle to the brave new world of deliberate chemicalization.

Any trade basis for the EEC embargo is unlikely, in view of tough regulations against hormones in European beef. Contrary to a "Public forum" piece by Dr. Rodney L. Preston in the Austin American Statesman, Feb. 22, EEC's 1985 Scientific Risk Assessment Committee recommended against continued use of synthetic hormones and emphasized the need to further evaluate natural hormones. Rather than finger-pointing at Europe, the embargo should prompt high-level investigation and reform of regulation and industry practices. The administration also raises problems of dual standard in view of its 1987 ban on Australian beef imports on grounds of excess residues of the carcinogenic pesticide heptachlor.

Hormonal and other carcinogenic additives should be banned immediately, as should be all additives absent evidence on efficacy and safety. Additives use and residue levels in meat products, including milk and eggs, should also be subject to explicit labeling requirements.

Until then, state initiatives, such as the "Texas Plan," establishing hormone-free certification for European shipments, should be applauded and extended domestically. Meanwhile, consumers should boycott chemicalized in favor of organic meat, and insist on the right to know which additives have been used and their residues. Consumers should further demand independent certification and verification for hormones and other additives, such as the California Nutri-Clean program for testing pesticide residues on fruits and vegetables, available in 600 supermarkets nationwide.

May 1, 1989

The Chemical Jungle

Today's Beef Industry

The United States is isolated among meat-exporting countries, such as Argentina and Australia, in threatening retaliatory sanctions and in accusing the European Economic Community (EEC) of unfair trade practices because of its January 1, 1989 ban of hormone-treated U.S. meat. The accusations ignore serious questions about the carcinogenic and other risks of hormonally contaminated meat that are of major concern to European consumers who, over two years ago, pressured the EEC into banning the use of all hormone additives.

Growth promoting hormone additives, fed or implanted in over 95 percent of U.S. cattle, are mostly synthetic non-steroids such as Zeranol, natural sex steroids such as estrogens, or pituitary hormones such as somatotropines. Although the carcinogenicity of the synthetic DES in test animals was known by 1938, its use as a feed additive was approved by the U.S. Department of Agriculture (USDA) and the Food and Drug Administration (FDA) in 1947. After repeated hearings on the hazards of diethystilbestril (DES), in 1958 Congress passed the Delaney Amendment to the Federal Food Drug and Cosmetic Act, banning the deliberate addition of any level of carcinogens into food. This law reflected the overwhelming scientific consensus, which still prevails, that there is no way of setting safe levels or tolerances for carcinogens. Nevertheless, the USDA and the FDA allowed continued use of DES on the alleged grounds that this did not result in detectable and illegal residues in meat products, and that the Delaney law could not be applied retroactively. By 1971, DES was being used in 75 percent of U.S. cattle. In spite of infrequent federal sampling and insensitive monitoring, DES residues were found in cattle and sheep at levels in excess of those inducing cancer experimentally. At about the same time, vaginal cancers were reported in the daughters of women treated with DES during pregnancy. Based on these findings, DES-treated meat was banned in more than 20 foreign countries, mostly European. However, misleading assurances of safety and stonewalling by the FDA and USDA, including the deliberate suppression of residue data, managed to delay a U.S. ban on DES until 1979.

The meat industry then promptly switched to other carcinogenic additives, particularly natural sex hormones, which are implanted in the ears of commercially raised feedlot cattle. Unlike the synthetic DES, whose residues can be monitored and whose use was conditional on a seven day pre-slaughter withdrawal period, residues of natural hormones are not routinely detectable because they cannot be differentiated from the same hormones produced by the body. Since 1983, the FDA has allowed virtually unregulated use of these natural additives right up to the time of slaughter, subject only to the non-enforceable requirement that residue levels in meat must be less than 1 percent of the daily hormonal production of children.

A dramatic warning of the dangers of growth-promoting additives was triggered by an epidemic of premature sexual development and ovarian cysts involving about 3,000 Puerto Rican infants and children from 1979 to 1981. These toxic effects were traced to hormonal contamination of fresh meat products, and were usually reversed by simple dietary changes. Using highly specialized research techniques, independent testing found that samples of the meat products were contaminated with estrogen residues more than ten-fold in excess of normal ranges. Additionally, elevated estrogen levels and the synthetic Zeranol were found in the blood of afflicted children. Increased rates of uterine and ovarian cancers in adult women were also associated with this epidemic.

More than a decade ago, Roy Hertz, then director of endocrinology of the National Cancer Institute and a world authority on hormonal cancer, warned of the carcinogenic risks of estrogenic feed additives, particularly for hormonally sensitive tissues such as breast tissue, because they could increase normal body hormonal levels and disturb delicately poised hormonal balances. Hertz pointed to evidence in innumerable animal tests and human clinical experience that such imbalance can be carcinogenic. Hertz also warned of the essentially uncontrolled and unregulated use of these extremely potent biological agents, no dietary levels of which could be regarded as safe. Even a dime-sized piece of meat contains billions of trillions of molecules of these carcinogens.

Virtually the entire U.S. population consumes, with-out any warning, labeling or information, unknown and unpredictable amounts of hormonal residues in meat products over their lifetimes. In 1986, as many as half of all cattle sampled in feed lots as large as 600 animals, were found to have hormones illegally implanted in muscle rather than the ear skin, to provide further increased growth. This resulted in very high meat residues which even the FDA admitted could produce "adverse effects." Left unanswered is whether such chronic and uncontrolled estrogen dosages are involved in increasing cancer rates (now striking one in three Americans), particularly the alarming 50 percent increase in the incidence of breast cancer since 1965. These questions are of further concern in light of recent evidence confirming the association between breast cancer and oral contraceptives, whose estrogen dosage over a fraction of a lifetime is known and controlled, in contrast with that from residues of growth hormones in meat products.

Hormonal feed contamination in America is only part of a much larger problem caused by the use of thousands of feed additives. These include antibiotics, tranquilizers, Beef in a packing plan pesticides, animal drugs, artificial flavors and industrial wastes, many of which are carcinogenic in addition to their other harmful effects. The runaway technologies of the meat—product and pharmaceutical industries are supported by an eager cadre of academic consultants, contractees and apologists, tremendous lobbying pressures and a revolving door between senior personnel in industry and regulatory agencies. This was personified by Reagan Administration agriculture secretaries John Block, a former Illinois hog farmer, and Richard Lyng, a former head of the American Meat Institute.

As clearly evidenced in a series of Government Accounting Office investigations and Congressional hearings, USDA inspection and FDA registration and residue-tolerance programs are in near total disarray, aggravated by brazen denials and cover-ups by these agencies. A January 1986 report, "Human Food Safety and the Regulation of Animal Drugs," unanimously approved by the House Committee on Government Operations, concluded that the "FDA has consistently disregarded its responsibility—has repeatedly put what it perceives are interests of veterinarians and the livestock industry ahead of its legal obligation to protect consumers—jeopardizing the health and safety of consumers of meat, milk and poultry." The great majority of feed additives are used in the absence of evidence of efficacy, practical and sensitive monitoring methods and minimal if any safety test data, apart from the widespread use of illegal and unapproved drugs. The hazards of U.S. meat have retrogressed from the random fecal and bacterial contamination of Upton Sinclair's *Jungle* to the brave new world of deliberate chemicalization.

Any possible trade basis for the EEC embargo is extremely unlikely, particularly in view of tough regulations and criminal sanctions against use of hormonal additives in European beef. Contrary to repeated assertions by the U.S. meat industry, the EEC's 1985 Scientific Risk Assessment Committee did not exculpate the use of hormonal additives, but recommended against the use of a synthetics and emphasized the need to further evaluate the safety of natural hormones. Rather than finger-pointing at Europe, the embargo should prompt a high-level, independent investigation and a drastic reform of meat industry practices and federal regulation to include the use of hormones in particular and feed additives in general. Immediate action, not further study, is well overdue. The U.S. position also reflects a disturbing double standard, since the administration banned imports of Australian beef in 1987 on the grounds of excess residues of the carcinogenic pesticide heptachlor.

All hormonal and other carcinogenic feed additives should be banned immediately, as should be all other animal additives in the absence of conclusive evidence of their efficacy and safety. Any additive use should be subject to explicit labeling requirements of use and of residue levels in all meat products, including milk and eggs.

Until then, initiatives at the state level, such as State Agriculture Commissioner Jim Hightower's "Texas Plan" to establish a hormone-free certification program for shipments to Europe, should be applauded and vigorously extended to the domestic market. Meanwhile, consumers should avoid chemicalized meat products in favor of organic ones. Consumers should also insist on their absolute right to know which additives have been used in their meat products, their residue levels and their known adverse effects. Finally, they should demand independent certification and verification for hormones and other feed additives, such as the California Nutri-Clean program for testing pesticide residues on fruits and vegetables that is now available in about 600 supermarkets nationwide.

January 22, 1992

USA Today

Risks of Radiation: Too Many Questions about Food Safety

The nation's first irradiated food, fresh fruit and vegetables, is soon to go on sale at a small Miami supermarket. This food was treated with massive doses of ionizing radiation (100,000 rads, roughly equivalent to 10 million medical x-rays) at large cobalt-60 facility, Vindicator Inc., which plans to treat 800 million tons of food a year for nationwide sale.

Food irradiation was the brainchild of the Atomic Energy Commission's efforts in the Eisenhower administration to find practical uses for the flood of radioactive wastes from nuclear weapons.

Atomic Energy of Canada (Nordion Ltd), with its virtual monopoly on cobalt-60 and with strong backing from the International Atomic Energy Agency, hopes to operate a chain of U.S. plants with U.S. irradiation companies.

Industry and the Food and Drug Administration insist that irradiated food has been thoroughly tested and is absolutely safe. However, New York, New Jersey and Maine have prohibited the sale and distribution of irradiated food, as have foreign governments, including Germany, Denmark, Sweden, Australia and New Zealand. Claims of safety are unproven at best. High-energy irradiation produces complex chemical changes in food with the formation of poorly characterized radiolytic products, including benzene, organic peroxides and carbonyls. Radiolytic products kill bacteria, molds and larvae and thus ensure spoilage-free food, a major attraction to the purveyors of marginal produce and contaminated poultry. However, concentrated extracts of these products have never been tested for cancer and other delayed adverse effects. The overdue need for such studies is further emphasized by numerous reports of chronic toxic effects in insensitive studies on test animal fed unextracted whole irradiated food. These include reproductive damage in rodents and chromosomal damage in rodents, monkeys and children.

Besides food safety, irradiation poses serious occupational and environmental hazards due to the transport and handling of radioactive materials. Accidents have already been reported in facilities sterilizing medical supplies by irradiation. Irradiation also reduces levels of essential nutrients in food, especially vitamins A, C, E and the B complex. Cooking irradiated food reduces these levels still further. The industry reluctantly admits this but suggests that the problem could be taken care of by vitamin supplements!

In spite of this substantial evidence, Food and Drug Administration approved food irradiation in 1986. The FDA based its decision on five questionable or allegedly negative tests and on theoretical estimates on cancer risk, which was claimed to be insignificant and "acceptable." This position is consistent with the administration's revocation of the Delaney law, which banned the deliberate contamination of food with any amount of cancer-causing chemicals, and its substitution by rubber number standards based on "acceptable" cancer risk. Cancer rates have now reached epidemic proportions, striking one in three and killing one in four, with 500,000 deaths last year. Further risks to the entire nation of cancer, besides other health effects, hardly seem justified by the narrow economic interest of a small industry supported by a highly politicized federal bureaucracy.

October 8, 1996

Europe's Ban on Hormone-Raised Beef Is Based on Sound Science

America's challenge to Europe's ban on hormone-raised beef will be heard by a World Trade Organization (WTO) Panel in Geneva on October 10.

"The cancer risks of meat from cattle fattened with sex hormones is based on sound science," said Samuel S. Epstein, M.D., professor of Environmental Medicine at the University of Illinois at Chicago, and chairman of the Cancer Prevention Coalition. Dr. Epstein has submitted a scientific affidavit to the European Union in support of its ban.

Nearly all cattle in U.S. feedlots are legally implanted under their ear skin with combinations of natural of synthetic sex hormones. The most commonly used is estradiol, which is as carcinogenic as DES, the banned hormone known to cause vaginal cancers in young women following administration to their mothers during pregnancy. Estradiol is also thousands of times more potent than estrogenic pesticides and other industrial food pollutants whose feminizing and male infertility effects are of increasing concern.

Confidential industry tests reveal that residues of estradiol and other natural hormones such as testosterone, are up to 30 times higher in implanted than unimplanted cattle. Still higher residues result from the not uncommon illegal practice of intra-muscular implantation. Furthermore, contrary to misleading FDA and USDA assurances, cattle are not monitored for hormone residues.

While reports from the Food and Agriculture Organization and the World Health organization (FAO/WHO) and the 1995 European Commission Conference, have falsely claimed that hormone-raised meat is safe, these committees are largely controlled by senior U.S. regulatory officials and veterinary and food scientists, with minimal expertise in public health and cancer prevention. Apart from the problems of conflict of interest, these committees largely rely on unpublished and confidential industry data.

"Residues of sex hormones in meat products poses series cancer and feminizing risks, especially to infants and young children in view of their

---

191

high sensitivity to hormones and carcinogens," continued Dr. Epstein. Such exposures have been incriminated in the sharply increased incidence of reproductive cancers in the U.S. since 1950-55% for breast, 100% for prostate, and 120% for testis.

Dr. Epstein concluded: "The Europeans have a strong basis for their concerns, which should be shared by American consumers."

March 24, 1997

Los Angeles Times

None of Us Should Eat Extra Estrogen

Instead of forcing Europe to open its markets to U.S. beef, why not just quit implanting hormones in American cattle? When U.S. and Canadian beef cattle go to feedlots, hormone pellets are implanted under the ear skin, a process that is repeated at the midpoint of their 100-day fattening period. The hormones increase the weight of the cattle, adding to profits by about $80 per animal.

The most common hormone in current use is estradiol, a potent cancer-causing and gene-damaging estrogen. The FDA maintains that residues of estradiol and other hormones in meat are within "normal" levels, and has waived any requirements for monitoring and chemical testing.

Europe, however, has rightly eyed U.S. claims with great skepticism and since 1989 the European Union has forbidden the sale of beef from hormone-treated cattle. The opening of global markets has placed that ban under attack.

On Feb. 17, a panel of World Trade Organization judges began closed hearings on a U.S. and Canadian challenge charging that the European ban is merely protectionist and is costing North America $100 million a year in lost exports.

The FDA's claims of safety were endorsed by a 1987 report of two U.N. bodies, the Food and Agriculture Organization and the World Health Organization, an endorsement that is the main basis of the U.S. and Canadian action against Europe. The joint committee that prepared the report, however, has minimal expertise in public health and high representation of veterinary scientists and senior FDA and U.S. Department of Agriculture officials. Relying heavily on unpublished industry information and outdated scientific citations, the committee claimed that hormone residues in legally implanted cattle are so low that eating treated meat could not possibly induce any hormonal or carcinogenic effects.

However, confidential industry reports to the FDA, obtained under the Freedom of Information Act, reveal high hormone residues in meat products even under ideal test conditions. Following a single ear implant in steers of Synovex-S, a combination of estradiol and progesterone, estradiol levels in different meat products were up to 20-fold higher than normal. The amount of estradiol in two hamburgers eaten in one day by an 8-year-old boy could increase his total hormone levels by as much as 10%, based on conservative assumptions, because young children have very low natural hormone levels.

In real life, the situation may be much worse. An unpublicized random USDA survey of 32 large feedlots found that as many as half the cattle had visible illegal "misplaced implants" in muscle, rather than under ear skin. This would result in very high local concentrations of hormones, and also elevated levels in muscle meat at distant sites. Such abuse is very hard to detect.

Responding to European concerns, the USDA recently claimed that, based on standard residue monitoring programs, drug levels in violation of regulations have not been detected in meat products. However, of 130 million livestock commercially slaughtered in 1993, not one was tested for estradiol or any related hormone.

The question we ought to be asking is not why Europe won't buy our hormone-treated meat, but why we allow beef from hormone-treated cattle to be sold to American and Canadian consumers. Untreated meat is currently hard to find and expensive; if it were widely produced and available, the price would come down. At the least, meat produced from hormone-treated animals should be explicitly labeled.

These hormones are linked ever more closely to the escalating incidence of reproductive cancers in the U.S. since 1950-55% for breast cancer, 120% for testicular cancer and 190% for prostate cancer. The endocrine-disruptive effects of estrogenic pesticides and other industrial food contaminants known as xenoestrogens are now under intensive investigation by federal regulatory and health agencies. But the contamination of meat with residues of the far-more-potent estradiol remains ignored.

The world trade judges ought to listen to one of the top FDA officials involved in meat safety, David Livingston. In Orville Schell's 1984 meat industry expose, "Modern Meat," Livingston is quoted as saying, "Well, if you're going to have enough inexpensive meat for everyone, you're going to have to use some of these drugs. But personally, I'd rather eat meat that was raised without them." In other words, what's good enough for the rest of us is not something he wants to eat.

February 2, 1998

New Challenges on the Safety Of U.S. Meat: Oprah Right for Other Reasons

The World Trade Organization (WTO) ruled in favor of the 1989 European ban on the use of sex hormones for growth promotion of cattle in feedlots prior to slaughter. While subject to further assessment before it can be made permanent, this ruling is a major victory for European consumers. It is also a major defeat for the United States and Canada which challenged the European ban claiming that it was "protectionist," costing over $100 million a year in lost exports, and that it reflected "consumerism versus science." The WTO ruling also raises serious concerns on the safety of U.S. meat, recently questioned on different grounds by Oprah Winfrey, based on the following considerations:

Confidential industry reports to the FDA, obtained under the Freedom of Information Act, reveal high residues of natural and synthetic sex hormones in meat products even under ideal test conditions. This is contrary to repeated and explicit assurances by the FDA and USDA.

Following legal implantation in the ear of steers of Synovex-S, a combination of estradiol and progesterone, estradiol levels in meat products ranged up to 20-fold in excess of the normal. Based on conservative estimates, the amount of estradiol in two hamburgers eaten by an 8-year-old boy could increase his hormone levels by 10%.

Much higher hormone residues are found in meat products following illegal implantation in cattle muscle which is commonplace in U.S. feedlots. The WTO ruled that such abuse alone would justify the European ban.

Contrary to repeated and explicit assurances by the FDA and USDA, none of the approximately 130 million U.S. livestock slaughtered annually are tested for residues of cancer-causing and gene-damaging estradiol or any related sex hormones. This misrepresentation has been confirmed by European Commission inspectors, in a November 1997 survey of U.S. control programs, who reported that there was no monitoring for residues of sex hormones nor for illegal animal drugs, including antibiotics, and that U.S. residue monitoring was totally inadequate to meet European standards.

Repeated assurances on the safety of hormonal meat by two World Health Organization bodies, the Food and Agriculture Organization and the Codex Alimentarius Commission (FAO/CODEX), reflect minimal expertise in public health, high representation of senior FDA and USDA officials and industry consultants, reliance on unpublished industry and outdated scientific information, and conflicts of interest. Paradoxically, the same Codex Commission which approved hormonal meat, explicitly warned over a decade ago that baby meat foods "shall be free from residues of hormones."

The endocrine-disruptive effects of estrogenic pesticides and other industrial food contaminants, known as xenoestrogens, are now under intensive investigation by U.S. regulatory and health agencies. But contamination of meat with residues of the thousands-fold more potent estradiol remains ignored.

Lifelong exposure to high residues of natural and synthetic sex hormones in meat products poses serious risks of breast and other reproductive cancers, whose incidence in the U.S. has sharply escalated since 1950-55% for breast cancer, 120% for testicular cancer, and 230% for prostate cancer. Those residues have also been incriminated in increasing trends of precocious sexual development.

Commenting on these facts, Samuel S. Epstein, M.D., Professor of Environmental Medicine at the University of Illinois Chicago, School of Public Health, stated: "The European ban on hormonal meat should serve as a long-overdue wake-up call for U.S. consumers to demand an immediate ban on hormone use or, minimally, the explicit labeling of hormonal meat products. It should also lead to a congressional investigation of the FDA and USDA for gross regulatory abdication besides suppression of information vital to consumer health. The dangers of U.S. hormonal meat can no longer be ignored."

May 4, 1999

Fao/Who's Joint Expert Committee on Food Additives Report on Hormonal Meat Is Scientifically Invalid and Fails to Warn Consumers of Cancer Risks

A February 1999 Joint Expert Committee on Food Additives (JECFA), report which has just become available, claims that the natural sex hormones, estradiol, progesterone and testosterone, can be safely used for growth promotion of cattle in feed lots without risks to consumers, particularly of breast and other reproductive cancers.

The report established "Acceptable Daily Intakes" (ADI's) or safe threshold tolerances for these natural hormones on the basis of "hormone-dependent parameters," which were accepted as the determinants of carcinogenicity. This novel proposal is scientifically invalid. It is also in diametric opposition to 1997 World Trade Organization (WTO) testimony opposing the EU ban on hormonal meat by US and Canadian experts, some of whom also authored the 1999 report.

> While the latest JECFA report admits that estradiol is a gene-damaging (genotoxic) carcinogen, it fails to recognize that this precludes the establishment of an ADI. Setting this ADI also contradicts illustrative WTO testimony by US/Canadian experts: "—chemicals which produce carcinogenicity through a clear genotoxic mechanism should be regulated as if a threshold dose cannot be derived and hence an—ADI—cannot be proposed"; and "—the ADI model does not predict quantitative risks and is not applicable to genotoxic carcinogens." Of related interest is recent confirmation by FDA scientists on the absence of a threshold for estradiol in experimental studies on estradiol-induced sex reversal.

The 1999 JECFA report emphasized that the carcinogenicity of estradiol is due to its hormonal effects "—which occur at much lower doses than other toxicological effects—," on whose basis ADIs were developed. However, the report ignores well documented and long-standing evidence that estradiol is carcinogenic in non-hormone dependent tissues including liver and skin (malignant melanoma) in humans, and bone, lymphoid, salivary and thyroid cancers in rodents.

Establishment of the estradiol ADI is in sharp variance with evidence on the extreme sensitivity of infants and pre-pubertal children to hormonal carcinogens. Furthermore, a growing literature on "hormonal imprinting" strongly suggests that exogenous hormonal influences in infancy and critical phases of sexual maturation determine hormonal responsiveness and carcinogenic risks in adult life.

Establishment of the 1999 ADI ignores evidence on additive and/or synergistic interactions between estradiol and other simultaneously implanted hormones. Illustrative are the synergistic effects of estradiol and progesterone in the induction of mammary tumors in mice and prostate cancer in rats. Failure to address these concerns also contrasts with 1997 testimony by a lead US/Canadian expert that "—studies relating to the genotoxicity or carcinogenicity of hormone combinations have not been carried out even though this is frequently the preferred method of use"; establishment of the ADI also ignores synergistic interactions between estrogens and other unrelated carcinogens.

JECFA 1999 admits that estradiol, besides progesterone and testosterone, residues are "statistically significantly higher than in corresponding values in concurrent controls." Nevertheless, JECFA concludes that monitoring for such excess residues is unnecessary.

JECFA appears unaware that ultrasensitive hormonal assays in pre-pubertal children, as reported in 1994, have shown that daily production rates of estradiol may have been over estimated by 100-fold. Thus, residues in organs/tissues of implanted cattle could be well in excess of ADI levels.

JECFA appears unaware of serious concerns on environmental contamination, particularly of drinking water, from fecal and urinary excretion of hormones by millions of cattle continuously processed through feed lots. Of equal concern is the reported sale to rendering plants of discarded ears of slaughtered cattle containing very high levels of residual hormones for potential uses including animal feed, pet food, and manufacture of gelatin and glycerol for cosmetics, foods and pharmaceutical products.

Finally, serious concerns persist with regard to the selection procedures, composition, scientific competence and conflicts of interest in JECFA, apart from their reliance on unpublished industry data and lack of procedural transparency.

May 31, 1999

The European Ban on Hormonal Meat Is Based on Valid Scientific Evidence

On May 14, U.S. Agriculture (USDA) Secretary Dan Glickman stated that "scientific study after study confirms that American beef is safe and threatened Europe with punitive duties. As the lead public health expert who testified in 1997 before the World Trade Organization (WTO) on the validity of European concerns on breast and other cancer risks from hormonal meat, I am unaware of any such studies on the basis of which Secretary Glickman has been led to rely. In fact, there is a wealth of published scientific evidence, to the contrary.

Contrary to misleading explicit assurance by the USDA, virtually none of the 130 million cattle slaughtered annually are monitored for residues in meat of estradiol or the other two natural sex hormones—progesterone and testosterone—or the three synthetic hormones—trenbolone, zeranol and melengesterol—implanted under the ear skin or fed to cattle in feedlots to increase their weight prior to slaughter. Furthermore, confidential New Animal Drug Applications (NADA's), submitted to the Food and Drug Administration by the animal drug industry since the 1980's, reveal substantial excess residues of these hormones following legal implantation under the ear skin. Illustratively, estradiol residues in meat range up to 20-fold in excess of natural background levels. While US and Canadian experts testified in 1997 before the WTO that such hormone residues are within physiological ranges, these same experts in a February 1999 report by FAO/WHO's Joint Expert Committee on Food Additives (JECFA) now admit that these residues are "statistically significantly elevated." Consumption of hormonal meat by pre-pubertal boys can expose them to excess estradiol at levels close to if not greater than their daily production rates, rather than less than one thousandth as testified by US and Canadian experts in 1997. It should further be stressed that much higher residues, than those reported in the NADA's, result from illegal or accidental implantation in muscle.

For the most commonly used cattle hormone estradiol, its carcinogenicity in reproductive and non-reproductive organs of rodents, relationship to breast and uterine cancers in women, and also gene-damaging (genotoxic) effects have been well established since the 1980's. However, this evidence on genotoxicity was strenuously denied in WTO testimony by US and Canadian experts who stated that safe thresholds or "Acceptable Daily Intakes" (ADI's) could not be established for genotoxic carcinogens. Yet, these same experts, as lead authors of the 1999 JECFA report, reversed themselves doubly by admitting the genotoxicity of estradiol while claiming that ADI's could nevertheless be established.

The high incidence of volatile residues in US certified hormone-free meat exported to the U.S. has raised recent concerns. Further concerns, unrecognized by the US, include environmental contamination, particularly of drinking water, from fecal and urinary excretion of hormones by millions of cattle continuingly processed through feedlots. Of related concern is the reported sale to rendering plants of discarded ears of slaughtered cattle containing very high residual levels of hormones for potential uses including animal feed, pet food, and manufacture of gelatin and glycerol for cosmetics, food and pharmaceutical products.

Finally, it should be stressed that there are serious concerns with regard to the transparency of proceedings, integrity, conflicts of interests, and lack of expertise of the membership of JECFA on the basis of whose reports US and Canadian WTO testimony and claims of safety have been, and remain, based. Illustratively, over half of the members of the 1999 JECFA report are US and Canadian regulatory officials and industry' consultants, none of whom have recognized expertise in public health, preventive medicine, and cancer prevention. These considerations have even broader implications with regard to global concerns and decision making on food safety.

June 6, 2000

The Cancer Prevention Coalition and Public Citizen Charge Congress with Proposing Deceptive Labeling of Irradiated Food, besides Ignoring Its Risks to Health and the Environment

Caving in to industry interests, the House and Senate Appropriations Committees have introduced legislation to exempt irradiated food from being labeled "irradiated" in favor of "electronically pasteurized." Support for this euphemistic absurdity comes from the Food and Drug Administration (FDA), whose approved 450,000 rads meat irradiation dosage is approximately equivalent to 150 million chest x-rays, which has capitalized on recent outbreaks of E. coli 0157 food poisoning to mobilize public acceptance of food irradiation and its safety. Further support comes from the U.S. Department of Agriculture (USDA), Nuclear Regulatory Commission (NRC) and Department of Energy (DOE).

This labeling initiative is reckless. Testing irradiated food by industry over the last four decades does not meet minimal toxicological standards which could justify industry and FDA safety claims. Furthermore, there is persuasive independent evidence of carcinogenic and genetic hazards of radiated food, apart from catastrophic risks of accidents from the over 1200 nationwide unregulated nuclear facilities envisaged for the potentially enormous radiation market.

Irradiated meat is a very different product from cooked meat. Irrespective whether radiated by X ray machines, linear accelerators, or radioactive isotopes, the resulting ionizing radiation produces highly reactive free radicals and peroxides from unsaturated fats, which can completely alter the natural chemical composition of meat and poultry. U.S. Army analyses in 1977 revealed major differences between volatile chemicals formed during radiation or cooking meat. Levels of the carcinogen benzene in radiated beef were some ten-fold higher than cooked beef. In addition, high concentrations of six poorly characterized Unique Radiolytic chemical Products (URPs), admittedly "implicated as carcinogens or carcinogenic under certain conditions," were also identified.

Based on these striking changes in the chemistry of irradiated meat, FDA's 1980 Irradiated Food Committee warned that safety testing should be based on concentrated extracts of irradiated foods, rather than on whole foods, to maximize the concentration of radiolytic products. This would enable development of sufficient sensitivity essential for routine safety testing. One of us (SE) more specifically warned in a 1984 letter to Science that: "Stable radiolytic products could be extracted from irradiated foods by various—solvents which could then be concentrated and subsequently tested. Until such fundamental studies are undertaken, there is little scientific basis for accepting industry's assurances of safety." However, FDA has still refused to require such testing on alleged grounds that it is inherently difficult and expensive. Instead, FDA has relied on some five studies selected from over 400 in the 1970's and early 1980's, on which its claims of safety remain based. However, Dr. Gemert, chair of FDA's Irradiated Food Task Committee which reviewed these studies, insists that none were adequate by 1982 standards, and even less so by 1993. Furthermore, detailed analysis of these studies, by Dr. Louria, Chairman of New Jersey University's Department of Preventive Medicine, has revealed that all are grossly flawed and non-exculpatory.

These results are hardly surprising since several independent studies prior to 1986 clearly identified mutagenic or carcinogenic radiolytic products in radiated food. Furthermore, earlier studies reported evidence of genetic damage in tests of radiated food. Noteworthy are studies in the 1970's by India's National Institute of Nutrition, knowingly misrepresented by FDA, which reported that feeding freshly radiated wheat to malnourished Indian children, monkeys, rats, and mice induced gross chromosomal damage in blood or bone marrow cells; dominant lethal mutations were also induced in rodents, as confirmed by others.

As reported by USDA's Agriculture Research Service, food radiation results in major micronutrient losses, particularly vitamins A, C, E, and the B complex. These losses are synergistically increased by cooking, resulting in "empty calorie" food. Radiation has also been used to clean up food unfit for human consumption, such as spoiled fish, by killing odorous contaminating bacteria.

While the USDA is promoting meat and poultry radiation, it has been moving to deregulate and privatize the industry by promoting a self-policing "Hazard Analysis and Critical Control Point" (HACCP) control program. Food radiation is also being aggressively promoted by the DOE's "Byproducts Utilization Program" to reduce disposal costs of spent military and civilian nuclear fuel by providing a commercial market for nuclear wastes.

In contrast to major nuclear power reactors, food radiation plants are: relatively small; unregulated; unlikely to be secure; vulnerable to sabotage or terrorist attacks; and require regular replenishment of radioactive isotopes, Cobalt (Co-60) or Cesium (Cs-137), entailing transportation hazards. The track record of the radiation industry is unimpressive. Apart from some 49 accidents including worker deaths prior to 1989, Robert Alvarez, former Senior Policy Advisor to the Secretary of Energy, recently warned that NRC files are bulging with unreported documents on radioactive spills, worker overexposures, and offsite radiation leakage. It must be further stressed that linear accelerators, limited by their ability to penetrate thick foods, or pelletized radioactive isotopes, are subject only to minimal regulation. Strangely, EPA still does not require an Environmental Impact Statement prior to the setting of food irradiation facilities.

Not surprisingly, the focus of the radiation and agribusiness industries has been directed to the lucrative cleanup of contaminated food rather than preventing of contamination. However, 0157 food poisoning could largely be prevented by long overdue improved sanitation. Feedlot pen sanitation, together with water chlorination and fly control, could drastically reduce cattle infection rates, which could be further reduced by feeding hay 7 days prior to slaughter. Sanitation could also prevent water contamination from feed lot run off, incriminated in recent outbreaks of 0157 poisoning; this would remain a continuing threat even if all meat were irradiated. Post-knocking (pre-slaughter) and post-evisceration sanitation at meat packing plants is also highly effective for reducing cattle infection rates. Testing of pooled carcasses for 0157 and Salmonella is economic, practical, and rapid. Costs would be trivial compared to those of radiation, which would be passed to consumers, apart from assuring its wholesomeness and safety, besides preventing nuclear accidents. Additional costs could result from the likelihood of a European, if not international, ban on imports of irradiated U.S. food.

The Cancer Prevention Coalition and Public Citizen charge that the House Appropriations Committee's "electronically pasteurized" label is a camouflaged denial of citizen's fundamental right-to-know. Rather than sanitizing the label in response to special interests, the Committee should focus on sanitizing food production in response to the public interest.

ENDORSERS:

Dr. Quentin Young
Past-president
American Public Health Association

Dr. Marvin Legator
Professor Preventive Medicine
University of Texas, Galveston

Dr. William Lijinsky
Former Director Chemical Carcinogenesis
Frederick Cancer Research Center

Dr. Barry Castleman
Environmental Consultant

Wenonah Hauter
Public Citizen

October 3, 2000

FDA Legalized Food Irradiation without Adequately Evaluating Its Risks, Dismissed Evidence of Serious Public Health Hazards

The U.S. Food and Drug Administration (FDA) has legalized the irradiation of fruit, vegetables, meat and eggs while ignoring federal safety regulations and relying on dozens of tests that the agency's own expert scientists have dismissed as invalid, a new report from Public Citizen and the Cancer Prevention Coalition reveals.

"For 17 years, the FDA has knowingly and systematically ignored its own testing protocols—protocols that must be followed before irradiated food can be legalized for human consumption," said Mark Worth, senior researcher for Public Citizen's Critical Mass Energy and Environment Program. "The FDA's record of regulating food irradiation is an utter embarrassment. The agency's failings should outrage everyone concerned about the wholesomeness of our food supply."

"The scientific sleight-of-hand perpetuated by the FDA—year after year, decision after decision—sets a new standard for governmental misfeasance," said Dr. Samuel Epstein, chair of the Cancer Prevention Coalition, and professor of environmental and occupational medicine at the University of Illinois Medical Center-Chicago. "The FDA should be held accountable for abdicating its regulatory mandate to comply with standard testing procedures, while ignoring substantive evidence of public health hazards.

"The day will soon come," Epstein said, "when international opposition to American exports of irradiated food will surpass that of genetically engineered food. If Congress fails to ban irradiated food, American farmers, ranchers and the economy could pay a devastating price."

The new report, *A Broken Record: How the FDA Legalized—and Continues to Legalize—Food Irradiation without Testing It for Safety* was released today by Public Citizen and the Cancer Prevention Coalition.

The report reveals how the FDA over the past 17 years has ignored its own rules for certifying the safety of irradiated food; relied on more than

100 occasions on research declared "deficient" by FDA toxicologists, and, along with other federal agencies, misled Congress about the safety of irradiated food.

Moreover, the FDA has systematically dismissed evidence that irradiated food may not be safe for human consumption. Much of this evidence suggesting that irradiated food can cause mutations of genetic material and be toxic resulted from government-funded research submitted to the FDA and members of Congress as early as 1968.

Public Citizen and the Cancer Prevention Coalition are calling for the revocation of all food irradiation permits and a full congressional investigation into the FDA's role in regulating irradiated food.

"FDA bureaucrats must abide by their legal and moral responsibilities to ensure that American families have safe food on their tables," said Wenonah Hauter, director of Public Citizen's Critical Mass Energy and Environment Program. "Regulatory systems at the FDA have broken down completely. It is no wonder that most Americans do not trust their government to do the right thing. We should never see another fiasco like this."

"This report underscores the need for a ban on the sale and distribution of irradiated food, which I have proposed in my home state," said New Jersey Assemblyman John Kelly (R-Essex). "I hope that other states—and Congress—will follow our lead."

April 8, 2001

Administration Proposal to Serve Irradiated Beef to School Children Poses Cancer, Genetic and Other Risks

The recent proposal by the Bush Administration to allow irradiated ground beef into the National School-Lunch Program will endanger the health of tens of millions of school children and should be withdrawn immediately.

"The government's assertion that irradiated food is safe for human consumption does not even pass the laugh test," states Samuel S. Epstein, M.D., emeritus professor of environmental medicine at University of Illinois School of Public Health, Chicago. "Exposing America's school children to the hazards of irradiated food is reckless negligence, compounded by the absence of any warning to parents."

Irradiated meat is a very different product than natural meat. This is hardly surprising as the Food and Drug Administration's (FDA) approved irradiation dosage of 450,000 rads is approximately 150 million times greater than that of a chest x-ray. Apart from high levels of benzene, new chemicals known as "unique radiolytic products" were identified in irradiated meat in U.S. Army tests in 1977 and recognized as carcinogenic. Later tests identified other chemicals shown to induce genetic toxicity. In sharp contrast to FDA's claims of safety, based on grossly inadequate testing which fails to meet the agency's minimal standards and which were explicitly rebutted by its own expert committees, there is well-documented scientific evidence that eating irradiated meat poses grave risks of cancer and genetic damage. Irradiated meat is also highly susceptible to cross-contamination with food poisoning bacteria.

Nevertheless, the meat and irradiation industries, with FDA's complicity, are lobbying aggressively to sanitize the agency's weak labeling requirements for irradiated meat and other food by eliminating the word "irradiated" in favor of "electronic (or cold) pasteurization." This euphemistic absurdity would circumvent consumer's fundamental right-to-know.

Furthermore, irradiation masks grossly unsanitary conditions in slaughterhouses and meat processing plants. Irradiation is thus a major disincentive to decades-long overdue basic sanitary practices essential for the prevention of Salmonella, E.coli O157, and other pathogenic food poisoning. While irradiation kills most bacteria in meat, pork and poultry, it does nothing to prevent gross fecal and other contamination.

Warnings on the hazards of irradiated food were endorsed in a recent publication, in the world's leading peer-reviewed public health journal, by a wide range of national and international experts including:

Dr. Neal Barnard, President, Physicians Committee for Responsible Medicine, Washington, D.C.

Dr. John Gofman, Emeritus Professor, Molecular and Radiation Biology, University of California, Berkeley, California

Dr. Jay M. Gould, Director, Radiation and Public Health Project, U.S.A.

Dr. Vyvyan Howard, Professor of Pathology, University of Liverpool, U.K.

Dr. David Kriebel, Professor of Epidemiology, University of Massachusetts, Lowell, Massachusetts

Dr. Marvin Legator, Professor of Preventive Medicine, University of Texas, Galveston, Texas

Dr. E. Lichter, Professor of Community Medicine, University of Illinois Medical School, Chicago, Illinois

Dr. William Lijinsky, former Director, Chemical Carcinogenesis, Frederick Cancer Research Center, Maryland

Dr. Sheldon Margen, Emeritus Professor of Public Health Nutrition, University of California, Berkeley, California

Dr. Vicente Navarro, Professor of Health and Public Policy, The Johns Hopkins University, Baltimore, Maryland, Professor of Political and Social Sciences, Universitat Pompeu Fabra, Spain

Dr. Herbert Needleman, Professor of Pediatrics and Psychiatry, University of Pittsburgh, Pittsburgh, Pennsylvania

Dr. Robert Rinehart, Emeritus Professor of Biology, San Diego State University, California

Dr. George Tritsch, Cancer Research Scientist, Roswell Park Memorial Institute, New York State Department of Health, New York

Dr. Quentin Young, past President, American Public Health Association, Chicago, Illinois

June 18, 2001

FDA, USDA Officials Dismiss Citizens' Concerns about Irradiated Food at Symposium

Squandering an opportunity to set the record straight, federal officials dismissed numerous concerns about the safety of irradiated food raised by citizens at a symposium held at the University of Illinois. Sponsored by the Cancer Prevention Coalition, Friday's event was the first occasion in recent years that officials from the Food and Drug Administration (FDA) and U.S. Department of Agriculture (USDA) met citizens face-to-face to discuss food irradiation.

Citizens in attendance sought explanations about why the FDA has legalized food irradiation despite well-documented problems associated with the process. Irradiation can deplete vitamins and nutrients, form chemicals that are known or suspected to cause cancer and birth defects, and corrupt the flavor, texture and odor of food. Dozens of experiments dating to the 1950s have revealed a wide range of serious health problems in animals fed irradiated food. Nonetheless, since 1983 the FDA has legalized the irradiation of beef, pork, poultry, fruit, vegetables, eggs, spices, juice and sprouting seeds.

Friday's symposium featured a presentation by Dr. Vijayalaxmi, whose experiments at India's National Institute of Nutrition during the 1970s revealed genetic damage, fetal deaths, weakened immune systems and low sperm counts in animals that ate irradiated wheat. In one of the few tests ever conducted on people, the Institute discovered genetic damage in children who ate bread made from irradiated wheat.

George Pauli of the FDA's Center for Food Safety and Applied Nutrition, and Donald Thayer of the USDA's Agricultural Research Service dismissed these and many other experimental findings that strongly suggest irradiated food is not safe for human consumption.

"It defies belief that our government can remain in such a severe state of denial," said Samuel Epstein, M.D., chair of the Cancer Prevention Coalition and emeritus professor of environmental medicine at the University of Illinois' School of Public Health. "Every man, woman and child who takes a bite of irradiated food increases their chance of getting cancer. It is no exaggeration to say that our government has turned the American people into guinea pigs."

Epstein co-authored an article that appeared earlier this year in the International Journal of Health Services in which 26 prominent doctors and researchers, as well as consumer, health and environmental protection leaders, issued an urgent warning about the dangers of irradiated food.

The article's other co-author, Wenonah Hauter, director of Public Citizen's Critical Mass Energy and Environment Program, said: "In the face of so much evidence that irradiated food could be harmful, one can hardly overstate the gross negligence that the FDA has displayed over the past 20 years. The FDA must stop rolling the dice with the health of the American people."

FDA and USDA officials dismissed many other concerns raised Friday, including:

Recent German studies found that a chemical formed in certain irradiated foods caused genetic damage in rats and in human cells. The chemical, called 2-DCB, is an irradiation byproduct of palmitic acid, a fat that virtually all foods contain. The chemical itself does not occur naturally in any food. Despite these and many other studies that have revealed hazardous chemical byproducts of irradiation, the USDA's Thayer denied the existence of such evidence.

One-third of the studies published in peer-reviewed scientific journals that looked at the question of genetic damage caused by irradiated food showed genetic damage in animals, humans or cell cultures.

The head of the FDA panel that reviewed more than 400 food irradiation studies in the 1980s later revealed that none of them were properly conducted. And, all seven of the key studies that the FDA relied upon to legalize food irradiation did not meet modern scientific protocols.

In addition to the studies conducted by Vijayalaxmi, the FDA has dismissed numerous other studies that revealed serious health problems in animals that ate irradiated food.

The synergy between irradiation and cooking can, in the words of a USDA report, result in "empty calorie" food.

Irradiation is being embraced by the food industry as a way to mask filthy conditions in factory-style slaughterhouses and processing plants. Because it greatly extends the shelf life of food, irradiation is also being embraced by multinational corporations as a way to move food production operations to developing nations, a trend that has already financially imperiled multitudes of American farmers and ranchers.

In one of the few instances in which citizens' concerns were acknowledged, a high-profile representative of the food irradiation industry said that irradiated food should be properly labeled. Michelle Marcotte of Ion Beam Applications, a Belgian company whose American subsidiary operates several irradiation facilities, said that consumers should have the right to know that food has been irradiated so that they can make informed buying decisions.

Also speaking were representatives from the Northeast Council of Food Inspection Locals and the Center for Food Safety. And, University of Virginia physics Professor Donal Day spoke about the potential that irradiation could induce radioactivity in food. Among the food industry representatives who declined invitations to speak were former Minnesota state epidemiologist Michael Osterholm and executives of Titan/SureBeam, a defense contractor that now sells irradiation equipment.

January 17, 2002

CPC and Illinois Food Safety Coalition Announce a Public Information Campaign to Warn of the Serious Dangers of Food Irradiation

The irradiation industry, with Food and Drug Administration (FDA) approval, claims that irradiating meat and other food is essential to preventing E.coli O157 and other serious bacterial food poisoning. In fact, this could readily be prevented by basic sanitary practices in feedlots and meat packing plants which the powerful meat and irradiation industries are unwilling to do. Furthermore, industry and the FDA claim that irradiated food is safe.

However, these claims are false. "There is well-documented scientific evidence on the cancer and other risks of irradiated food," emphasizes Dr. Samuel Epstein, Chairman of the Cancer Prevention Coalition (CPC). Furthermore, Paul Fehribach, Director of the Illinois Food Safety Coalition (IFSC) states: "The posters will warn of the risks to Schaumburg and Glendale Heights communities where irradiation plants have been recently constructed."

In order to inform unsuspecting consumers, the CPC and IFSC are displaying 46″ x 30″ posters (see attached), at two platforms in each of the four major Chicago Transit Authority (CTA) stations—the Washington and Jackson Red Lines, and the Washington and Jackson Blue Lines—for up to five weeks from today. Additionally, mini-versions of the posters will be distributed at locations including select CTA stations outside downtown.

These warnings are endorsed by 20 statewide citizen and consumer groups including: Alden Ponds Foundation, Chicago Diner, EarthSave, Families Against Rural Messes (F.A.R.M.), Food Animal Concerns Trust (F.A.C.T.), Global Resource Action Center for the Environment (GRACE), Illinois Greens, Illinois Peace Action, Illinois Stewardship Alliance, Lake Michigan Interleague Group of the League of Women Voters (LMILG), Living Upstream, Media Watch, Natural Needs, Nuclear Energy Information Service (NEIS), Nukewatch, Nutrition for Optimal Health Association (NOHA), Organic Consumers Association, and Organic Food Network.

ENDORSERS:

Paul Fehribach
Director
Illinois Food Safety Coalition

March 8, 2002

Food Irradiation Threatens Public Health, National Security

Iowa Senator Tom Harkin's last minute provisions in the Senate farm bill allowing irradiated beef to be labeled "pasteurized," instead of the Food and Drug Administration's small print "treated by irradiation" label, is a surprising denial of consumers' fundamental right-to-know.

Consumers are wary of irradiated food, and with good reason even if they don't understand the dangers involved. Irradiated meat is a very different product from cooked meat. Irrespective of whether radiated by radioactive cobalt pellets or rods, x-ray machines or electron beams, the current permissible radiation dosage is about 200 million times greater than a chest x-ray.

As well documented since the 1960s, these massive doses of ionizing radiation produce profound chemical changes in meat. These include elevated levels of the carcinogenic chemical benzene, and also the production of unique new chemicals, known as radiolytic products, some of which have been implicated as carcinogenic.

Additionally, irradiated food has been shown to induce genetic damage in a wide range of studies, including tests on malnourished children by India's National Institute of Nutrition.

Of particular concern in this regard, are a group of readily detectable unique chemicals known as cyclobutanones which have recently been shown to cause chromosomal damage in intestinal cells of rats and humans.

The Food and Drug Administration (FDA) and the U.S. Department of Agriculture (USDA) have ignored the strong evidence on the cancer and genetic risks of irradiated food. Instead, they have relied on a group of five studies, selected from a total of over 400 studies prior to 1980, on which their current claims of safety are based.

The FDA has persisted in these claims even though its own expert Irradiated Food Committee warned that the tests are grossly flawed and inadequate.

Furthermore, as admitted by USDA's Agricultural Research Service, irradiation results in major losses of vitamins, particularly A, C, E and the B complex. These losses are substantially increased by cooking, resulting in empty calorie food, a concern of major importance for the malnourished. Radiation has also been used to clean up food unfit for human consumption, such as spoiled fish, by killing odorous contaminating bacteria.

While the USDA is actively supporting meat and poultry radiation, it has been moving to deregulate and privatize the industry by promoting self-policing programs. Irradiation is also aggressively promoted by the Department of Energy's Byproducts Utilization Program to reduce disposal costs of spent military and civilian nuclear fuel by providing a commercial market for nuclear wastes.

Food irradiation plants pose grave dangers to national security. They are relatively small, unregulated, and unlikely to be secure. As such, they are highly vulnerable to sabotage.

Of particular current concern are terrorist attacks to steal radioactive cobalt pellets. These could be mixed with conventional explosives to produce so-called "dirty bombs," whose effects could be devastating.

These plants pose additional dangers to local communities by generating high levels of ozone, a very toxic atmospheric pollutant when it is close to ground level instead of high in the stratosphere where it protects the Earth from ultraviolet radiation.

Not surprisingly, the focus of the radiation and agribusiness industries has been directed to the lucrative cleanup of contaminated food, rather than preventing contamination at its source. However, bacterial food poisoning, particularly with E.coli O157, which can be dangerous and lethal to young children, can be largely prevented by long overdue improved sanitation, apart from thorough cooking of meat.

Sanitation in cattle feedlots, including reducing overcrowding, drinking water disinfection and fly control, would drastically reduce cattle infection rates.

Moreover, O157 infection rates could be virtually eliminated by feeding hay seven days prior to slaughter, which the industry is unwilling to do because of higher costs. Sanitation would also prevent drinking water contamination from feedlot run off, incriminated in recent outbreaks of O157 poisoning; this would remain a continuing threat even if all meat were irradiated.

Pre-slaughter and post-evisceration sanitation at meat packing plants are also highly effective for reducing carcass contamination rates. Practical techniques are available for rapid individual or pooled carcasses for fecal and bacterial contamination.

The expense of producing sanitary meat would be trivial compared to the high costs of irradiation, which would be passed on to consumers, apart from assuring its wholesomeness and safety, besides preventing nuclear accidents and terrorism.

Rather than sanitizing the label in response to special interests, Congress should focus on sanitation, not irradiation of the nation's food supply.

For further information on food irradiation, see the recently published article "Preventing Pathogenic Food Poisoning: Sanitation, Not Irradiation," endorsed by over 20 leading international experts, "International Journal of Health Services," volume 31(1):187-192, 2001.

November 1, 2002

USDA'S Allowing Schools to Serve Irradiated Meat Is Reckless

USDA claims that irradiated food is safe, and that low levels of radiation are used do not even pass the laugh test," warns Samuel S. Epstein, M.D., Chairman of the Cancer Prevention Coalition. The Parent Teacher Association, nationally, regionally and locally, and parents are urged to boycott irradiated food, and protect children from serious risks to future health and life.

Irradiated meat is a very different product than natural meat. This is hardly surprising as the approved irradiation dosage of 450,000 rads. is some 200 million times greater than a chest x-ray. Apart from high levels of benzene, new chemicals known as "unique radiolytic products" have been identified in irradiated food since the 1970's. Contrary to USDA assurances, which have been rejected by a high level expert FDA committee in addition to independent scientists, these pose risks of cancer, and genetic damage, as demonstrated in test tube, animal tests and also children. Furthermore, as admitted by a USDA report, cooking irradiated food depletes its vitamin content, resulting in "empty calorie food."

Irradiation is now being aggressively promoted by the food industry to divert attention from grossly unsanitary conditions in factory style feedlots, slaughterhouses and packing plants, and to sterilize meat contaminated with feces. The recklessness of the industry is encouraged by recently leaked UDSA instructions which discourage federal meat inspectors from preventing fecal contamination of meat: "Remember YOU are accountable for the very serious responsibility of stopping the company's production for the benefit of food safety."

Our warnings on the dangers of irradiated food are endorsed by some 25 independent national and international experts, and by Public Citizen and other consumer groups.

Sanitation, but not irradiation, is the answer to preventing food poisoning.

December 4, 2002

Jewel-Osco's Sale of Surebeam's Irradiated Meat Threatens Consumer Health

On November 29 Chicago Tonight TV, meat industry representatives admitted that irradiated meat can taste like "Wet Dog," while supporting Jewel-Osco and SureBeam claims that the meat is safe. "However, these claims don't even pass the laugh test," states Samuel S. Epstein, M.D., Professor emeritus of Environmental Medicine at the University of Illinois School of Public Health, Chicago, and Chairman of the Cancer Prevention Coalition.

SureBeam's claim that its electron-beam irradiation technology destroys food poisoning bacteria just "like thermal pasteurization" of milk is a euphemistic absurdity, and its claim that the technology just "uses ordinary electricity" is deceptive in extreme. The technology, originally designed to zap incoming missiles for President Reagan's "Star Wars Program," shoots meat with a stream of electrons traveling at the speed of light. This results in an irradiation dosage of 450,000 rads, approximately 150 million times greater than that of a chest x-ray.

Not surprisingly, irradiated meat is a very different product than natural meat. Apart from high levels of benzene, new chemicals known as "unique radiolytic products" have been identified in irradiated food since the 1970's.

Contrary to FDA assurances, which were rejected in 1981 by its own high level expert committee and also by independent scientists, these pose risks of cancer, and of genetic damage, as demonstrated in test tube and animal tests, and in children. Furthermore, as admitted by an internal USDA report, cooking irradiated food depletes its vitamin content, resulting in "empty calorie food."

Irradiation is now being aggressively promoted by the meat industry to divert attention from grossly unsanitary conditions in factory style feedlots, slaughterhouses and packing plants, and to sterilize meat contaminated with feces. The recklessness of the industry is actively encouraged by recent USDA instructions which discourage federal meat inspectors from preventing fecal contamination of meat: "Remember YOU are accountable for the very serious responsibility of stopping the country's production for the benefit of food safety."

Warnings on the dangers of irradiated food have been endorsed by some 25 leading national and international scientists and by Public Citizen and other consumer groups. Sanitation, but not irradiation, is the answer to preventing food poisoning.

May 23, 2003

Beware of Irradiated Dietary Supplements

In an April 16 notice in the Federal Register, the Food and Drug Administration [FDA] announced that Steris Corporation had filed a petition requesting "the safe use of ionizing radiation" for sterilizing dietary supplements, and ingredients used in their manufacture. In support of the petition, FDA reassured "that this action . . . does not . . . have a significant effect on the human environment."

However, in spite of industry and FDA assurances, irradiated dietary supplements are nutritionally inferior. Worse still, they are even dangerous.

The irradiation dosage proposed by Steris ranges to as high as one billion times greater than that of a single chest x-ray, and about six times greater than that allowed by FDA for the sterilization of fresh meat. Such high doses of ionizing radiation produce profound changes in the chemical composition of the fats in nutritional ingredients. These include the production of high levels of benzene, and also a group of unique chemicals, some of which are highly stable. These chemicals, and irradiated food, have been incriminated as causing cancer. They have also been shown to cause genetic damage in test tube experiments, rodents, monkeys, and young children.

Of still further concern, irradiation results in major losses of vitamins, particularly A, C, E, and the B complex.

The Steris petition for sterilizing nutritional supplements with high dose radiation raises serious concerns regarding the likelihood of bacterial contamination of mainstream industry products. Accordingly, the public should be so informed by explicit labeling.

For further details, see the Cancer Prevention Coalition February 2003 "Stop Cancer Before It Starts Campaign" report at www.preventcancer. com; the report has been endorsed by over 100 scientific experts in cancer prevention, and representatives of environmental, consumer, and other activist groups.

July 1, 2003

McDonald's Is Leading the Way, but Hasn't Gone Far Enough Yet

Commendably responding to growing concerns that the routine use of antibiotics in meat production has resulted in their decreased effectiveness for treating infectious diseases, McDonald's Corporation has demanded that its suppliers phase out antibiotic growth promoters by the end of 2004. This trailblazing initiative is backed by Burger King, Wendy's, and KFC, and by Elanco, the nation's largest veterinary drug company. However, McDonald's initiative excludes hormonal growth promoters.

When beef cattle enter feedlots, hormone pellets are implanted under the ear skin, a process that is repeated at the mid-point of their 100-day pre-slaughter fattening period. The hormones increase cattle weight, adding about $80.00 profit per animal.

The commonest hormone in current use is the potent cancer-causing, and gene-damaging estradiol. Other hormones include progesterone, testosterone, and their synthetic variants. However, the FDA and USDA claim that residues of these hormones in meat are within "normal" levels, and could not possibly induce any harmful effects. However, of 130 million livestock slaughtered annually, few, if any, have been monitored for residues of estradiol or any other hormone.

In sharp contrast, confidential industry reports to the FDA, obtained under the Freedom of Information Act, have revealed high hormone residues in meat under idealized test conditions. Following a single implant in a steer of Synovex-S, a combination of estradiol and progesterone, estradiol levels in different meat products were over 20-fold higher than normal. The amount of estradiol in two hamburgers eaten daily by an 8-year-old boy would increase his hormone residues by at least 10 percent over very low natural levels.

However, the situation may be much worse in real life. An unpublicized random USDA survey of 32 large feedlots found that as many as half the cattle had illegal "misplaced implants" in muscle, rather than under the ear skin. This would result in very high local concentrations of hormones, and in meat all over the body. Besides such abusive practice, accidental implantation of hormone pellets in neck muscle, rather than under ear skin, is not uncommon and would also result in high residues in meat.

These sex hormones, particularly estradiol, are linked ever more closely to the escalating incidence of reproductive cancers since 197354 percent for post-menopausal breast cancer, 67 percent for testicular cancer, and 105 percent for prostate cancer. Of particular concern also is the increasing incidence of premature puberty in young girls, which has been linked to hormonal meat.

The endocrine disruptive effects of estrogenic industrial chemicals, including pesticides, cosmetic ingredients, and food contaminants, are now under intensive investigation by federal regulatory and health agencies. But the contamination of meat with residues of the much more potent estradiol, besides other sex hormones, remains ignored.

Europe has been highly skeptical of U.S. claims on the safety of hormonal meat, and banned its sale and import since 1989. In 1997, the U.S. and Canada appealed this ban before the World Trade Organization (WTO) on the grounds that it was discriminatory trade practice, and not scientifically justified. The WTO ruled in favor of the appeal on the narrow and arguable technical grounds that the European Commission (EC) had not undertaken a formal quantitative "health risk assessment," and imposed financial penalties on the EC.

The EC then requested a "Scientific Committee" of nine independent experts, including four from the U.S., to undertake a comprehensive risk assessment of all growth-promoting hormones. By 1999, the Committee concluded that the risk to consumers had been clearly established, and that safe exposure levels could not be identified for any of these hormones. They further warned that exposure to even small traces in meat posed carcinogenic, endocrine, and genetic risks, especially for pre-pubertal children because of their "extremely low level" of production of sex hormones. In striking contrast, despite the EC's repeated requests, the U.S. has failed to produce any scientific information or publications on which they still base their claims of safety.

The EC went further by funding 17 comprehensive studies on hormone residues in meat. All these, most already published in peer-reviewed scientific journals, further document the carcinogenic, genetic, and other risks of hormonal meat.

McDonald's should further strengthen its "Social Responsibility" campaign by extending concerns on the dangers of growth-promoting agents, from the antibiotic to the hormonal.

November 7, 2005

More Than One Reason for the Threatened Beef Boycott

Threats by Consumers Union of Japan to boycott U.S. beef because of risks of mad cow disease (BSE) are well based. While Japan routinely tests all the 1.3 million beef carcasses it processes annually, the U.S. tests only about 1 in 2,000 cattle, largely restricted to cattle over 30 months old with BSE symptoms. Of additional concern, the U.S. still has no tracking system which would allow tracing infected cattle back to their herds.

Reinforcing and extending the basis for the threatened boycott is the fact that U.S. beef is heavily contaminated with sex hormones. When U.S. beef cattle enter feedlots, sex hormone pellets are implanted under the ear skin, a process that is repeated at the midpoint of their 100-day pre-slaughter fattening period. These hormones increase the weight of the cattle, adding to profits by about $80 per animal.

The hormones in past and current use include the natural—estradiol, progesterone, and testosterone—and the synthetic—zeranol, trenbolone, and melengesterol. The U.S. Food and Drug Administration (FDA) and the U.S. Department of Agriculture (USDA) have maintained and still maintain that residues of these hormones in meat are within "normal levels," and have waived any requirements for residue testing.

Europe, however, has rightly viewed U.S. claims with considerable skepticism, and since 1989 the European Union has banned the sale of beef from hormone-treated cattle. The U.S., and also Canada, have challenged that the European ban is protectionist, and is costing North America $100 million annually in lost exports.

However, confidential industry reports to the FDA, obtained under the Freedom of Information Act, have revealed high hormone residues in meat products. Following a single ear implant in steers of Synovex-S, a combination of estradiol and progesterone, residues of these hormones in meat were found to be up to 20-fold higher than normal. The amount of estradiol in two hamburgers eaten in one day by an 8-year-old boy could increase his total hormone levels by as much as 10%, particularly as young children have very low natural hormone levels.

Increased levels of sex hormones are linked ever more closely to the escalating increase of reproductive cancers in the U.S., 37% for post-menopausal breast cancer, 46% for testicular cancer, and 88% for prostate cancer, since 1975. The endocrine disruptive effects of estrogenic pesticides and phthalate contaminants in food, besides phthalate and paraben ingredients in cosmetics and toiletries, are now well recognized. However, the contamination of meat with residues of the much more highly potent estradiol, zeranol, and other sex hormones remains virtually unrecognized.

These concerns have been strongly reinforced by recent evidence, from researchers at Ohio State University, that meat and blood from cattle implanted with zeranol have powerful hormonal effects, which resist cooking. This is evidenced by strong stimulatory effects on normal and cancerous human breast cells in laboratory tests.

It is well recognized that American women have about a five-fold greater risk of breast cancer than Japanese. However, as recently confirmed by studies of cancer rates in Los Angeles County, the most highly populated and ethnically diverse county in the U.S., the low risk in Japanese women increases sharply in immigrants to the U.S. after one to two generations. This, and a wide range of other studies in migrant populations, is strongly supportive of avoidable, dietary, and possibly other "Westernized" lifestyle, causes of breast cancer.

Based on these considerations, Japanese consumer groups should consider extending their concerns on the dangers of U.S. beef from BSE to hormonal contaminants.

April 10, 2006

National School Lunches: Unsafe at Any Eating

On April 6, a bipartisan Congressional group, with strong support in both Houses, announced plans to introduce legislation amending the National School Lunch Act. This would prohibit the sale in schools of sugary or fatty junk foods, notably soft drinks and French fries.

This welcomed initiative officially endorses longstanding efforts by many school districts to provide only healthy foods, and hopefully reduce the growing incidence of childhood obesity and related diseases.

Enforcement of this initiative would be the responsibility of the U.S. Department of Agriculture (USDA), which is in charge of the current Public School Lunch Program. This extended authority was applauded by the Center for Science in the Public Interest, a national food safety activist group, stating that "The Agency has done a good job with the official school lunch and could do a good job with all other foods." This endorsement may well be warranted nutritionally. However, it certainly is not warranted by the USDA's failure to disclose well-documented scientific evidence on the risks to health of the two school lunch staples, milk and meat.

Much of the nations milk supply comes from cows injected with a genetically engineered variant of their natural growth hormone, technically known as rBGH (recombinant Bovine Growth Hormone). Manufactured by Monsanto, and sold to dairy farmers under the trade name POSILAC. Injection of the hormone forces cows to increase their milk yield by about 10 percent, while making them sick in the process.

Monsanto and the USDA insist that rBGH milk is indistinguishable from natural milk, and that it is safe for children and other consumers. This is scientifically and medically untrue. rBGH milk makes cows sick. Monsanto has been forced to admit to some 20 toxic veterinary effects on its POSILAC (rBGH) label. These include mastitis, resulting in pus cells in milk, and antibiotics used to treat the mastitis. rBGH milk is also chemically, and nutritionally different than natural milk, and is supercharged with excess levels of a natural growth factor (IGF-1), which is readily absorbed through the intestines into the blood. Of major concern is a wealth of longstanding scientific evidence incriminating these excess levels as delayed causes of breast, colon, and prostate cancers.

Reacting to the fully documented scientific evidence on the dangers of rBGH milk, a wide range of nations including all of Europe, Canada, Australia, New Zealand and Japan have all banned rBGH milk.

U.S. beef is heavily contaminated with sex hormones. When U.S. beef cattle enter feedlots, sex hormone pellets are implanted under the ear skin, a process that is repeated at the midpoint of their 100-day pre-slaughter fattening period. These hormones increase the weight of the cattle, adding to profits by about $80 per animal.

The hormones in past and current use include the natural estradiol, progesterone, and testosterone, and their more potent synthetic counterparts, zeranol, trenbolone, and melengesterol. The FDA and USDA have both maintained and still claim that residues of these hormones in meat are safe and within normal limits.

October 21, 2009

Hormones in U.S. Beef Linked to Increased Cancer Risk

Beef produced in the United States is heavily contaminated with natural or synthetic sex hormones, which are associated with an increased risk of reproductive and childhood cancers, warns Dr. Samuel S. Epstein, Chairman of the Cancer Prevention Coalition.

"Increased levels of sex hormones are linked to the escalating incidence of reproductive cancers in the United States since 1975-60% for prostate, 59% for testis, and 10% for breast," Dr. Epstein says.

The hormones in past and current use include the natural estrogen, progesterone and testosterone, and the synthetic zeranol, trenbolone, and melengesterol.

When beef cattle enter feedlots, pellets of these hormones are implanted under the ear skin, a process that is repeated at the midpoint of their 100-day pre-slaughter fattening period, Dr. Epstein explains. These hormones increase carcass weight, adding over $80 in extra profit per animal.

Also, Dr. Epstein says, "Not surprisingly, but contrary to longstanding claims by the U.S. Food and Drug Administration (FDA) and the U.S. Department of Agriculture (USDA), residues of these hormones in meat are up to 20-fold higher than normal."

"Still higher residues result from the not uncommon illegal practice of implantation directly into muscle. Furthermore, contrary to misleading assurances, meat is still not monitored for hormone residues," Dr. Epstein emphasizes.

Nevertheless, he points out, the FDA and USDA maintain that hormone residues in meat are within "normal levels," while waiving any requirements for residue testing.

Following a single ear implant in steers of Synovex-S, a combination of estrogen and progesterone, residues of these hormones in meat were found to be up to 20-fold higher than normal.

The amount of estradiol in two hamburgers eaten in one day by an 8-year-old boy could increase his total hormone levels by as much as 10%, particularly as young children have very low natural hormone levels.

Not surprisingly, Dr. Epstein says, the incidence of childhood cancer has increased by 38% since 1975.

These concerns are not new. As evidenced in a series of General Accountability Office investigations and Congressional hearings, FDA residue-tolerance programs and USDA inspections are in near total disarray, aggravated by brazen denials and cover-ups.

A January 1986 report, "Human Food Safety and the Regulation of Animal Drugs," unanimously approved by the House Committee on Government Operations, concluded that "the FDA has consistently disregarded its responsibility—has repeatedly put what is perceives are interests of veterinarians and the livestock industry ahead of its legal obligation to protect consumers, thus jeopardizing the health and safety of consumers of meat, milk and poultry."

On January 1, 1989, the European Community placed a ban on meat imports from animals treated with growth inducing hormones. This had a direct impact on the U.S. beef industry, which uses hormones in more than half of the cattle sent to market each year.

Twenty-years later, on May 6, 2009, the European Union and the United States settled their long-running dispute over hormone-treated beef. Under terms of the four-year deal the EU will be permitted to maintain its ban on hormone-fed beef. In return, the EU has agreed to increase the amount of hormone-free beef that can be imported from the U.S. without duty.

It is well recognized that American women have about a five-fold greater risk of breast cancer than women in countries that do not permit the sale of hormonal beef.

However, as recently confirmed by studies of cancer rates in Los Angeles County, the most highly populated, ethnically diverse county in the U.S., the low risk in Japanese women in Japan increases sharply in Japanese immigrants to the United States after one to two generations.

This, and a wide range of other studies in migrant populations, is evidence that avoidable causes of breast cancer include adoption of Western dietary habits, particularly the consumption of hormone—laced beef.

February 2, 2010

A Ban on Hormonal Meat Is Three Decades Overdue

On January 29, 2010, with three other scientific experts, Samuel S. Epstein, M.D., Chairman of the Cancer Prevention Coalition, filed a Food and Drug Administration (FDA) Petition seeking an urgent ban on hormonal meat, as it poses unrecognized risks of hormonal cancers.

The Petition requests the FDA to take the following action:

Require producers of hormonal meat to label it with an explicit warning such as "Produced with the use of sex hormones, and poses increased risks of breast, prostate, and testis cancers.

Prohibit the routine implantation of sex hormone pellets under the ear skin of cattle on entry into feedlots 100 days prior to slaughter. The object of the implants is to increase meat production by about 50 pounds per animal, and profitability by about 10%.

Ban hormonal meat. The hormones in past and current use include the natural: testosterone, estrogen, and progesterone; and the synthetic: trenbolone, zeranol, and melengesterol.

STATEMENT OF GROUNDS

Based on the scientific literature, besides World Health Organization (WHO) reports, there is explicit evidence that the use of sex hormones to increase meat production poses serious dangers to consumers," Dr. Epstein warns in the Petition.

"Of particular concern are the increased risks of hormonal cancers since 1975: breast by 23%, prostate by 60%, and testes by 60%," he emphasizes.

For these reasons, the Petition urges the FDA to take the following actions, now decades overdue:

Recognize that hormonal meat poses "imminent hazards" to the total U.S. population.

Take prompt, and decades overdue, regulatory action to eliminate the use of sex hormones in meat production.

Dr. Epstein explains that some three decades ago, Dr. Roy Hertz, then Director of Endocrinology of the National Cancer Institute and world authority on breast and other hormonal cancers, warned of cancer risks due to the use of estrogenic cattle implants, particularly for the breast.

Dr. Hertz emphasized that these implants increase normal hormonal levels, and that such imbalance causes reproductive cancers. Hertz also warned of the essentially uncontrolled and unregulated use of these extremely potent biological agents, no levels of which can be regarded as safe.

"These warnings are even more apt today, particularly in view of the FDA's longstanding and reckless failure to ban hormonal meat," Dr. Epstein declares.

The misleading assurances since 1979, by the FDA and United States Department of Agriculture (USDA) on the safety of hormonal meat remain unchanged, Dr. Epstein declares. Of further concern are longstanding problems linked to conflicts of interest in senior agency personnel and their consultants. As clearly evidenced in a series of General Accountability Office investigations and Congressional hearings, the USDA and FDA have failed to take any regulatory action to protect the public from the dangers of hormonal meat, Dr. Epstein points out.

Dr. Epstein cites a 1986 report, "Human Food Safety and Regulation of Animal Drugs," unanimously approved by the House Committee on Government Operations, which concluded that the "FDA has consistently disregarded its responsibility—has repeatedly put what it perceives are interests of veterinarians and the livestock industry ahead of its legal obligation to protect consumers—jeopardizing the health and safety of consumers meat, milk, and poultry."

In response to questions on hormonal meat raised in February 1996 by the European Commission, the USDA responded with assurances that less than 0.25% of animals tested annually proved positive for "residue violations." Dr. Epstein asserts, "These criticisms remain equally appropriate today. In fact, meat is still not monitored for sex hormone levels by the U.S. Department of Agriculture or the U.S. Food and Drug Administration.

ENDORSERS:

Nicholas Ashford, PhD, JD
Professor of Technology and Policy
Massachusetts Institute of Technology

Ronnie Cummins
Executive Director
Organic Consumers Association

Quentin D. Young, M.D.
Chairman, Health & Medicine Policy Research Group
Past President, American Public Health Association

D.
Cosmetics and Personal Care Products

Cosmetics and Personal Care Products

Newspaper Articles, Press Releases, and Huffington Post Blogs

Citizen Petition Seeking Carcinogenic Labeling on All Cosmetic Talc Products

November 17, 1994

David A. Kessler, M.D.
Commissioner

This Petition is based on scientific papers dating back to the 1960s which warn of increased cancer rates resulting from frequent exposure to cosmetic grade talc.

The undersigned submits this petition to request the Commissioner of Food and Drugs to require that all cosmetic talc products bear labels with a warning such as Talcum powder causes cancer in laboratory animals. Frequent talc application in the female genital area increases risk of ovarian cancer.

A. AGENCY ACTION REQUESTED

This petition requests that FDA take the following action: Immediately require cosmetic talcum powder products to bear labels with a warning such as Talcum powder causes cancer in laboratory animals. Frequent talc application in the female genital area increases the risk of ovarian cancer.

B. STATEMENT OF GROUNDS

Ovarian cancer is the fourth deadliest women's cancer in the U.S., striking approximately 23,000 and killing approximately 14,000 women this year. Ovarian cancer is very difficult to detect at the early stages of the disease, making the survival rate very low. Only three percent of ovarian cancer cases can be attributed to family history. One of the avoidable risk factors for ovarian cancer is the daily use of talcum powder in the genital area.

Research done as early as 1961 has shown that particles, similar to talc and asbestos particles, can translocate from the exterior genital area to the ovaries in women. These findings provide support to the unexpected high rate of mortality from ovarian cancer in female asbestos workers. Minute particles, such as talc are able to translocate through the female reproductive tract and cause foreign body reactions in the ovary.

241

There is a large body of scientific evidence, dating back thirty years, on the toxicity and mineralogy of cosmetic talc products. As early as 1968, Cralley et al. Concluded:

All of the 22 talcum products analyzed have a . . . fiber content . . . averaging 19%. The fibrous material was predominantly talc but probably contained minor amounts of tremolite, anthophyllite, and chrysotile [asbestos-like fibers] as these are often present in fibrous talc mineral deposits . . . Unknown significant amounts of such materials in products that may be used without precautions may create an unsuspected problem.

As a follow-up to previous findings, Rohl, et al., examined 21 samples of consumer talcums and powders, including baby powders, body powders, facial powders and pharmaceutical powders between 1971-1975. The study concluded:

". . . cosmetic grade talc was not used exclusively. The presence in these products of asbestiform anthophyllite and tremolite, chrysotile, and quartz indicates the need for a regulatory standard for cosmetic talc . . . We also recommend that evaluation be made to determine the possible health hazards associated with the use of these products."

Talc is a carcinogen, with or without the presence of asbestos-like fibers. In 1993, the National Toxicology Program published a study on the toxicity of non-asbestiform talc and found clear evidence of carcinogenic activity.

Recent cancer research in the United States has found conclusively that frequent talcum powder application in the genital area increases a woman's risk of developing ovarian cancer. Cramer, et al, suggested that talc application directly to the genital area around the time of ovulation might lead to talc particles becoming deeply imbedded in the substance of the ovary and perhaps causing foreign body reaction (granulomas) capable of causing growth of epithelial ovarian tissue.

Harlow, et al, found that frequent talc use directly on the genital area during ovulation increased a woman's risk *threefold*. That study also found:

"The most frequent method of talc exposure was use as a dusting powder directly to the perineum (genitals) . . . Brand or generic 'baby powder' was used most frequently and was the category associated with a statistically significant risk for ovarian cancer."

In Harlow's report, arguably the most comprehensive study of talc use and ovarian cancer to date, 235 ovarian cancer cases were identified and compared to 239 controls, women with no sign of ovarian cancer or related health problems. Through personal interviews, Harlow, et al, found that 16.7% of the control group reported frequent talc application to the perineum. This percentage is useful in estimating the number of women in the general population exposed to cosmetic talc in the genital area on a regular basis. Harlow, et al, concludes:

". . . given the poor prognosis for ovarian cancer, any potentially harmful exposures should be avoided, particularly those with limited benefits. For this reason, we discourage the use of talc in genital hygiene, particularly as a daily habit."

Clearly, large numbers of women—an estimated 17%—are using cosmetic talc in the genital area and may not be adequately warned of the risk of ovarian cancer from daily use.

C. CERTIFICATION

The undersigned certifies, that, to the best knowledge and belief of the undersigned, this petition includes all information and views on which the petition relies, and that it includes representative data and information known to the petitioner which are unfavorable to the petition.

This petition, based on 18 scientific references, was submitted by:

Samuel S. Epstein, M.D.
Chairman, Cancer Prevention Coalition
Professor Occupational and Environmental Medicine
University of Illinois School of Public Health, Chicago

Jill A. Cashen

Michael E. Deutsch, Esq., Legal Director, Center for Constitutional Rights, New York

APPENDIX I: Results of an informal survey of talc products in Chicago drug stores

BABY POWDERS

Johnson & Johnson Baby Powder. Contains: TALC, fragrance.

Osco Brand Baby Powder. Contains: TALC, fragrance.

Jean Nate Perfumed Talc. Contains: TALC, kaolin, magnesium carbonate, fragrance.

Shower to Shower. Contains: TALC, cornstarch, sodium bicarbonate, fragrance, polysaccarides.

Ammens Medicated Powder. Contains: Zinc oxide, cornstarch, fragrance, isostearic acid, PPG-20, methyl glucose ether, TALC.

Cashmere Bouquet Perfumed Powder. Contains: TALC, magnesium carbonate, zinc stearate, fragrance.

Gold Bond Medicated Powder. Contains: Menthol, zinc oxide, boric acid, eucalyptol, methyl salicylate, salicylic acid, TALC, thymol, zinc stearate.

FEMININE PRODUCTS

Vaginex Feminine Powder. Contains: Zinc oxide, cornstarch, fragrance, 6-hydroxquinoline, 8-hydroxquinoline sulfate, isostearic acid, PPG-20, methyl glucose ether, TALC.

Vagisil Feminine Powder. Contains: Cornstarch, aloe, mineral oil, magnesium stearate, silica, benzethonium chloride, fragrance.

Summer's Eve Feminine Powder. Contains: Cornstarch, tricalcium phosphate, oxoxynol-9, benzethonium chloride, fragrance.

FDS Feminine Deodorant Spray. Contains: Isobutane, isopropyl myristate, cornstarch, mineral oil, fragrance, lanolin alcohol, hydrated silica, magnesium stearate, benzyl alcohol.

Citizen Petition Seeking to Ban the Use of Lindane (Gamma-Hexachlorocyclohexane) as Treatment for Lice and Scabies

January 17, 1995

David A. Kessler, M.D.
Commissioner

This Petition is based on recent scientific information on risks of brain cancer in children resulting from the use of lindane shampoo, other evidence of carcinogenicity, and evidence of haematoxicity and neurotoxicity.

The undersigned submits this petition to request the Commissioner of the Food and Drug Administration (FDA) to immediately ban the use of lindane as a treatment for lice and scabies.

A. AGENCY ACTION REQUESTED

This petition requests that FDA take the following action:

Immediately ban the use of lindane as a treatment for lice and scabies.

B. STATEMENT OF GROUNDS

Lice and scabies are endemic among the population. An estimated six million Americans, mainly children, are infested with lice each year. Most children are treated with pesticide-containing products marketed as shampoos. Lindane (gamma-hexachlorocyclohexane) is one of the most widely prescribed treatments for lice and scabies.

In a recent case-control study, Davis, et al. reported a statistically significant increase of brain cancer in children following treatment with lindane shampoo. ". . . use of Kwell®, [lindane] was significantly associated with childhood brain cancer in comparison to friend controls (OR = 4.6; 95% CI = 1.0-21.3)."

These findings are of particular significance in relation to the striking increase, 38%, in the incidence of brain and nervous system cancers in children from 1973-1991S.

Further evidence on carcinogenicity is provided by two epidemiological studies by the National Cancer Institute. Statistically significant increases, up to six-fold, in the incidence of non-Hodgkin's lymphoma were reported in farmers exposed to lindane.

In addition to these epidemiological data, series of case reports on blood disorders, including aplastic anemia, with case fatality rates of some 50%, and leukemia have appeared in the literature over the last three decades. Of related interest is recent evidence on the high toxicity of lindane to human red blood stem cells.

These epidemiological data are further supported by experimental evidence on the carcinogenicity of lindane. Lindane is classified as Group 2B by the International Agency for Research on Cancer, and as 2B/C by the Environmental Protection Agency. The EPA has restricted lindane's use as an agricultural pesticide. Agricultural and other uses of lindane and other isomers of hexachlorocyclohexane have been severely restricted or banned by other countries.

The neurotoxic effects of lindane are well known. A 1976 FDA alert was issued to warn physicians of such risks. Numerous case reports have documented seizures and brain damage following lindane exposure. Recent studies have emphasized that recommended dosages of lindane may cause seizures:

"Therefore, given the extremely narrow range of safety of this drug and the risk imposed by the kindling effects, which potentiates convulsive seizures, and that this potentiation may be carried on for a considerable period of time, there is no good reason to use lindane in children or adults when other perfectly effective, safer pediculides are available."

Lindane is readily absorbed through the skin. After topical application to the adult skin without washing for 24 hours, almost 10% can be recovered from urine. Absorption is further increased when lindane is administered in warm water or followed by oil-based hair care preparations.

This petition, based on fifteen scientific references, was submitted by:

Samuel S. Epstein, M.D.
Chairman, Cancer Prevention Coalition
Professor emeritus Occupational and Environmental Medicine
University of Illinois School of Public Health, Chicago

Jill A. Cashen

Quentin D. Young, M.D., Chairman, Health and Medicine Policy Research Group, Past President of the American Public Health Association

Peter Orris, M.D., Professor and Chief of Service, University of Illinois at Chicago Medical Center

Michael Deutsch, Esq., Legal Director, Center for Constitutional Rights, New York

Citizen Petition Seeking Cancer Warning on Cosmetics Containing DEA

October 22, 1996

David A. Kessler, M.D.
Commissioner

This Petition requests that all cosmetic products containing diethanolamine (DEA) bear labels with a warning: "Caution—This product may contain N-nitrosodiethanolamine, a known cancer—causing agent."

A. AGENCY ACTION REQUESTED

This petition requests that FDA takes the following action:

Issue a regulation under the Federal Food, Drug and Cosmetic Act, Section 601(a), stating that "All cosmetics containing diethanolamine (DEA), a constituent of diethanolamide soaps that may react with nitrosating agents to form N-nitrosodiethanolamine (NDEA), bear a label as an adulterated product containing poisonous and deleterious substances which may render it injurious to users under the conditions of use prescribed in the labeling thereof, or under such conditions of use as are customary or usual: that which contains DEA also bears the following legend conspicuously displayed thereon: 'Caution—This product may contain N-nitrosodi-ethanolamine, a known cancer-causing agent.'"

B. STATEMENT OF GROUNDS

1. Widespread Contamination of Cosmetics with DEA and NDEA

Diethanolamine (DEA) is a high production chemical used in a wide range of cosmetic pro-ducts, including shampoos, lotions and creams. In the presence of long-chain fatty acids DEA reacts to form neutral ethanolamide soaps, which are used as wetting agents in cosmetics. These soaps contain unreacted DEA. Triethanolamine (TEA), also used widely in cosmetics, may also be contaminated with DEA. According to the Cosmetics, Toiletries and Fragrance Association,

Cocamide DEA, Lauramide DEA, Linoleamide DEA and Oleamide DEA are fatty acid diethanolamides which may contain 4 to 33 percent diethanolamine. These ingredients are used in cosmetics at concentrations of <0.1 percent to 50 percent, with most products containing percent to 25 percent diethanolamide.

As of 1980, FDA reported that approximately 42 percent of all cosmetic products were contaminated with NDEA at the following concentrations: facial cosmetics from .042 to 49 mg/kg, lotions from less than .010 to .140 mg/kg, shampoos from less than 10 to 160 mg/kg. In two surveys of cosmetics, 27 out of 29 American products contained up to 48 mg/kg NDEA. A more recent FDA analysis (1991-1992) found that NDEA is present in some products at mg/kg concentrations.

2. DEA Is a Precursor of NDEA

N-nitrosodiethanolamine (NDEA), is readily formed in cosmetic by nitrosation of DEA. Even small amounts of DEA in cosmetics can react with nitrosating agents to form nitrosamines. According to the Cosmetics, Toiletries and Fragrance Association: Nitrosamine contamination of diethanolamine and fatty acid diethanolamides, and nitrosamine formation are potential problems in using these diethanolamides. The diethanolamides used in cosmetic products should be free of nitrosamines, and the finished product should not contain nitrosating agents as ingredients.

Nitrosating agents are added to cosmetics in one of three ways: (a) Nitrites are added directly as anti-corrosive agents; (b) Nitrites are released by the degradation of 2-nitro-1,3-propanediol (BNDP); and (c) Nitrites are contaminants in the raw materials or resulting from the exposure of cosmetics to air. Secondary amines, such as DEA, are rapidly nitrosated by nitrogen oxides. Nitrosamines formation from nitrite and amines is accelerated under specific conditions by formaldehyde, paraformaldehyde, thiocyanate, nitrophenols and certain metal salts (e.g., ZnI_2, $CuCl$, $AgNO_3$, $SnCl_2$ and $HgCl_2$).

Cosmetics remain on store shelves and in cabinets of consumers for long periods of time, allowing nitrosamines to form. If DEA is present, nitrosamines can continue to form throughout storage, especially at elevated temperatures.

Acidic pH is an optimal reaction condition for nitrosamine formation. Although cosmetics generally have neutral pH, N-nitrosamines can be formed at neutral or alkaline pH by the reaction of a nitrosating agent with an amine in the presence of carbonyl compounds such as formaldehyde. Formaldehyde is present in cosmetics either from in situ formaldehyde-releasing agents, such as BNDP, or from its use as a preservative.

3. Dermal Absorption of NDEA

There is substantial evidence of the dermal absorption of NDEA in both rodents and humans. "[NDEA] is a known carcinogen in laboratory animals; it is absorbed through the skin. The absorption rate is a function of the nature of the cosmetic; absorption is fastest in nonpolar vehicles." Dermal absorption of NDEA was demonstrated by Lijinsky et al. In 1981. As a fat-soluble chemical NDEA can be absorbed dermally in rats and humans.

4. NDEA Increases Cancer Risk

There is substantial evidence of potent carcinogenicity of NDEA in a wide range of animal species. According to the International Agency for Research on Cancer (IARC).

There is sufficient evidence of a carcinogenic effect of N-nitrosodiethanolamine—. In view of the widespread exposure to appreciable concentrations of N-nitrosodiethanol-amine, efforts should be made to obtain epidemiological information.

The National Toxicology Program similarly concluded: There is sufficient evidence for the carcinogenicity of N-nitrosodiethanolamine in experimental animals. Of over 44 different species in which N-nitroso compounds have been tested, all have been susceptible. Humans are most unlikely to be the only exception to this trend.

In 1978, the IARC concluded that "although no epidemiological data were available, nitrosodiethanolamine should be regarded for practical purposes as if it were carcinogenic to humans." In 1987 the IARC further confirmed the carcinogenicity of NDEA.

Based on early evidence of the carcinogenicity of NDEA and evidence of cutting fluid contamination, 20 years ago NIOSH recommended that action be taken to protect workers including elimination of nitrosamines from the fluids. More recently, NIOSH published a hazard review of cutting fluids used in metal working that contain NDEA among other nitrosamines. This hazard review indicates that, based on epidemiological evidence in human beings, "Increased cancer risk has been generally attributed to worker exposure to nitrosamine or PAH (polyaromatic hydrocarbon) contaminants in metal working fluids."

5. The Failure of the FDA to Take Appropriate Regulatory Action

In the Federal Register of April 10, 1979, the FDA called for industry "to take immediate measures to eliminate to the extent possible [NDEA] and any other N-nitrosamines from cosmetic products," and further insisted that "cosmetic products may be analyzed by FDA for nitrosamine contamination and that individual products could be subject to enforcement action."

FDA has taken no subsequent enforcement actions despite the limited compliance with this Federal Register order. According to the FDA officials Don Havery and Hardy Chou in 1994.

In the United States . . . the personal care industry has invested resources in understanding both the mechanisms of N-nitrosamine formation in cosmetic systems and the means of inhibiting N-nitrosamine formation. However, there is still room for improvement. New products containing nitrosatable amines with formaldehyde and nitrite-releasing preservatives are still appearing on the U.S. market. Manufacturers have a responsibility to be aware of the potential for N-nitrosamine formation and to take steps necessary to keep N-nitrosamine levels as low as possible as part of their good manufacturing practices.

The goal of good manufacturing practices is to reduce "human exposure to N-nitrosamines to the lowest level technologically feasible by reducing levels in all personal care products. With the information and technology currently available to cosmetic manufacturers, N-nitrosamine levels can and should be further reduced in consumer products."

The FDA has failed to act on the Federal Register recommendations made in 1979. More recently, the FDA has not fully recognized the consumer hazards of this carcinogen. Measurements have not been made to determine total daily exposure to nitrosamines and it is inappropriate to quantify exposures without such data.

6. Cosmetic Industry Response to FDA Action

In response to the FDA Federal Register order, the Nitrosamine Task Force of the Cosmetics, Toiletries and Fragrance Association failed to eliminate the use of DEA, but rather, they investigated ways to inhibit the formation of NDEA.

There are no known nitrosation inhibitors that eliminate nitrosamine contamination. Inhibitors have failed for the following reasons:

The compound a-tocopherol has been used as an inhibitor but this compound is useful only when the nitrosating agent is nitrite itself. It is not effective against nitrogen oxide, a gas found in polluted air. It has also been shown to be ineffective in some cosmetic systems.

Many cosmetics make inhibition of nitrosamine formation more difficult. If they are two-phase emulsion systems the inhibitor must be soluble in both hydrophilic and hydrophobic media to be effective as an inhibitor.

Ascorbic acid, sodium bisulfite, butylated hydroxyanisole (BHA), butylated hydroxytoluene (BHT) sodium ascorbated, ascorbyl palmitate and a-tocopherol have all been used in attempts to inhibit nitrosamine formation. None of these inhibitors have been adequate against all possible nitrosation agents to which a shelved cosmetic is exposed.

Industry has had no success in reducing NDEA below 1984 levels. As a result, in 1996 the Cosmetics, Toiletries and Fragrance Association stated in 1996, "These chemicals [Cocamide DEA, Lauramide DEA, Linoleamide DEA, and Oleamide DEA] should not be used as ingredients in cosmetic products containing nitrosating agents." Nevertheless, DEA is still widely used by major cosmetic manufacturers.

In contrast, some other manufacturers such as Aubrey Organics, have ceased to use diethanolamide soaps entirely. According to Aubrey Hampton of Aubrey Organics, None of our products perform less effectively because they do not contain DEA. There are many alternative soap bases available without DEA that can be used by cosmetic manufacturers. In short, the removal of DEA does not pose a manufacturing problem to the cosmetic industry. There is no reason for high levels of NDEA to be found in cosmetic products. With safe alternatives available, the elimination of DEA should not be an economic burden for the cosmetic industry.

7. Response of National Institutes for Occupational Safety and Health

In striking contrast to the FDA's position on NDEA, The National Institutes for Occupational Safety and Health (NIOSH) has issued two reports, one as early as 1976, stating that protective measures should be taken when workers are exposed to levels of NDEA similar to those found in cosmetics.

8. Response of German Industry and European Union

The German Federal Health Office issued a request to eliminate all secondary amines from cosmetics in 1987 and in response, the German manufacturers 'association has voluntarily complied and sharply reduced the use of secondary amines in cosmetics and toiletries. Included in the specifications of the German Federal Health Office were that fatty acid diethanolamides contain as low as achievable contamination by unreacted diethanolamine. Eisenbrand et al. explained:

Commercially available products from the German market analyzed six to 18 months after the recommendation had been issued showed that only 15 percent were contaminated with [NDEA] or NDHPA . . . . The overall results of this study demonstrate however, a strong downward trend in both levels and frequency of contamination. They prove that nitrosamine contamination of cosmetics can be minimized by simple preventive measures.

The European Union has stated specific maximum allowable concentrations of inadvertently formed N-nitrosodialkanolamine. In legislation that was most recently amended in 1993, the European Union asserted that monoalkanolamines and trialkanolamines must be stored in nitrite free containers, cannot be used in nitrosating systems, must have purity of at least 99% and can contain no more than .5% secondary alkanolamine. With regards to N-nitrosodialkanolamine specifically, the maximum content that the EU allows is 50 micrograms per kilogram

(50ppb). In comparison, U.S. cosmetic levels for NDEA as high as 2,960 parts per billion were reported in 1992.

9. Conclusion

There is strong evidence proving: the widespread use of DEA in cosmetics, nitrosation of DEA to form NDEA, contamination of cosmetics with NDEA, the potent carcinogenicity of NDEA, and the availability of alternatives to DEA. The FDA should take prompt action to require labels on all products containing DEA that reads: "Caution—This product may contain N-nitrosodi-ethanolamine, a known cancer-causing agent."

This petition, based on fifty-one scientific references, was submitted by:

Samuel S. Epstein, M.D.
Chairman, Cancer Prevention Coalition
Professor Occupational and Environmental Medicine
University of Illinois School of Public Health, Chicago

Michael Deutsch, Esq., Legal Director, Center for Constitutional Rights, New York

FDA RESPONSE (FEBRUARY 13, 1997)

FDA has not been able to reach a decision because of "the limited availability of resources and other agency priorities."

Citizen Petition Seeking a Cancer Warning on Cosmetic Talc Products

May 13, 2008

Mike Leavitt
Secretary of Health and Human Services
U.S. Department of Health and Human Services

Andrew C. von Eschenbach, M.D.
Commissioner of Food and Drugs

This Petition requests the Commissioner of Food and Drugs to require that all cosmetic talc products bear labels with a warning such as, "Frequent application of talcum powder in the female genital area substantially increases risk of ovarian cancer."

A. AGENCY ACTION REQUESTED

This petition requests that FDA take the following action:

1. Immediately require cosmetic talcum powder products to bear labels with a warning such as: "Frequent application of talcum powder in the female genital area substantially increases risk of ovarian cancer."

B. STATEMENT OF GROUNDS

On November 17, 1994, the Cancer Prevention Coalition and the New York Center for Constitutional Rights submitted a Citizen Petition to the Commissioner of the FDA, "Seeking Carcinogenic Labeling on all Cosmetic Talc Products." The Petition was endorsed by Quentin Young, M.D., Chairman of The Health and Medicine Policy Research Group, Peter Orris, M.D., Director of Health Hazard Evaluation, Cook County Hospital, and Professor of Medicine, University of Illinois Medical School, Chicago, Nancy Nelson, Chair of the Ovarian Cancer Early Detection and Prevention Foundation, and subsequently by Senator Edward Kennedy. In a 1997 statement to the Senate, he requested the FDA to place a cancer warning on the label of talc products, besides other products containing known carcinogens. However, over a decade later his warning remains ignored.

The 1994 Petition was supported by 15 scientific publications. These included nine, from 1983 to 1992, on the major risks of ovarian cancer from the frequent application of brand or generic talc "baby powder" to the genital area of women without any warning of the risks involved. Two of these publications also reported that the genital application of talc could result in its translocation to the ovary.

The scientific basis of the 1994 Petition was further supported by J. Mande, Acting Associate Commissioner for Legislative Affairs of the Department of Health and Human Services. On August 25, 1993, he admitted that "We are aware that there have been reports in the medical literature between frequent direct female perineal talc dusting over a protracted period of years, and an incremental increase in the statistical odds of subsequent development of certain ovarian cancers . . . (However) at the present time, the FDA is not considering to ban, restrict or require a warning statement on the label of talc containing products."

The scientific basis of the 1994 Petition was also admitted by the industry. In an August 12, 1982, article in the *New York Times*, Johnson & Johnson, the manufacturer and retailer of talc dusting powder, stated it was aware of a publication which concluded that frequent genital application of talc was responsible for a three-fold increased risk of ovarian cancer. Warnings of these risks were emphasized by the Cancer Prevention Coalition in November 19, 1994, in letters to Mr. Ralph Larsen, CEO of Johnson & Johnson, and Mr. C.R. Walgreen, Chairman and CEO of Walgreens. Johnson & Johnson was urged to substitute cornstarch, a safe organic carbohydrate, for talcum powder products, and also to label its products with a warning on cancer risks.

In spite of the scientific evidence, and admission by Johnson & Johnson, the Petition was denied by Dr. John Bailey, FDA's Director of the Office of Cosmetics and Colors, on the basis of the "limited availability" (of Agency's resources) and on alleged scientific grounds. Dr. Bailey is currently Director of the industry's Personal Care Products Council.

Evidence for the May 2008 Petition is supported by Edward Kavanaugh, President of the industry's Cosmetic Toiletry and Fragrance Association. In 2002, he admitted that talc is "toxic," that it "can reach the human ovaries," and that prior epidemiological investigations concluded that its genital application increased the risk of ovarian cancer. Further evidence for this Petition is based on 12 publications since 1995, cited below. These confirm the causal relation between genital application of talc and ovarian cancer, and the protective effect of tubal ligation or hysterectomy, preventing the translocation of talc to the ovary.

As Dr. Andrew C. von Eschenbach, former Director of the National Cancer Institute, is aware, the mortality of ovarian cancer for women over the age of 65, has escalated dramatically since 1975, by 13% for white and 47% for black women. There are about 15,300 deaths from ovarian cancer each year. This makes it the fourth most common fatal cancer in women after colon, breast, and lung.

A case-control study, the largest to date, confirmed the relation between the perineal use of talc and ovarian cancer. This has also been confirmed by other reports. In view of the strength of this evidence, "formal public health warnings" were urged in 1999. An analysis of 16 pooled studies confirmed a statistically significant 33% increased risk of ovarian cancer associated with the perineal use of talc. A report by 19 scientists in eight nations worldwide, under the auspices of the International Agency for Research on Cancer, concluded that eight publications confirmed a 30-60% increased risk of ovarian cancer following the perineal application of talc. This risk has been confirmed in other reports.

The protective effects of tubal ligation or hysterectomy, preventing the translocation of talc from the perineum to the ovary, have also been confirmed.

This petition, based on twelve scientific references, was submitted by:

Samuel S. Epstein, M.D.
Chairman, Cancer Prevention Coalition
Professor emeritus Occupational and Environmental Medicine
University of Illinois School of Public Health, Chicago

November 17, 1994

Dusting with Cancer: Coalition Urges Chicago Drug Stores to Label Talc

According to the Cancer Prevention Coalition, the regular use of talc increases the risk of ovarian cancer. The Cancer Prevention Coalition (CPC) will announce its plans for a talcum powder labeling initiative here in Chicago at a Thursday, November 17, 1994 press briefing.

Speakers at the press briefing will include CPC Chair Dr. Samuel Epstein, CPC Board members Dr. Quentin Young and Dr. Peter Orris, and an ovarian cancer survivor. The speakers will explain why a labeling initiative is important to residents of Chicago, and will also answer questions from the press.

Recently, CPC sent letters to the Chicago corporate offices of Osco and Walgreen drug stores urging that they provide customers with information on the dangers associated with the use of talc. Additionally, CPC is filing a petition with the FDA requesting that talc products be explicitly labeled.

The use of talc poses a serious risk of ovarian cancer. Estimates are that up to 17% of American women regularly use talc in the genital area. Women have been compelled through advertisements of the cosmetic industry, to dust themselves to mask odors. Talcum powder has historically been a symbol of freshness, cleanliness and purity. Talc is even more commonly used on infants.

Ovarian cancer is a silent killer. It causes 38 deaths daily among American women—totaling 14,000 deaths annually. It is the fourth highest women's cancer death rate in the U.S. Over 60% of ovarian cancer victims die within five years of diagnosis.

"Studies seem to indicate that talc poses an increased risk factor for ovarian cancer, thus I would support a warning label to alert women to this possible risk," stated Diane Farrell, a Chicago resident who has been fighting ovarian cancer for the last two years.

According to Dr. Samuel Epstein, of the Cancer Prevention Coalition, "A wide range of scientific studies over the last three decades have clearly linked regular talc use by women and ovarian cancer."

The talc labeling project is the first phase of a "Consumer Labeling Initiative" that will inform citizens of the presence of undisclosed carcinogenic ingredients and contaminants in cosmetics, other consumer products, and food and how to avoid them.

January 15, 1995

Lice Won't Kill You but Its Treatment Can

Experts Call For Ban on Lindane Shampoos

According to scientific experts, commonly prescribed lice shampoos can cause fatal childhood cancer. The Cancer Prevention Coalition (CPC) will inform the public of this danger at a press briefing on January 17, 1995 at 12 noon.

About six million Americans, mainly children, are infested with lice each year. A common treatment for lice is a shampoo containing the pesticide lindane. Recent epidemiological studies have reported high rates of brain cancer in children treated with lindane shampoos. These findings are significant in light of the dramatic 38% increase of childhood brain and nervous system cancer rates from 1973 to 1991.

Additional evidence comes from recent studies linking lindane exposure to increased risks of non-Hodgkin's lymphoma, and also from long-standing evidence on fatal blood diseases including aplastic anemia and leukemia. These findings are supported by experimental evidence of carcinogenicity confirmed by the World Health Organization, the Environmental protection Agency, and the Department of health and Human Services; on the basis of such hazards, the EPA and several other countries have restricted lindane's use in agriculture, and other countries have banned it. Additionally, lindane is a known neurotoxin—resulting in seizures and brain damages at dose levels used in the shampoos.

CPC has sent letters to the Chicago Board, and to other local and state authorities urging that they warn parents of the dangers of lindane shampoo and to encourage them to seek out safer treatments. CPC has also filed a citizen petition with the Food and Drug Administration calling for a ban of lindane-based shampoos.

Speakers at the press conference will include Chair Dr. Samuel Epstein, CPC Board members Dr. Quentin Young and Dr. Peter Orris, parent Community Council President Mr. James Deanes, and Legal Director of the New York-based Center for Constitutional Rights, Michael Deutsch. The speakers will discuss the public health implications of these data and will offer information about safer alternatives.

Commenting on the widely-prescribed use of lindane, Dr. Quentin Young, CPC Board member said, "It is a serious medical tragedy when these products are used with such good intentions and can have such tragic outcomes."

ENDORSER:

Michael Deutsch, Legal Director, Center for Constitutional Rights

September 21, 1995

Cancer Group and Ralph Nader Release First Annual "Dirty Dozen" Consumer Product List

The Cancer Prevention Coalition (CPC) and Ralph Nader will release tomorrow a "Dirty Dozen" list of consumer products used in most American homes, and manufactured by giant U.S. corporations. Brand named "Dirty Dozen" products include: Ajax Cleanser®, Clairol® Nice n' Easy Haircolor and Lysol® Disinfectant.

The "Dirty Dozen" products contain a wide-range of carcinogenic and other toxic ingredients and contaminants to which most of us are exposed daily.

CPC Chairperson Samuel Epstein, M.D., and investigative journalist, David Steinman, compiled the "Dirty Dozen" from data on over 3,500 consumer products analyzed and ranked in their recently published The Safe Shopper's Bible. The good news is that safer alternatives are available for all the "Dirty Dozen."

Nader and CPC urged the manufacturers of the "Dirty Dozen" to reformulate their products with non-toxic alternatives. "Ironically, some "Dirty Dozen" manufacturers also market safer alternatives," said Dr. Epstein.

"What is particularly galling about the "Dirty Dozen," emphasized Ralph Nader, "is that these toxic chemicals don't have to be there. Yet these corporations continue to expose people to health hazards unnecessarily."

Current product labeling provides no warning for cancer and other chronic health risks. Food is labeled for cholesterol, but not for carcinogens. Cosmetics are labeled for major ingredients, but not for those that form carcinogens or contain carcinogenic contaminants. Except for pesticides, household products contain no information on their ingredients.

Cancer rates are skyrocketing. Currently, more than one-third of all of us will develop cancer in our lifetime, and one-fourth will die from the disease. Many cancers are due to avoidable exposures to industrial carcinogens in the food we eat, and the cosmetics and household products we use.

"Americans have a fundamental right-to-know about hazardous chemicals in all consumer products they buy, and the cancer and other risks of those chemicals—information that remains hidden in government and industry files," concluded Dr. Epstein. "With this knowledge, consumers can protect themselves by voting with their shopping dollars and buying safer alternatives."

October 22, 1996

They Make You Smell, Feel, and Look Good. But Can Cosmetics Increase Your Risk Of Cancer?

Tough standards are essential for phasing out diethanolamine (DEA) from cosmetics and toiletries.

In a petition to the Food and Drug Administration (FDA) released today, the Cancer Prevention Coalition (CPC) urged the labeling or phasing out of DEA in cosmetic products. DEA is a precursor of nitrosodiethanolamine (NDEA), a proven carcinogen as recognized by four Federal agencies and institutions and the World Health Organization. The proposed label would read, "Caution—This product may contain N-nitrosodiethanolamine, a known cancer-causing agent."

DEA-based detergents are widely used in shampoos, lotions and creams. Since 1976, workers exposed to NDEA in metal working fluids, at levels similar to those in cosmetics, have been warned of cancer risks and steps are taken to protect them.

Aubrey Hampton, founder of Aubrey Organics, noted that DEA is not an essential ingredient in hair and skin care products. There are natural, safe and effective alternatives to DEA that pose no financial hardship for the manufacturer or the consumer"

In 1979, the FDA urged the cosmetics industry to take "immediate action to eliminate" NDEA in cosmetics. However, the FDA has taken no subsequent action while industry remains unresponsive. In striking contrast, the EEC has sharply reduced permissible uses of DEA. German cosmetic industry has also resolved this problem by phasing out DEA detergents, thereby preventing the formation of NDEA

Dr. William Lijinsky, leading international nitrosamine researcher, emphasized, "The continued use of DEA is unacceptable especially in view of the overwhelming scientific evidence of its cancer risks and the availability of safe alternatives."

Samuel S. Epstein, M.D., professor of environmental and occupational medicine at the University of Illinois School of Public Health and chairman of the Cancer Prevention Coalition said that, "Faced with escalating cancer rates, the FDA and other health agencies should take overdue action to reduce avoidable exposures to carcinogens. NDEA in cosmetics, used by many million consumers for many decades, is a prime example of such an avoidable carcinogen.

February 22, 1998

Major Cosmetic and Toiletry Ingredient Poses Avoidable Cancer Risks, Warns Professor of Environmental Medicine at University of Illinois School of Public Health

As reported on CBS Morning News today, the National Toxicology Program (NTP) recently found that repeated skin application to mouse skin of diethanolamine (DEA), or its fatty acid derivative cocamide-DEA, induced liver and kidney cancer. Besides this "clear evidence of carcinogenicity," NTP also emphasized that DEA is readily absorbed through the skin and accumulates in organs, such as the brain, where it induces chronic toxic effects.

High concentrations of DEA-based detergents are commonly used in a wide range of cosmetics and toiletries, including shampoos, hair dyes and conditioners, lotions, creams and bubble baths, besides liquid dishwashing and laundry soaps. Lifelong use of these products thus clearly poses major avoidable cancer risks to the great majority of U.S. consumers, particularly infants and young children.

Further increasing these cancer risks is longstanding evidence that DEA readily interacts with nitrite preservatives or contaminants in cosmetics or toiletries to form nitrosodiethanolamine (NDELA), another carcinogen as well recognized by Federal agencies and institutions and the World Health Organization, which, like DEA, is also rapidly absorbed through the skin. In 1979, FDA warned that over 40% of all cosmetic products were contaminated with NDELA and called for industry "to take immediate action to eliminate this carcinogen from cosmetic products." In two 1991 surveys, 27 out of 29 products were found to be contaminated with high concentrations of this carcinogen, results which were subsequently confirmed by the FDA. Based on this information, the European Union and European industry have both taken strong action to reduce or eliminate DEA and NDELA from cosmetics and toiletries. In sharp contrast, the FDA has taken no such action, nor has it responded to a 1996 petition from the Cancer Prevention Coalition to phase out the use of DEA or to label DEA-containing products with an explicit cancer warning. The mainstream U.S. industry has been similarly unresponsive, even to the extent of ignoring an explicit warning by the Cosmetics, Toiletries and Fragrance Association to discontinue uses of DEA. Such reckless intransigence is in strong contrast to the responsiveness of the growing safe cosmetic industry.

Tom Mower, CEO of Neways Inc., a major distributor of carcinogen-free cosmetics, emphasizes: "I see no reason at all to use DEA, as there are safe and cost-effective alternatives which we have been using in a wide range of our cosmetics and toiletries for the last decade."

Faced with escalating cancer rates, now striking more than one in three Americans, FDA should take immediate action to prevent further exposure to the avoidable carcinogens DEA and NDELA in cosmetics, toiletries and liquid soaps. Safe and effective alternatives to DEA are readily available.

January 7, 2000

New Initiatives in Personal Care Product Safety

Fragrances and Perfumes:

As emphasized in the Safe Shopper's Bible, fragrances and perfumes in mainstream cosmetics and toiletries, besides in soaps and other household products, are leading causes of allergy, sensitization, and irritation. Their toxicity is also in serious question as is their contribution to indoor air pollution.

The National Institute of Occupational Safety and Health has reported that the fragrance industry uses up to 3,000 ingredients, predominantly synthetic, some 900 of which were identified as toxic. However, the industry is not required to disclose ingredients of fragrances and perfumes on their labels due to trade secrecy considerations. The FDA supports this non-disclosure on the grounds that "consumers are not adversely affected—and should not be deprived of the enjoyment" of these products.

An analysis of six different mainstream perfumes by Scientific Instrument Services, released in November 1998, identified over 800 ingredients with distinctive patterns for each perfume. These ingredients include a wide range of volatile and semi-volatile organic chemicals, which are thus significant contributors to indoor pollution.

On May 11, 1999, the California Environmental Health Network filed a Citizen Petition with the FDA requiring warning labels on all fragrances which are marketed without prior adequate safety testing. Additionally, the petition requested the FDA to take administrative action and declare Calvin Klein's "Eternity eau de parfum" as "misbranded." This petition has been supported and endorsed by the CPC. While Eternity perfume was based on recent analysis of the perfume by two independent laboratories, Scientific Instrument Services and the cosmetic industry's Research Institute of Fragrance Materials Laboratory. Of all 41 ingredients identified, no toxicity data are available on some, data on most are inadequate, and others are known to be toxic to the skin, mucous membranes, respiratory tract, and reproductive and nervous system by routes including skin absorption and inhalation. Additionally, two ingredients (phenylmethyl acetic acid ester and 2,6-bis (1,1-dimethylethyl)-4-methyl-phenol) were identified as carcinogens.

The FDA has 180 days to respond to this petition. However, any positive response is most unlikely.

Neways International, a leading alternative safe consumer products company, has taken a precedential initiative in the area of fragrance safety. The few fragrances used in Neways personal care products contain less than 10 ingredients, most of which are natural. As importantly, none of the few synthetics used are known to be toxic or carcinogenic. In the near future, these products will be labeled accordingly.

Surfactants:

A wide range of personal care products including shampoos, hair conditions, cleansers, lotions, and creams, besides household products such as soaps and cleaning products, contain surfactants or detergents such as ethoxylated alcohols, polysorbates, and laureths. These ingredients are generally contaminated with high concentrations of the highly volatile 1,4-dioxane, which is both readily inhaled and absorbed through the skin. The carcinogenicity of dioxane in rodents was first reported in 1965 and subsequently confirmed in other studies including by the National Cancer Institute in 1978; the predominant sites of cancer were nasal passages in rats and liver in mice. Epidemiological studies on dioxane-exposed furniture makers have reported suggestive evidence of excess nasal passage cancers. On the basis of such evidence, the Consumer Product Safety Commission concluded, "the presence of 1,4-dioxane, even as a trace contaminant, is a cause of concern." These avoidable risks of cancer in numerous personal care, besides other consumer products, is inexcusable, particularly as the dioxane is readily removed from surfactants during their manufacture by a process known as "vacuum stripping."

Again, Neways now stands alone in certifying and labeling the surfactants in its personal care products as "dioxane-free," and thus sets an important precedent to the entire personal care products industry.

February 7, 2000

Perfume: Cupid's Arrow or Poison Dart

Lovers looking for the perfect Valentine's gift should think twice before giving a bottle of toxic chemicals to their sweethearts. Recent analysis of Calvin Klein's "Eternity Eau de Parfum" (Eternity) by an industry laboratory specializing in fragrance chemistry revealed 41 ingredients. These include some known to be toxic to the skin, respiratory tract, nervous, and reproductive systems, and others known to be carcinogens; no toxicity data are available on several ingredients, while data on most are inadequate. Additionally, some ingredients are volatile and a source of indoor air pollution. Since 1995, several consumers have complained to the Food and Drug Administration (FDA) of neurological and respiratory problems due to Eternity.

The analysis was recently commissioned by the Environmental Health Network (EHN) as many members had complained of asthma, migraine, sensitization, or multiple chemical sensitivity when exposed to Eternity. Based on this analysis, EHN filed a Citizen Petition with the FDA on May 11, 1999, which was subsequently endorsed by the Cancer Prevention Coalition. The petition requests that the FDA take administrative action and declare Eternity "misbranded" or "adulterated" since it does not carry a warning label as required by the terms of the Food, Drug, and Cosmetic Act and the Fair Packaging and Labeling Act. Grounds for requesting the warning label include FDA regulation 21CFR Sec. 740/10: "Each ingredient used in a cosmetic product and each finished cosmetic product shall be adequately substantiated for safety prior to marketing. Any such ingredient or product whose safety is not adequately substantiated prior to marketing is misbranded unless it contains the following conspicuous statement on the principal display panel: Warning: the safety of this product has not been determined."

Since May, over 700 consumers with health problems from exposure to various mainstream fragrances have written to the FDA supporting EHN's petition. The FDA responded on November 30 to the effect that they had been unable to reach a decision on the grounds of "other priorities and the limited availability of resources." The petition is thus still open for further public complaints and endorsements.

A wide range of mainstream fragrances and perfumes, predominantly based on synthetic ingredients, are used in numerous cosmetics and toiletries, and also soaps and other household products. Currently, the fragrance industry is virtually unregulated. Its recklessness is abetted and compounded by FDA's complicity. The FDA has refused to require the industry to disclose ingredients due to trade secrecy considerations, and still takes the position that "consumers are not adversely affected—and should not be deprived of the enjoyment" of these products. The Cancer Prevention Coalition and EHN take the unequivocal position that the FDA should implement its own regulations and act belatedly to protect consumer health and safety.

Valentine sweethearts should switch to organically grown (pesticide-free) roses or other flowers as safe alternatives to mainstream perfumes.

ENDORSER:

Amy Marsh
President of the Environmental Health Network
Larkspur, California

January 15, 2001

Undisclosed Carcinogens in Cosmetics and Personal Care Products Pose Avoidable Risks of Cancer

Government scientists recently identified a group of toxic chemicals known as phthalates in urine of adults, with highest levels in premenopausal women, resulting from inhalation and skin exposure to volatile parent ingredients used extensively as solvents and plasticizers in personal care and cosmetic (PCC) products. These include perfumes, shampoos, hair sprays and nail polishes. These findings raise major concerns in view of documented evidence, dating back to 1985, that these phthalates induce birth defects, low sperm counts, and other reproductive toxicity in experimental animals. The Food and Drug Administration (FDA), authorized by the 1938 Food, Drug and Cosmetics Act to ban unsafe PCC products, responded that it will now "consider" this longstanding information. While obviously important, the phthalate findings merely reflect the tip of an iceberg of more fundamental problems which have received minimal, if any, attention, from Congress, the media and the public.

The FDA's relaxed response reflects reckless regulatory abdication matched by unresponsiveness of mainstream industries. A 1990 report by the U.S. General Accounting Office charging that the FDA commits no resources for assessing PCC safety had no impact on the agency's policies. The agency's sole requirement is restricted to ingredient labeling of PCC products, with the exception of fragrances and perfumes. With rare exceptions, such as children's bubble baths, the FDA has never required industry to label PCC products with any warning of well-documented toxic or cancer risks, nor has it banned the sale of unsafe products to an unsuspecting public.

Black and dark brown permanent hair dyes contain numerous ingredients, such as diaminoanisole and FD&C Red 33, recognized as carcinogens in experimental animals. This evidence is supported by studies establishing that regular use of these dyes poses major risks of relatively rare cancers— non-Hodgkin's lymphoma, Hodgkin's disease and multiple myeloma.

Cosmetic grade talc is carcinogenic in experimental animals. Also, frequent genital dusting with talc, routinely practiced by some 17% of women, increases risks of ovarian cancer.

A group of widely used preservatives, such as quaternium15 and bronopol, widely used in baby products, though not carcinogenic themselves, break down to release formaldehyde, a potent irritant and carcinogen.

Lanolin, widely used on babies' skin and nipples of nursing mothers, is commonly contaminated with DDT and other carcinogenic pesticides.

Commonly used PCC detergents and foaming agents, such as polysorbates and PEG, are usually contaminated with the volatile carcinogen dioxane, although this could be easily removed by vacuum stripping during manufacture.

DEA, another widely used chemical detergent, has been known since 1975 to combine with nitrite preservatives or contaminants in PCC products to form a highly carcinogenic nitrosamine. Furthermore, recent government studies showed that DEA itself is also carcinogenic following application to mouse skin.

Citizen petitions to the FDA by the Cancer Prevention Coalition in 1994 and 1996 detailing evidence on the cancer risks of talc and DEA-containing products, respectively, and "Seeking Carcinogenic Labeling" on these products, met with no substantive response.

Concerns on cancer risks from PCC products are emphasized by: lifelong use of multiple products by the majority of the U.S. population; the ready skin absorption of carcinogenic ingredients, further increased by detergents, especially when left on the skin for prolonged periods; and by decades-long suppression of information by the FDA and industry, abetted by a roll-over media, in flagrant denial of consumers' right-to-know. Mainstream industry products thus pose major risks of avoidable cancer. Their role in the escalating incidence of cancer, now striking one in two men and one in three women in their lifetimes, remains largely unrecognized by our apparently health conscious society. Armed with such information, consumers should protect themselves by shopping for safe alternative products available from the growing non-mainstream industry.

July 11, 2002

Phthalates in Cosmetics Are Suspect, but Carcinogens Even More So

The Environmental Working Group, Coming Clean, and Health Care Without Harm groups are to be warmly commended for their stellar July 10 report on unlabelled phthalate ingredients in common cosmetics and personal care (CPC) products.

In October 2000, the Centers for Disease Control and Prevention and other federal scientists reported on the identification of phthalates in the urine of adults, with highest levels in premenopausal women. The FDA responded that it would "consider" this information. This response was and remains reckless, in view of well-documented evidence since 1985 that phthalates induce birth defects, low sperm counts, and other reproductive toxicity in experimental animals.

A critical 1990 report by the U.S. General Accounting Office, charging that the FDA committed no resources for assessing CPC products safety, had no impact on the agency's reckless policies. The agency's sole requirement is restricted to ingredient labeling of products, except fragrances and perfumes.

However, with rare exceptions such as children's bubble baths, the FDA has never required the industry to label its products with any warning of well—documented risks, particularly reproductive and cancer; nor has the FDA banned the sale of unsafe products to an unsuspecting public, although so explicitly authorized by the 1938 Food, Drug and Cosmetics Act. Examples of carcinogenic products and ingredients include:

Black and dark brown permanent hair dyes contain "coal tar" dye ingredients recognized as carcinogens in experimental animals. This evidence is supported by studies establishing that regular use of these dyes poses major risks of relatively rare cancers-non-Hodgkin's lymphoma, Hodgkin's disease, and multiple myeloma.

Cosmetic grade talc is carcinogenic in experimental animals. Also, frequent genital dusting with talc, routinely practiced by some 17% of premenopausal women, increases risks of ovarian cancer.

A group of widely used preservatives, such as quaternium 15 and bronopol, commonly used in baby products, though not carcinogenic themselves, break down to release formaldehyde, a potent irritant and carcinogen.

Lanolin, widely used on babies' skin and nipples of nursing mothers, is commonly contaminated with DDT and other carcinogenic pesticides. n Commonly used detergents and foaming agents, such as polysorbates and PEG, are usually contaminated with the volatile carcinogens dioxane and ethylene oxide, although they could readily be removed by vacuum stripping during manufacture.

DEA, another widely used detergent, has been known since 1975 to combine with nitrite preservatives or contaminants in CPC products to form a highly carcinogenic nitrosamine. Furthermore, in 1997, DEA itself was shown to be carcinogenic following application to mouse skin.

Citizen petitions to the FDA by the Cancer Prevention Coalition in 1994 and 1996 detailing evidence on the cancer risks of talc and of DEA-containing products, respectively, and "Seeking Carcinogenic Labeling" on these products, met with no substantive response.

Concerns on cancer risks from CPC products are emphasized by: the unrecognized presence of over 50 carcinogenic ingredients in these products; lifelong use of multiple products by the majority of the U.S. population; the ready skin absorption of many carcinogenic ingredients, further increased by detergents, especially when left on the skin for prolonged periods; and by decades-long suppression of information by FDA and the industry in denial of consumers' democratic right-to-know.

Mainstream industry products thus pose significant public health risks, particularly reproductive and cancer. The role of these avoidable exposures in the escalating incidence of cancer, now striking nearly one in two men and over one in three women in their lifetimes, remains largely unrecognized by our apparently health conscious society. Armed with such information, consumers should protect themselves by shopping for safe alternative products available from the growing non-mainstream industry. Finally, Congress should belatedly and aggressively ensure that the FDA obeys the law.

August 15, 2002

Groups Call for Labeling of Cosmetics and Toiletries, Citing Cancer and Other Health Risks

Senator Edward Kennedy (D-MA) is to be commended for his May 2002 bill (S. 2499) requiring consumer-friendly food label warnings for allergens, to which roughly 7 percent of the U.S. population are sensitive. Today, a coalition of public health and environmental organizations are requesting Senator Kennedy to consider legislation mandating similar labels for cosmetics and toiletries containing ingredients that pose serious, irreversible health risks.

Millions of Americans are sensitive to allergens in cosmetics, particularly in fragrances and perfumes. However, in addition to allergens, cosmetics and toiletries contain numerous other hazardous ingredients, including almost 100 carcinogens and 15 endocrine (hormonal) disruptors, particularly phthalates.

"These ingredients pose risks of cancer, genetic damage, and reproductive toxicity (including infertility) to unsuspecting consumers, and their infants and children," said University of Illinois School of Public Health Emeritus Professor Samuel Epstein, M.D.

These risks are high. This is due to: the virtual lifelong use of many cosmetic products, such as shampoos and lotions; their routine daily application to large areas of skin; the ready skin absorption of some ingredients, facilitated by detergents in most products; the inhalation absorption of volatile ingredients or their contaminants; and the additive or synergistic interactions between multiple carcinogenic or otherwise toxic ingredients.

Strong concerns on these risks were expressed by Senator Kennedy at hearings on the 1997 FDA cosmetics reform bill. "Our message is that cosmetics can be dangerous to your health. The American people have a right to full and fair information about the actual and potential dangers of the products they use every day."

Despite these considerations, FDA denies consumers their right-to-know by refusing to require label warnings on the risks of cosmetic ingredients.

This failure violates the 1938 Federal Food, Drug and Cosmetic Act which mandates that "each ingredient used in a cosmetic product—shall be adequately substantiated for safety prior to marketing," and which authorizes FDA to recall and seize unsafe products. Nevertheless, the Agency merely requires a listing of the complex chemical names or their abbreviations of the 10 to 20 ingredients on product labels. However, this information is incomprehensible to consumers, let alone their physicians.

A November 1994 citizen petition to the FDA requested the agency to require that cosmetic talc products be labeled with a warning that frequent application to the genital area significantly increases risks of ovarian cancer. FDA declined to act on this petition on grounds of the "limited availability of resources and other agency priorities."

An October 1996 citizen petition to the FDA requested the agency to require that cosmetics containing the common detergent diethanolamine (DEA) be labeled with a cancer warning, as DEA reacts with nitrites present in many products to form a potent (nitrosamine) carcinogen. DEA itself was also subsequently shown to be carcinogenic when applied to mouse skin. FDA similarly declined to act on this petition.

More seriously, FDA has declined to request Congressional authority to require label warnings on black and dark brown coal tar hair dyes, which are technically exempt from the 1938 Cosmetic Act. This reflects disregard of a series of studies over the last three decades incriminating prolonged use of these dyes with breast and bladder cancers, and non-Hodgkin's lymphoma and multiple myeloma.

FDA policies and those of the Cosmetic, Toiletry and Fragrance Association (CTFA), the U.S. trade association, which represents the multi-billion dollar cosmetic industry, are mutually supportive. The major priority of the CTFA is to prevent "new and unnecessary" label warnings.

Label warnings are even more critical in view of the escalating incidence of cancer, now striking nearly one in two men and more than one in three women in their lifetimes. Still sharper increases are anticipated in coming decades.

Informed by user-friendly labels, consumers could reduce their avoidable risks of cancer and other disease by shunning unsafe products and shopping for safer alternatives. While currently limited, their availability will rapidly increase with increasing demand; this is well exemplified by the organic food industry which has escalated to its current $8 billion market share over the last decade. Legislative action by Senator Kennedy would not only protect consumers, but also stimulate overdue recognition by the $20 billion mainstream petrochemical cosmetic industry that safety sells.

In striking contrast to FDA policies, the Scientific Committee on Cosmetic Products of the European Union recently called for a blanket ban on all carcinogenic, gene-damaging and reproductive toxic ingredients in cosmetics.

Finally, FDA's failure to require the cosmetic industry to disclose information on risks of their products to U.S. consumers is at least as critical as SEC's failure to require disclosure of information on corporate accountability to public investors. Clearly, the FDA is a lap dog, rather than watchdog, of the cosmetic industry.

ENDORSERS:

Mark Helm, Director
Media Relations
Friends of the Earth

Bryony Schwan
National Campaigns Director
Women's Voices for the Earth

Larry Bohlen
Friends of the Earth

Alise Cappel
Center for Environmental Health

Gary Cohen
Environmental Health Fund

Mary Lamielle
National Center for Environmental Health Strategies, Inc.

David Monk
Oregon Toxics Alliance

Barbara Wilkie
Environmental Health Network

Janet Zeller
Blue Ridge Environmental Defense League

July 1, 2004

Environmental Working Group Report on Personal Care Products: Ambitious, but Flawed

The Environmental Working Group (EWG) should be commended for its June "Skin Deep" report on personal care products. EWG should also be commended for its FDA petition to recall or issue "warning labels on 356 personal care products" that, as admitted by the industry's Cosmetic Ingredient Review safety panel, "lack sufficient data to support their safe use in personal care products." Regrettably, however, EWG's report is confusing and scientifically flawed.

EWG emphasizes that "only 11 percent of 10,500 personal care products, identified by the industry's trade association, have been publicly assessed for safety." However, this seems an overstatement. Such "suspect" ingredients include: purified water; sodium chloride (table salt); citric acid; natural amino acids; natural botanicals; FDA-approved colorants; and many food additives approved in 1958 by the FDA as "Generally Recognized as Safe."

Moreover, EWG is apparently unaware that substantial information on a wide range of carcinogenic ingredients, carcinogenic contaminants in other ingredients, and ingredients causing dermatitis in most products, marketed by most major companies, has been widely available for nearly a decade. The Safe Shopper's Bible (Macmillan, 1995), which I co-authored, details such information on these unsafe products. The book also provides information on safer products, marketed by smaller companies.

Furthermore, EWG's claim that "consumers and government officials have no way of knowing of ingredients that can be contaminated with impurities linked to cancer" is questionable. This information is admitted, although trivialized, by the Cosmetic Ingredient Review, with particular reference to a large group of detergents (ethoxylates) which, unless purified, are contaminated with potent carcinogenic impurities. More disturbingly, officials of the federal National Cancer Institute are fully aware of such long-standing information, of which they have failed to inform consumers; the American Cancer Society goes still further by virtually dismissing any cancer risks from cosmetics.

EWG's listing of "Carcinogens in Personal Care Products" identifies eight "known and probable human carcinogens." However, no reference is made to talc, identified as a lung carcinogen, following inhalation tests in rodents by the National Toxicology Program in 1993. This is of particular importance in view of the common use of talcum baby powders. Of greater importance are several publications, in leading medical journals since 1982, reporting that frequent use of talc as a genital dusting powder, practiced by about 17% of women, increases risk of ovarian cancer by four-fold.

Based on these concerns, the Cancer Prevention Coalition and the Center for Constitutional Rights filed a 1994 petition to the FDA seeking "Carcinogenic Labeling on all Cosmetic Talc Products." The FDA has remained unresponsive.

EWG's computerized "Skin Deep" report is detailed in two major searchable sections, Find Products You Use, and Customer Shoppers Guide. The Find Products section evaluates 7,500 products sold by many leading cosmetic companies. These products are evaluated on the basis of "Health Concerns," including: cancer; pregnancy problems; safety violations; harmful impurities; penetration enhancers (ingredients which increase skin absorption of other ingredients); unstudied ingredients; and allergies and other health concerns. Products in 25 different categories are each evaluated on the basis of "Top Five Ingredients of Concern."

However, these evaluations are marred by errors of omission and commission:

"Ingredients of Concern," incriminated as posing risks of cancer in different products, include: tocopherol (vitamin E); hydrogen peroxide; acetone; menthol; sodium borate; boric acid; zinc sulfate; propylene glycol; and parabens. However, there is no evidence on the carcinogenicity of these ingredients, although there has been such speculation for parabens.

More puzzling are the Top Five Ingredients incriminated as posing risks of "Allergies and Other Health Problems." These include sodium borate; boric acid; tocopherol; acetone, and silica. However, none of these are known allergens. Also, contrary to EWG, a fragrance is not an ingredient, nor as implied, necessarily allergenic. In fact, fragrances contain mixtures of ingredients, many of which pose no risks of allergy. Moreover, no information is provided as to nature of the unspecified "Health Problems."

Inexplicably, the report omits any reference to ingredients known to induce genetic damage (mutagens), such as aminophenol, hydroquinone, and crotonaldehyde, even though these have been clearly incriminated in recent European Scientific Committee reports.

EWG unfavorably rates all products containing "penetration enhancer" ingredients, which facilitate absorption of other ingredients through the skin. However, this rating extends to most products, as these contain water, and oil or fatty ingredients. These ingredients are necessarily mixed together to form stable solutions, by the addition of detergent (surfactant) ingredients. There are two main types of detergents, sodium or ammonium lauryl sulfate, and a wide range of unrelated ingredients, known as ethoxylates. Most companies avoid the use of sulfate detergents, as they irritate or damage the skin. While purified ethoxylates are not irritants, they are safe "penetration enhancers." However, this is of no concern, unless the product also contains toxic ingredients.

August 6, 2004

High Time to Label Fragrance Allergens

On July 20, the U.S. House of Representatives passed the "Food Allergen Labeling and Consumer Protection Act of 2003," requiring explicit labeling of eight major allergens in food products. This will make life much safer for about 11 million Americans with food allergies. But why has no such action yet been taken to protect more than twice the number of Americans who develop allergies from unlabeled allergens in fragranced products?

Exposure to these allergens can result in "allergic contact dermatitis" (ACD). This can range from mere itching and transient redness of the skin, to swelling, blistering, and ulceration. ACD is usually localized to the immediate area of the allergen-exposed skin. However, it may spread extensively, and require treatment with antihistamines and cortisone, and even hospitalization; fatal anaphylactic shock has been reported as a rare complication. Inhalation exposure to highly volatile fragrance allergens is also recognized as a cause of asthma in children and adults, particularly those with sensitive airways.

Over 5,000 fragrance ingredients, predominantly synthetic, are commonly used in a wide range of products. These include: household products, such as soaps, cleansers, toilet blocks, sanitary wipes and pads, air fresheners and even pesticides; common toiletries, such as shampoos, aftershave, and cologne, particularly for men, and sunscreens, eye, nail products, hair dyes, and perfumes, particularly for women; and formaldehyde or other preservatives in virtually all fragrances and cosmetics.

Some cosmetics, and other fragranced products, are misleadingly labeled "fragrance-free" if they contain fragrance ingredients, but not the whole fragrance itself. Also, some companies misleadingly label their cosmetics as "hypoallergenic" if they do not contain any of the more common allergens.

However, while the "hypoallergenic" label, and other labels such as "allergy tested" and "safe for sensitive skin," have considerable promotional value, they can mean just whatever any particular company wants them to mean. Manufacturers of these products are not required to do any skin testing to validate such claims, nor to substantiate them to the Food and Drug Administration (FDA). It should, however, be recognized that the Food,

Drug and Cosmetic Act authorizes the FDA to declare any product "misbranded" if there is evidence that it contains harmful ingredients.

According to recent U.S. and Danish surveys, the incidence of ACD has increased by about 10 percent over the last decade. This reflects the burgeoning number of cosmetic and fragranced products being marketed, and their increasing use on infants and children, and by men.

Representative Jan Schakowsky, D-Ill., has reintroduced legislation, "The Safe Notification and Information for Fragrances (SNIFF) Act," to amend the Food, Drug, and Cosmetic Act. This requires that allergens in fragranced products be labeled accordingly. More explicitly, the European Parliament has recently proposed that all products containing 26 well-known allergens should be labeled.

In a damage control response to these legislative initiatives, the industry's International Fragrance Association has agreed that information on allergenic ingredients should be made available, but only on request, to dermatologists for diagnostic purposes. However, this "Fragrance On Call List" action continues to deny the public its undeniable right-to-know of major avoidable causes of ACD. Furthermore, the Association has failed to respond to repeated requests for labeling of fragranced products, stating that they contain no known allergens.

Finally, it should be emphasized that allergens represent the tip of the iceberg of a wide range of other unlabeled toxic ingredients in cosmetics and toiletries. While the effects of allergens are almost immediate and obvious, those of carcinogens, gene-damaging and hormonal ingredients can be delayed for decades. As such, they are poorly, if at all, recognizable. Clearly, corrective legislation is well overdue for other toxic ingredients, besides allergens.

October 14, 2004

Europe Leads the Way in Cosmetic Product Safety

At UNESCO Headquarters on Friday, The French Association for Research on Treatments Against Cancer is convening a trans-Atlantic group of leading cancer specialists to present scientific evidence on the role of environmental pollutants as major causes of cancer and other diseases.

Foremost on the agenda is the proposed new chemicals policy for the European Union, known as REACH—Registration, Evaluation and Authorization of Chemicals—an unprecedented complex of regulations for industrial chemicals.

First outlined by the European Commission in 2001, REACH was opposed by the European and U.S. chemical industries, and also by the Bush Administration. A weaker version was offered in 2003, but in view of the drastic rise in deaths from avoidable causes of cancer such as industrial chemicals, the distinguished scientists at this Colloquium will present evidence to show that REACH needs to be strengthened, not weakened.

As the world's largest chemical market, Europe has the ability to act as a catalyst for reform of global legislative policies on the regulation of industrial chemicals. The U.S. government and chemicals industry is closely watching the progress of REACH on its path through the European legislative process. At this critical moment, the experts meeting at UNESCO are engaged in a life and death struggle with cancer and the chemicals that cause this constellation of diseases.

The Colloquium opens with an address by distinguished French oncologist Lucien Israel, M.D., who has spent nearly 60 years in the cancer field. He will share the podium with renowned French virologist Dr. Luc Montagnier, best known for his 1983 discovery of the human immunodeficiency virus (HIV), which has been identified as the cause of AIDS.

From the American side of the Atlantic comes Samuel Epstein, M.D., professor emeritus of environmental and occupational medicine at the University of Illinois at Chicago School of Public Health, and a winner of the Right Livelihood Award who chairs the Cancer Prevention Coalition.

Dr. Epstein will give the introductory morning talk on cancer prevention, which will emphasize the escalating incidence of non-smoking related cancers, such as testicular, brain and childhood cancers.

Boston University Professor of Environmental Health Dr. Richard Clapp will offer his perspective on the epidemiological approach to the links between cancer and the environment. Founder of the Massachusetts Cancer Registry, he now sits on the Governing Council of the International Society for Environmental Epidemiology.

The Colloquium, organized by Dr. Dominique Belpomme of Pesticides Action Network Europe, will hear from representatives of American, Belgian, British, French, and Spanish scientific and citizens' groups such as the Royal Commission on Environmental Pollution, Greenpeace Europe, the WWF, and the European Environmental Bureau, which represents 143 member organizations in 31 countries.

Paul Lannoye of Belgium, a Member of European Parliament representing the Green Group, will address the issues of a Europe facing environmental pollution, and lawyer Corinne LePage of France will advance the idea that polluting is a crime against humanity.

Cancers resulting from occupational exposure, cancer and foods, chemicals in consumer products—a full spectrum of chemical causes of cancer will be considered with the precautionary principle as well as the principle of prevention in mind.

"We have developed a very high dependence on chemicals," European Environment Commissioner Margot Wallstrom told the Second US-EU Chemicals Conference in Charlottesville, Virginia on April 26. "Yet this is not matched by sufficient knowledge about their potential risks and long-term effects, for which we are paying a high price."

"This is not just an issue for European countries," she said. "Chemical safety is a global concern. Countries all over the world are paying a high price for failures to address chemical safety."

Wallstrom has been the point person for the REACH program, which she said is designed to provide the information and safety Europe needs but in a way that is integrated with international efforts. "To facilitate transfer of information, we will be implementing the Globally Harmonised System, which is the UN system for classification and labeling of dangerous substances," she said.

But experts at the Colloquium strongly believe that the current version of REACH is too weak to be effective, and that it has been deliberately weakened at the behest of the chemicals industry on both sides of the Atlantic.

In a detailed 40 page report, "REACH: An Unprecedented European Initiative for Regulating Industrial Chemicals," Dr. Epstein writes, "In striking contrast to EU governments, which have maintained neutral positions, the Bush Administration has encouraged industry to take aggressive opposition to REACH."

Citing articles in the "New York Times," "Environmental Health Perspectives," and other respected publications, Dr. Epstein presents evidence that the Bush Administration is doing its best to undermine the precautionary principle on which REACH is founded, a principle accepted by the European Commission as a "full fledged and general principle of international law."

"Secretary of State Colin Powell, in a March 2002 U.S. "Nonpaper on EU Chemical Policy," warned that the Precautionary Principle would result in "politically motivated bans" of U.S. chemical products, which account for over 20 percent of all U.S. exports.

Dr. John Graham, administrator of the U.S. Office of Information and Regulatory Affairs, and former director of the industry-funded Harvard University Center for Risk Analysis, in a May 18, 2003 speech to EU regulators, stated that the Administration considers the Precautionary Principle "to be a mythical concept, perhaps like a unicorn."

Confidential documents obtained under the U.S. Freedom of Information Act, have revealed that the U.S. State and Commerce Department, the Environmental Protection Agency, and Office of the U.S. Trade Representative, have formed an alliance with Dow Chemical to fight REACH, as reported in the "Wall Street Journal" on September 9, 2003.

"These tactics, however, may backfire," Dr. Epstein writes. "Senator Frank Lautenberg (D-NJ), with other influential Congressional Democrats, is drafting a proposal to overhaul U.S. regulations to resemble the EU's proposed reforms."

The mainstream industry opposition has been mobilized by the American Chemistry Council and the European Chemical Industry Council, each accounting for approximately 30 percent of the world's chemical production. The Trans-Atlantic Business Dialogue has been established to coordinate industry opposition to REACH, Dr. Epstein notes.

A leaked American Chemistry Council memo made public by the Washington, DC based Environmental Working Group in November 2003 revealed aggressive and well-funded plans to fight laws and regulations based on the precautionary principle, observes Dr. Epstein.

The Council's public relations campaign is being handled by the firm of Nichols-Dezenhall, which, Dr. Epstein writes, "has hired former FBI and CIA agents to create phony front groups, and spy on environmental activists, including digging through their trash in efforts to smear them."

The industry is fighting against regulation of highly toxic industrial chemicals that REACH would impose.

Under REACH, certain classes of industrial chemicals are regarded as of Very High Concern. They are:

- carcinogens, mutagens, and reprotoxins which are either known or very likely to be toxic to humans
- chemicals that can become widely disseminated in the environment, and which are persistent, bioaccumulative, and toxic, particularly persistent organic pollutants
- chemicals that are very persistent and very bioaccumulative in humans and wildlife for which toxicity data are still unavailable

Many of these chemicals are ingredients or contaminants in pesticides, and in consumer products, including food, cosmetics and household products.

Under REACH, when a company intends to produce or import new and existing chemicals it would be required to prepare a Chemical Safety Report to notify the European Chemicals Bureau, a new body which would be responsible for the classification and labeling of dangerous substances.

The report would include—data on the identity of each chemical; toxicological, and ecotoxicological properties of intended uses; estimated human and environmental exposures; production quantity; proposed classification and labeling; safety data sheet; preliminary risk assessment; and proposed risk management.

This information would be entered into a publicly available database to be managed by the European Chemicals Bureau.

The chemicals notified would be evaluated by testing, and authorization will be granted for a limited number of chemicals of very high concern.

Chemical companies would be required to pay fees for each submission. Overall costs are estimated at: registration: €300 million; testing of 30,000 high production volume chemicals: €2.1B for a total of: €2.4 billion. Administrative costs of approximately €0.4 billion would be recovered on a fee based system.

The first formalized critique of REACH was detailed by the American Chemistry Council in July 10, 2003. "REACH is impractical and too costly," the Council said, and should be replaced by a "risk-based approach." The high costs of REACH would impose a negative impact on innovation and competitiveness of EU industry, the Council warned.

Dr. Epstein says the chemical industry is making exaggerated claims about the costs of REACH, which he says are only 0.05 percent of the chemical industry's €417 billion turnover in 2000. He maintains that these costs are "likely to be dwarfed by costs of poorly recognized public health and environmental impacts to which REACH makes the briefest reference."

The latest REACH proposal "fails to recognize the much higher public health and environmental costs of its drastically weakened regulations," Dr. Epstein warns. He points to "significantly increased . . . incidence of testicular cancer in young men, and allergies over the last decades, for which the underlying reasons have not yet been identified."

The American Chemistry Council objects that REACH is trade restrictive and incompatible with World Trade Organization objectives and international chemical regulations. The Council and its European counterpart say the EU should rely on existing registration and risk management, rather than on REACH.

The opposition to REACH by European and U.S. industry was so strong that the EU was forced to make substantial concessions, which were formalized in its October 2003 legislative proposals. These were jointly developed by Wallstrom and EU Enterprise Commissioner Erkki Liikanen.

Key among these concessions was the reduction of the number of high production volume chemicals for which comprehensive safety testing would be required from 30,000 to 10,000, in spite of what Dr. Epstein calls "minimal available test data on most of them."

Chemicals produced in smaller amounts, from one to 10 metric tons, were exempted from the requirements to produce data on reproductive toxicity and environmental persistence.

But people are getting sick and dying in increasing numbers from exposure to the very chemicals REACH is designed to regulate, chemicals that they are exposed to not just one at a time, but in combination.

This is one of the most serious weaknesses of the latest REACH proposal writes Dr. Epstein. "REACH focuses on the carcinogenic and other toxic effects of individual chemicals," particularly chemicals classified as of Very High Concern, "to the exclusion of well-documented evidence on additive and unpredictable synergistic interactions between individual carcinogens."

Formaldehyde, styrene, and atrazine each is toxic alone, for instance, but when a person is exposed to them at once, their combined toxicity is even greater.

REACH should be strengthened by emphasis that the right-to-know "is an inalienable democratic principle, with the exception of sensitive national security concerns," writes Dr. Epstein. "This right clearly extends to information on avoidable risks of disease and death, and environmental contamination, due to industry practices."

"These rights override claims of trade secrecy and confidentiality," he writes. "It should, however, be recognized that the right-to-know in the EU, besides other nations, is more honored in the breach than the observance. REACH should explicitly acknowledge this right, and detail the mechanism for its widest implementation."

Workers are at greatest risk of high level exposure to industrial chemicals of Very High Concern, and Dr. Epstein is calling on industry to recognize workers' right-to-know information on all such life threatening dangers. Workers must have specific information on the chemical and common name of each carcinogen, and carcinogenic process, he says, and specific information on precautions that can be taken to avoid inhalation and skin exposures.

Among many other recommendations for strengthening the REACH legislation, Dr. Epstein is calling for "independent audits of industry chemical safety dossiers prior to registration under REACH, and independent auditing of industry claims for waiving authorization of chemicals classed as of Very High Concern, based on no "right to concern," or that risks can be "adequately controlled."

"All advisory committees should include representatives of independent expert stakeholders, and meetings should be open to the public," he advises, and "all committee members should fully disclose their conflicts of interest."

He challenges the existing estimated health benefits, of €50 billion over 30 years, saying they do not reflect the escalating incidence of cancer, nor early life exposures due to industrial chemicals.

The environmental benefits should be estimated and recognized, and industry benefits from technological innovation stimulated by REACH also should be estimated and recognized, Dr. Epstein says.

The very existence of the REACH proposal has emphasized the inadequacies of the 1976 U.S. Toxic Substances Act, Dr. Epstein will tell the Colloquium. These U.S. regulations still require testing of only about five percent of chemicals in commerce. "Reflecting such concerns, exacerbated by the deregulation policies of the Bush Administration, progressive Congressional Democrats are now drafting a proposal to overhaul U.S. regulations to conform with those of REACH," he says. These initiatives may extend to state level, and the city of San Francisco is already moving in this direction.

Considering the wide range of exposure of the public to high production volume chemicals, Dr. Epstein is not surprised that many have been identified, particularly in the United States as body burden contaminants in fat and blood of the general population.

These chemicals are in the fat and blood of Europeans too, and European Environment Commissioner Wallstrom is no exception. The results of her personal blood test are now public knowledge and she shared them with participants in the Second US-EU Chemicals Conference.

"Among all the talk of costs, trade barriers, bureaucracy," she said, "the results of the test underline the urgency of cleaning out the chemicals stable."

"A couple of years ago, a British doctor told me that each of us have roughly 300-400 synthetic substances in our bodies, and that these were not present in our grandparents' generation. This got me curious," Wallstrom said.

"Last summer I participated in a limited screening involving three groups of man-made substances brominated flame retardants, PCBs and organo chlorine pesticides," she said. "Of the 77 looked for in this screening, I had 28 in my body, including PCB and DDT, which have been banned in Europe for several decades."

"I was told that my result was below the average of the group tested," Wallstrom said. "The result certainly made me concerned, particularly since I also was told that some of the chemical burden in my body was transferred to my children when I was breast feeding them. And, synthetic chemicals are certainly not something that I want to leave as a legacy with them!"

Dr. Epstein puts it even more strongly. "Reckless industry practices are violations of human rights, and white collar crime," he says, and under REACH authorization of chemicals of Very High Concern should be denied if safe alternatives are available.

If public support for REACH is forthcoming when it is introduced to the new European Parliament of 25 member states after the May elections, it will be none too soon for the scientists and nongovernmental organizations at the Paris Colloquium. Cancer is now a leading cause of disease and death in France and the United States, striking nearly one in two men and more than one in three women in their lifetimes.

February 28, 2005

Time to Protect Babies from Dangerous Products

From shortly after birth, mothers tenderly wash and pamper their infants with a wide range of baby products. These include soaps, shampoos, lotions, and dusting powders, some of which are used several times daily.

However, how would mothers react if they discovered that these baby products contain a witch's brew of dangerous ingredients? Hopping mad could be a reasonable understatement.

Most disturbing are three groups of widely used ingredients known as "hidden carcinogens"—ingredients which are contaminated by carcinogens, or which break down to release carcinogens, or which are precursors of carcinogens—to which infants are about 100 times more sensitive than adults.

The largest group of hidden carcinogens includes dozens of wetting agents or detergents, particularly PEGs, Laureths, and Cetearaths, all of which are contaminated with the potent and volatile carcinogens ethylene oxide and dioxane. These carcinogens could readily be stripped off during ingredient manufacture, if the industry just made the effort to do so. Another hidden carcinogenic ingredient is lanolin, derived from sheep's wool, most samples of which are contaminated with DDT-like pesticides.

The second group includes another detergent, Triethanolamine (TEA) which, following interaction with nitrite, is a precursor of a highly potent nitrosamine carcinogen.

The third group includes Quaterniums and Diazolidinyl urea preservatives which break down in the product or skin to release the carcinogenic formaldehyde.

Of additional concern is another group of common preservatives, known as Parabens. Numerous studies over the last decade have shown that these are weakly estrogenic. They produce abnormal hormonal effects following application to the skin of infant rodents, particularly male, resulting in decreased testosterone levels, and urogenital abnormalities. Parabens have also been found to accumulate in the breasts of women with breast cancer.

The common use of Talc dusting powder can result in its inhalation, resulting in acute or chronic lung irritation and disease (talcosis), and even death. Additionally, Talc is a suspect cause of lung cancer, based on rodent tests.

Fragrances, containing numerous ingredients, are commonly used in baby products for the mother's benefit. However, over 25 of these ingredients are known to cause allergic dermatitis.

A final ingredient of particular concern is the harshly irritant sodium lauryl sulfate. A single application to adult human skin has been shown to damage its microscopic structure, increasing the penetration of carcinogenic and other toxic ingredients.

Most disturbing is the ready availability of safe alternatives for all these dangerous ingredients (longstanding information on which is detailed on the Cancer Prevention Coalition website, http://www.preventcancer.com). So, why is it that the multibillion-dollar cosmetic and toiletry industry has not acted on this information? The answer is that the major priority of the industry's trade association is "to protect the freedom of the industry to compete in a fair market place." At the same time, the association pursues a highly aggressive agenda against what it claims are "unreasonable or unnecessary labeling or warning requirements." As Senator Edward M. Kennedy (D.MA) stated at 1997 Hearings on the FDA Reform bill: "The cosmetics industry has borrowed a page from the playbook of the tobacco industry by putting profits ahead of public health."

Astoundingly, the interests of industry remain reinforced by the regulatory abdication of the Food and Drug Administration (FDA), in spite of its authority under the 1938 Federal Food, Drug and Cosmetics (FD&C) Act. Clearly, the FDA is the lap dog, rather than the watchdog, of the industry.

Of even greater concern is the reckless failure of the federal National Cancer Institute and the "non-profit" American Cancer Society to inform the public of the avoidable risks of cancer from the use of baby products, especially in view of the escalating incidence of childhood cancers over recent decades. However, the silence of the American Cancer Society is consistent with its over $100,000 annual funding from about a dozen major cosmetic and toiletry industries.

The protracted failure of Congress to enforce FDA's compliance with the FD&C Act has evoked the growing concern of State legislatures. Assemblywoman Judy Chu (D-Monterey Park) of the California Senate Health Committee, recently introduced landmark legislation that requires disclosure of all carcinogenic, hormonal, and otherwise toxic ingredients in cosmetics. Strongly backed by a coalition of consumer, women's, occupational, and church groups, but opposed by powerful mainstream industry interests, the Bill failed to pass. However, this shot over the bows of the reckless mainstream industry marks the beginning of nationwide State initiatives to protect consumers and their babies from undisclosed dangerous products and ingredients. Safe alternative products and ingredients, including organic, are becoming increasingly available from non-mainstream companies.

ENDORSER:

Ronnie Cummins
National Director
Organic Consumers Association

December 27, 2006

Estee Lauder's Conflicted Marketing Strategies

Origins, one of the giant Estee Lauder companies, has recently launched a new line of cosmetic products. They are claimed to be "a totally integrative approach to skin care . . . to help your skin be as healthy as possible, (and) optimize its defenses against age accelerators."

However, review of these products reveals the following dangerous ingredients.

> Limonene, a well-known carcinogen, rated as such in 1990 by the National Toxicology Program.

> A large group of surfactants or emulsifiers, such as PEG-100 and ceteareth 20, known as ethoxylates. Unless readily purified, and appropriately labeled as such, these ingredients are contaminated with high concentrations of the potent carcinogen ethylene oxide, and also dioxane.

> Parabens, which even at very low concentrations, produce toxic hormonal effects, known as endocrine disruptive, especially in male embryos and infants.

> Bisabolol, technically known as a "penetration enhancer," increases the deep penetration of cosmetic ingredients through the skin.

> Butylene glycol, related to the anti-freeze ethylene glycol, is a skin irritant.

Communication of these concerns to the CEO of Origins was met with frank response that she was uninformed of these "scientific technicalities," and that she would communicate them to ther parent company, Estee Lauder. However, a subsequent response from a senior Estee executive attempted to challenge evidence on the carcinogenicity of Limonene on the irrelevant grounds that a European Council Directive, relating to the allergenic effects of Limonene, made no reference to carcinogenicity. Concerns on the other toxic ingredients were also not addressed. Nor was there any evidence, based on standard clinical trials, supporting the claimed anti-aging effects of the Origins products.

Of further interest, Estee explained that "the reason for the ingredient listing on a U.S. product is a business decision which allows us to sell the product globally. I fully support that decision, but will defer to the Brand (Origins) President if she feels otherwise . . . ." This policy is also consistent with an August 26, 2005 letter from Estee Lauder Japan's Manager of Regulatory Affairs, assuring that "There is no concerns in the Japanese public about Japanese cosmetic safety. Japanese and non-Japanese companies don't have made any special effort at improving safety of products."

In sharp contrast to Origins, another U.S. Estee company, Aveda, has taken active steps to phase out a wide range of hazardous ingredients, including those in Origins products.

Estee's dual national and international marketing policies are clearly conflicted with regard to ingredient safety. This is surprising, particularly in view of the credo of Fred Langhammer, Estee's previous President, that "safety sells."

June 28, 2007

The *New York Times* Ignores Information on Dangers Of Sunscreens

On June 19, the *New York Times* published an article "Saving Young Skin From the Sun's Perils," by its regular columnist Jane Brody. Brody warned that sunscreen "is a must for everyone starting at age six months . . . and should be reapplied every two hours," especially for children. However, Brody is unaware of the dangers of sunscreens.

Six ingredients are commonly used in sunscreens, at concentrations of up to 10%, in order to reduce risks of sunburn from exposure to short wave ultraviolet (UVB) solar radiation. It should, however, be emphasized that these ingredients fail to block the more dangerous long wave (UVA) radiation.

A series of recent studies have raised serious concerns on the dangers of sunscreens. Contrary to reassurances on safety, based on label claims for a high Skin Protection Factor (SPF), most light skinned people use sunscreens to protect against sunburn due to UVB radiation.

However, this common practice, particularly in children, results in high levels of cumulative exposure to the more dangerous UVA radiation. This penetrates into the deep layers of the skin without any warning of sunburn, breaks down the protein and collagen which keep the skin firm and plump, and is responsible for the classic signs of skin aging, including wrinkling and discoloration.

More seriously, UVA radiation is well recognized as the major cause of malignant melanoma. This is now the fastest rising cancer in the world whose incidence in the U.S. over recent decades has increased dramatically by about 130%, and whose mortality has increased by about 25%.

Of additional concern are the hormonal effects of sunscreens. Their ingredients belong to a family of hormone-damaging chemicals, known as endocrine disruptors. These stimulate uterine growth of infant rats following painting their skin with concentrations similar to those in sunscreens. Furthermore, there is well-documented evidence that sunscreen ingredients accumulate in the human body as evidenced by their detection in breast milk.

These dangers of sunscreens can be readily avoided by the use of conventional zinc oxide and/or titanium dioxide sunblocks. These are highly effective against the dangerous UVA radiation. Their only disadvantage is that they whiten skin, depending on the amount used and frequency of application.

Finally, my June 21 letter to the *New York Times* warning of the dangers of sunscreens and the safety of sunblocks remains unpublished.

March 24, 2008

The FDA Still Ignores the Lethal Risks of Talcum Powder

Up to 20 percent of U.S. pre-menopausal women regularly dust their genital area, sanitary pads or contraceptive diaphragms with cosmetic grade talcum powder.

Manufactured by Johnson & Johnson, and widely distributed by Osco and Walgreens, besides other drug stores, women have been persuaded by advertisements to dust themselves to mask alleged genital odors. Not surprisingly, talcum powder has become a symbol of freshness and cleanliness for over five decades.

On November 17, 1994, the Chicago-based Cancer Prevention Coalition and the New York Center for Constitutional Rights submitted a Citizen Petition to the FDA, "Seeking Carcinogenic Labeling on all Cosmetic Talc Products." The Petition was endorsed by Dr. Quentin Young, Chairman of The Health and Medicine Policy Research Group, by the Ovarian Cancer Early Detection and Prevention Foundation, and subsequently by Senator Edward Kennedy. In a 1997 statement to the Senate, he requested the FDA to place a cancer warning on the label of talc products, besides other products containing known carcinogens. However, over a decade later this warning remains ignored.

Based on 15 publications in leading scientific journals dating back to the 1960's, the Petition explicitly warned of "increased rates of ovarian cancer resulting from frequent exposure to cosmetic grade talc." After over a year's delay, the Petition was rejected by Dr. John Bailey, FDA's past Director of the Office of Cosmetics and Colors, and currently Director of the industry's The Personal Care Products Council. Since then, the strong relation between the genital use of talc powder and ovarian cancer has been endorsed by over 40 further scientific publications. These have reported increased risks ranging from 35% to 90%.

Of particular interest is a 1971 report on the identification of talc particles in ovarian cancers, a finding contested by Dr. G.Y. Hildick Smith, Johnson & Johnson's medical Director. However, a subsequent publication in the prestigious The Lancet warned that "The potentially harmful effects of talc . . . in the ovary . . . should not be ignored." This warning was further supported by a 2004 report on the major risk of ovarian cancer in talc users. However, there was no such risk in women whose fallopian tubes had been tied, blocking the access of talc dust to the ovaries.

Not surprisingly, the mortality of ovarian cancer for women over the age of 65, a relatively rare cancer at any age, has escalated dramatically over the last three decades, by 12% for white, and 32% for black women. It should further be noted that there are about 15,300 deaths from ovarian cancer each year. This makes it the fourth most common fatal cancer in women, after breast, colon and lung.

Nevertheless, the industry and, worse still the FDA, remain recklessly unresponsive to these dangers. The FDA has neither banned the genital use of talcum powder, nor required industry to label it with explicit warnings. This is all the more inexcusable since cosmetic grade starch powder is a readily available safe alternative.

ENDORSER:

Quentin Young, M.D., MACP
Chairman, Health and Medicine Policy Research Group

May 15, 2008

Talcum Powder Can Provoke Deadly Ovarian Cancer

What could be more benign than body powder, right? Some of Chicago's most highly placed doctors would say, wrong. They are part of a coalition of public health experts, medical doctors and consumers organizations that is petitioning the federal government for warning labels on cosmetic talcum powder products used by many women as part of their personal care regime—a warning that frequent use is linked to ovarian cancer.

The petition addresses Secretary of Health and Human Services Mike Leavitt, and Commissioner of Food and Drugs Andrew C. von Eschenbach, M.D., a former director of the National Cancer Institute.

The group seeks labels with a warning such as, "Frequent application of talcum powder in the female genital area substantially increases the risk of ovarian cancer," on all talc products.

The petitioners also seek a public hearing at which evidence can be presented that the genital application of talc can result in its translocation to the ovaries.

Ovarian cancer is known as particularly deadly because it is a silent cancer that shows few symptoms until it is well advanced.

Prevention is as easy as discontinuing the use of talcum powder, says lead petitioner Dr. Samuel Epstein, who chairs the Cancer Prevention Coalition, based in Chicago.

"As Dr. Andrew C. von Eschenbach, former director of the National Cancer Institute, is aware," said Dr. Epstein in a statement today, "the mortality of ovarian cancer for women over the age of 65, has escalated dramatically since 1975, by 13% for white and 47% for black women.

"There are about 15,300 deaths from ovarian cancer each year," he said. "This makes it the fourth most common fatal cancer in women after colon, breast and lung."

These figures are found in the National Cancer Institute's own SEER Cancer Statistics Review, 2005, posted three years after publication, in 2008.

Dr. Epstein suggests substituting "cornstarch, a safe organic carbohydrate, for talcum powder products."

Others, even women who have had a tubal ligation or hysterectomy, either of which prevents the transfer of talc from the perineum to the ovary, would not be affected by talc application, scientists have confirmed.

One of the studies cited by the petitioners even suggests that women may be dying from exposure to talc on condoms.

"Possible morbidity in women from talc on condoms," C.S. Kasper and P.J. Chandler Jr. is the title of a letter published in the Journal of the American Medical Association back in March 1995.

The term talc covers a wide range of natural rocks and minerals, most of which are magnesium silicates. Talc is characterized by softness, hydrophobic surface properties, chemical inertness and a slippery or soapy feeling.

The Citizen Petition is submitted on behalf of:

Samuel S. Epstein, M.D., Chairman, Cancer Prevention Coalition, and Professor emeritus Occupational and Environmental Medicine, University of Illinois at Chicago School of Public Health;

Peter Orris, M.D., Professor and Chief of Service, University of Illinois at Chicago Medical Center;

Quentin Young, M.D., Chairman, Health and Medicine Policy Research Group, Chicago;

Rosalie Bertell, PhD, International Association for Humanitarian Medicine, Scientific Advisor to the International Institute of Concern for Public Health, Toronto, and the International Science Oversight Board of the Organic Consumers Association, Washington, D.C.; and

Ronnie Cummins, National Director of the Organic Consumers Association.

This is the second petition application from Dr. Epstein and the Cancer Prevention Coalition on the issue of the health risks of talc. The first, submitted in November 1994, did not succeed.

Still, Epstein says the scientific basis of the 1994 Petition has been admitted by the industry. In an August 12, 1982, article in the New York Times, Johnson & Johnson, the manufacturer and retailer of talc dusting powder, stated it was aware of a publication which concluded that frequent genital application of talc was responsible for a three-fold increased risk of ovarian cancer.

The petition is supported by such heavyweights as Peter Orris, M.D., Director of Health Hazard Evaluation, Cook County Hospital, and Professor of Medicine, University of Illinois Medical School, Chicago.

The petitioners point to an analysis of 16 pooled studies that confirmed a statistically significant 33 percent increased risk of ovarian cancer associated with the perineal use of talc.

Yet another report, this one by 19 scientists in eight nations under the auspices of the International Agency for Research on Cancer, concluded that there is a 30-60 percent increased risk of ovarian cancer following the perineal application of talc. This risk has been confirmed in two other research reports cited by the petitioners.

Commercial talc properties can be identified by their chemistry and mineralogy. Not all deposits are suited for all applications.

Some commercial talc may be harder than cosmetic talc because of the presence of impurities and associated minerals such as dolomite, calcite, tremolite and quartz.

Talc is a mineral that may be dangerous for another reason—asbestos, although this is not the subject of the petition. The federal Agency for Toxic Substances says, "Tremolite asbestos may occur in deposits of chrysotile, vermiculite, and talc."

Another source suggests the possibility that some commercial talc products may contain asbestos.

"Some commercial talc may be harder because of the presence of impurities and associated minerals such as dolomite, calcite, tremolite and quartz," says talc producer Specialty Minerals Inc., a wholly owned subsidiary of Minerals Technologies Inc.

Talc is used commercially in the automobile and appliance industries. Its resistance to heat, electricity and acids make it an ideal surface for lab counter tops and electrical switchboards. It is also a filler material for paints, rubber and insecticide

May 19, 2008

CPC Submits Petition Seeking a Cancer Warning on Cosmetic Talc Powder Products

On May 13, 2008, the Cancer Prevention Coalition, endorsed by leading national authorities, submitted this Petition to the FDA. This updates scientific information detailed in a November 17, 1994, Citizen Petition which was denied by the FDA. It also documents prior knowledge of the FDA and industry of the cancer risks of cosmetic talc.

The scientific basis of the 2008 Petition is detailed in 11 reports in leading national and international scientific journals. These document the increased risks of ovarian cancer, ranging from 30% to 60%, from genital dusting with talc powder. In view of the strength of this evidence, a 1999 publication by a leading national expert urged that "formal public health warnings" should be made against the genital use of talcum dusting powder. Of further relevance is well-documented scientific evidence that ligation of the fallopian tubes or hysterectomy is protective against the dangers of talc by preventing its access to the ovaries.

It should further be emphasized that cornstarch, an organic carbohydrate, powder is a safe and effective alternative to talcum powder products.

As the Petition states, FDA Commissioner Dr. Andrew C. von Eschenbach, former Director of the National Cancer Institute, is or should be aware, that the mortality of ovarian cancer for women over the age of 65, has escalated dramatically since 1975, by 13% for white and 47% for black women. There are now about 15,300 deaths from ovarian cancer each year. This makes it the fourth commonest fatal cancer in women after colon, breast and lung. Yet Dr. von Eschenbach has failed to mandate a cancer warning label on talc powder, let alone ban its continued use.

Information on the cancer risks of talc dusting powder is not new to the FDA, nor to the industry.

As stated in the Petition, J. Mande, Acting Associate Commissioner for Legislative Affairs of the Department of Health and Human Services, admitted in August 1993 that "We are aware that there have been reports in the medical literature between frequent direct female perineal talc dusting over a protracted period of years, and an incremental increase in the statistical odds of subsequent development of certain ovarian cancers . . . (However) at the present time, the FDA is not considering to ban, restrict or require a warning statement on the label of talc containing products."

More reckless is the admission, in an August 12, 1992, New York Times article by Johnson & Johnson, the manufacturer and retailer of talc dusting powder, that frequent genital dusting with talc increases risks of ovarian cancer by three-fold. This risk was belatedly admitted this year by the industry's Cosmetic Toiletry and Fragrance Association.

Finally, Senator Edward Kennedy, in a 1997 statement to the Senate, requested the FDA to place a cancer warning on the label of talc products, besides other products containing known carcinogens. Nevertheless, over a decade later this warning remains ignored.

ENDORSERS:

Quentin Young, M.D.
Chairman, Health and Medicine Policy Research Group
Past President, American Public Health Association

Peter Orris, M.D.
Professor and Chief of Service
University of Illinois at Chicago Medical Center

Rosalie Bertell, PhD
International Association for Humanitarian Medicine

Ronnie Cummins
National Director of the Organic Consumers Association.

August 7, 2008

FDA Remains Asleep at the Wheel on the Dangers of Sunscreens, Besides Other Cosmetics and Personal Care Products

Since 1978, sunscreens have been regulated and labeled by the Food and Drug Administration (FDA) on the basis of their SPF (Skin Protection Factor).

On August 23, 2007, the FDA proposed new regulations for more informative labeling of sunscreens. However, almost a year later, they still remain pending.

In response to FDA's inaction, and mounting concerns on the unreliability of the SPF, Connecticut Attorney General Richard Blumenthal wrote to the FDA on July 24 criticizing its failure to regulate the sunscreen industry, and prevent it from making "dangerously misleading claims" on the safety and effectiveness of its products.

A week later, Senator Jack Reed (D-Ri) and Christopher Dodd (D-Ct) introduced the "Sunscreen Labeling Act of 2008." This gave the FDA six more months to finalize comprehensive rules, otherwise the Act would become law.

Sunscreens pose scientifically well documented risks. While well known for over a decade, they remain unregulated by the FDA, and ignored by the industry.

Sunscreens are based on six ingredients, some of which actively penetrate the skin, accumulate in the body, and have been identified in urine and breast milk.

More ominously, these ingredients have toxic hormonal effects, known technically as "endocrine disruptive." Evidence for these effects has been well documented over the last decade. This includes stimulation of human breast cancer cells in test tube experiments, and increased uterine growth in immature female rats following skin painting or feeding.

Sunscreens block short wave ultraviolet light (UVB), which is responsible for sunburn. This encourages prolonged exposure, particularly of children. Moreover, sunscreens are ineffective against long wave ultraviolet light (UVA), which is responsible for malignant melanoma, the fastest growing known cancer. As a result, its incidence has increased by 130%, and its mortality has increased by 26% since 1975. FDA's continuing regulatory failure in this regard reflects the reckless indifference to consumer product safety of its Commissioner Dr. Andrew von Eschenbach, former director of the National Cancer Institute.

Of major concern, and still ignored by the FDA, is the increasing addition to sunscreens of unlabeled atom or molecule size zinc oxide or titanium dioxide particles. Technically known as nanoparticles, they increase the durability and effectiveness of these products. However, as reported in over two dozen scientific publications since 2003, including those by an Environmental

Protection Agency research team and the International Center for Technology Assessment, nanoparticles can penetrate the skin, invade blood vessels, and produce devastating distant toxic effects.

FDA's regulatory failure extends from sunscreens to a wide range of other dangerous ingredients in cosmetics and personal care products. Of illustrative concern is FDA's reckless failure to respond to November 1994 and May 2008 Citizen Petitions, by the Cancer Prevention Coalition, "Seeking a Cancer Warning on Cosmetic Talc Products," used for feminine hygiene. As detailed in these Petitions, talc is a major avoidable cause of ovarian cancer, a relatively rare cancer at any age, whose incidence has escalated dramatically by 12% for white and 32% for black women, with about 15,000 deaths annually. This makes it the fourth most common fatal cancer after breast, colon and lung.

The "Sunscreen Labeling Act" should be the first step to developing a comprehensive "Cosmetics and Personal Care Products Labeling Act." This could be modeled along the lines of California's precedential 2007 Safe Cosmetics Act.

As warned by Senator Edward Kennedy (D-Ma) at September 10, 1997 Hearings on the FDA Reform Bill, "The cosmetics industry has borrowed a page from the playbook of the tobacco industry by putting profits ahead of public health." This warning remains recklessly unheeded by the FDA.

309

August 18, 2008

Responsibility of the FDA and National Cancer Institute for Cosmetics Related Escalating Cancer Rates

In November 1994, the Cancer Prevention Coalition and the Center for Constitutional Rights submitted a Petition to the FDA calling for "Cancer Labeling of Talc Products." Talc products are regularly used by up to 17% of women for genital hygiene.

Supported by about 15 references in the scientific literature, the Petition warned that talc posed major fatal risks of ovarian cancer. These could be avoided by the use of cornstarch powder as a safe alternative. However, the Petition was rejected.

In May 2008, the Coalition submitted a further Petition updating the evidence for the major cancer risks of genital talc products, as detailed in 11 leading national and international scientific journals. This Petition was endorsed by leading national scientific authorities including Dr. Quentin Young, Chairman of the Health and Medicine Policy Research Group, and past president of the American Public Health Association; Dr. Peter Orris, Chief of Services, University of Illinois at Chicago Medical Center; Ronnie Cummins, National Director of the Organic Consumers Association; and more recently the National Congress of Black Women. However, the FDA has failed to respond to the Petition.

As FDA Commissioner Dr. Andrew von Eschenbach, former Director of the National Cancer Institute, must be aware, the mortality from ovarian cancer for women over the age of 65 has escalated dramatically since 1975, by 13% for white and 47% for black women. There are now about 15,300 deaths from ovarian cancer each year. This makes it the fourth commonest fatal cancer in women after colon, breast and lung. Yet, Dr. von Eschenbach has failed to mandate a cancer warning label on talc powder, let alone ban its continued use.

Dr. von Eschenbach's reckless indifference to cancer prevention extends to sunscreens. Sunscreens pose scientifically well-documented risks of cancer, besides toxic hormonal effects. While well known for over a decade, they remain unregulated by the FDA, and ignored by the industry.

Sunscreens block short wave ultraviolet light (UVB), which is responsible for sunburn. This encourages prolonged exposure, particularly of children. Moreover, sunscreens are ineffective against long wave ultraviolet light (UVA), which is responsible for malignant melanoma, the fastest growing known cancer. As a result, its incidence has increased by 130%, and its mortality has increased by 26% since 1975.

Of further concern is FDA's failure to issue new regulations for informative labeling of sunscreens as proposed in August 2007. In response to FDA's inaction, Connecticut Attorney General Richard Blumenthal wrote to the FDA on July 24 this year criticizing its failure to regulate the sunscreen industry, and prevent it from making "dangerously misleading claims" on the safety and effectiveness of its products. A week later, Senators Jack Reed (D-RI) and Christopher Dodd (D-CT) introduced the "Sunscreen Labeling Act of 2008." This gave the FDA six more months to finalize comprehensive rules, otherwise the Act will become law.

Talc products should be banned immediately. The "Sunscreen Labeling Act" should be the first step to developing a comprehensive "Cosmetics and Personal Care Products Labeling Act." This could be modeled along the lines of California's precedential 2007 Safe Cosmetics Act.

As warned by Senator Edward Kennedy (D-MA) at September 10, 1997, Hearings on the FDA Reform Bill, "The cosmetics industry has borrowed a page from the playbook of the tobacco industry by putting profits ahead of public health." This warning remains recklessly unheeded by the FDA. Clearly, Dr. von Eschenbach is unable or unwilling to protect the public against other avoidable risks of cancer from cosmetics. These include over 20 known carcinogens, and a similar number of "hidden" carcinogens or carcinogen precursors.

March 27, 2009

America's Beauty Show Challenges Toxic Salons

America's Beauty Show, March 28-30 in Chicago, is dedicated to safe and healthy beauty salons. By doing so, the Show raises serious and decades overdue concerns on the dangers of conventional nationwide salons.

Salon products are generally dispensed from bulk containers without labeled ingredients. Of particular concern is the cumulative contamination of air, particularly in poorly ventilated salons, with volatile ingredients and fine particles, particularly from hair sprays. Known as aerosols, these can penetrate deeply into the lungs of clients, and even more so their stylists working a usual five-day week.

Products used in the great majority of nationwide salons contain a wide range of toxic ingredients, including carcinogens, hormonal ingredients, and allergens. Exposure to them poses hidden dangers to clients, and much more so their stylists.

Stylists, particularly in small hair and beauty salons, tend to drift in and out of their jobs. So formal long-term studies to investigate dangers to their health, known as epidemiological, are not feasible. Moreover, there is substantial and long standing evidence on a wide range of toxic effects in salon workers, particularly hairdressers and beauty stylists. These include nausea, sleep disorders, fatigue, and numbness and pain in the fingers. They also include allergic dermatitis, acute lung irritation, asthma, and chronic bronchitis.

An additional poorly recognized danger from salon and personal use relates to hair straighteners based on thioglycolic acid. Besides causing hair to become brittle and break, they can also irritate the scalp and cause pustular and allergic reactions.

Of particular concern are hair dyes. About 35 percent of women and 10 percent of men are regularly exposed to these dyes in salons or by personal use. Black and dark brown permanent and semi-permanent dyes contain carcinogens, particularly those known as phenylenediamines. These have been shown to cause cancers, particularly non-Hodgkin's lymphoma, Hodgkin's disease, and multiple myeloma, besides breast and bladder cancers. However, in spite of this long standing evidence, stylists, let alone their clients, remain unaware of these avoidable risks of sometimes lethal cancers. In sharp contrast to the U.S., these dyes have been banned in Europe.

The continued use of these dangerous hair dyes is all the more reckless. Safe certified organic dyes, particularly those marketed by Logona, a German company, are now available in the U.S. These dyes achieve stable and long-lasting colors, ranging from brown to black.

A recently recognized concern relates to the potent carcinogen vinyl chloride, a propellant in some pressure sprays, which has been incriminated as a cause of fatal liver cancer. Another recent concern relates to hormonal phthalates in sprays to which pregnant women may be exposed, and have been incriminated as a cause of congenital abnormalities in their male infants. Of critical importance is the protection of clients and, even more so, their stylists by establishing efficient ventilation of salons, and their workstations. The efficiency of this ventilation should conform to certified national standards.

Information on all ingredients in all products used in salons, including their risks and recommended safety precautions, should be detailed and made readily available to all stylists in standard Material Safety Data Sheets. This information is legally required by the Occupational Safety and Health Administration for all workplaces with ten or more employees. However, this requirement is observed more in the breach than the performance. This information should also be made readily available to clients.

Pressure sprays should be banned. They release very fine particles which are readily inhaled into the depths of the lungs and can irritate and cause toxic effects. Pump spray products are very much safer as their particles are at least tenfold larger, and large enough to be filtered out through the nose. Polyvinyl pyrrolidine, a common ingredient in hair sprays, is designed to increase smoothness and flexibility of the hair. However, it can cause chronic lung damage and should be banned.

Finally, eyeliners, skin lightening creams, and some brands of mascara used in salons, besides being available for purchase in beauty supply stores, contain mercury as a preservative. However, even small doses of mercury accumulate and can cause neurological damage following long term exposure.

April 2009

What You Don't Know Can Hurt You . . . In Fact, It Already Is

A groundbreaking new book, Toxic Beauty: How Cosmetics and Personal-Care Products Endanger Your Health . . . And What You Can Do About It, issues a long-overdue wake-up call to the public on the dangers of ingredients in common cosmetics and personal-care products whose safety most people naively take for granted.

"We are all playing Russian roulette with toxic-laden cosmetics and personal-care products that we apply to our skin, and to the skin of our infants and children, everyday," warns author Samuel S. Epstein, M.D.

How many women know of the risks to their health by using lipstick, moisturizers or deodorants? Why do so few mothers know of the risks to their infants and children from using personal-care products, including sunscreens? How can the cosmetic and personal care products industry recklessly continue to ignore these dangers?

Toxic Beauty is a fully documented exposé which reveals the wide range of avoidable health risks, some even life threatening, that Americans are unknowingly exposed to in their everyday cosmetic and personal-care products. "But there is also good news. These toxic exposures are 100 percent avoidable by taking just a few basic precautions," says Epstein.

Toxic Beauty is written by Dr. Samuel S. Epstein, an internationally recognized expert on avoidable causes of cancer, besides other toxic-related diseases, and investigative reporter Randall Fitzgerald. And besides chronicling the pervasive marketing of dangerous products, Toxic Beauty also informs readers on the growing availability of safe products.

In the pages of *Toxic Beauty*, you'll find:

- The five categories of common toxic ingredients in cosmetics and personal-care products.
- Toxic ingredients in these products have been incriminated in a wide range of diseases,

- particularly cancers. These include malignant melanoma of the skin, and lethal ovarian cancer. They also include birth defects in male infants.
- Safe synthetic and certified organic products as alternative to dangerous products.
- Dangerous exposures to employees from prolonged exposures to toxic ingredients in unlabeled
- Tear-out sheets listing all major categories of toxic ingredients; also tables on five major classes of toxic ingredients that can be downloaded from the Cancer Prevention Coalition Web site, www.preventcancer.com.

Epstein warns, "Unbelievably, the FDA has recklessly failed to protect us from toxic ingredients in cosmetics and personal-care products for the last six decades. What's more, the mainstream industry has remained criminally indifferent to the dangers of their products. In sharp contrast, European regulations ban all products containing toxic ingredients."

So, the reality is that protecting yourself and your family unfortunately is still entirely up to you. Toxic Beauty shows you just how.

July 20, 2009

Prevent Cancer: Phase Out Toxics in Cosmetics and Personal Care Products

The Cancer Prevention Coalition (CPC), and other concerned scientists and consumer advocates, are calling on the federal government to require a phase out of carcinogenic and other toxic ingredients in cosmetics and personal care products.

As the Obama Administration works with Congress to pass comprehensive health care reform legislation this year, the CPC notes that President Barack Obama told reporters at the July 10 Group of 8 news conference, "We have to bend the cost curve on health care, and there are some very specific ways of doing that—game changers that incentivize quality as opposed to quantity, that emphasize prevention."

Most cosmetics and personal care products on store shelves today contain five major categories of toxic ingredients, warns the CPC. These toxics are: frank carcinogens; precursors of or "hidden" carcinogens; endocrine or hormonally disruptive; penetration enhancers; and allergens.

Tables listing these five categories of toxic ingredients are available on the CPC website at http://www.preventcancer.com/consumers/cosmetics/Tables_cospcp.htm.

There are only a few exceptions to products containing these toxic ingredients, notably those that are certified organic by the U.S. Department of Agriculture.

The tables, compiled by Dr. Samuel Epstein and Randy Fitzgerald, are published in their new book, "Toxic Beauty: How Cosmetics and Personal Care Products Endanger Your Health . . . And What You Can do About It."

"Our skin is highly permeable," cautions Dr. Epstein in "Toxic Beauty." Less than one-tenth of an inch thick, skin is a porous membrane that is highly sensitive to toxic chemicals. What we put on our skin affects our health just as much, if not more, than what we put in our mouths."

Some toxic ingredients "illegally remain unlabeled," warns Dr. Epstein. "Of particular concern are hormonal phthalates, and synthetic "aroma boosters" which strongly intensify organic fragrances."

Expressing concerns on carcinogenic products, U.S. Senator Edward Kennedy of Massachusetts, in 1997 Senate Hearings on the U.S. Food and Drug Administration (FDA) Reform Bill, warned that, "The cosmetics industry has borrowed a page from the playbook of the tobacco industry by putting profits ahead of public health."

This is a major understatement, warns Dr. Epstein, who points out that tobacco products are labeled with explicit warnings on cancer risks, which relate only to late adolescents and adults.

In striking contrast, there are no warnings whatsoever on cosmetics and personal care products, yet their ingredients pose unrecognized lifelong dangers to the entire U.S. population, including the fetus, following maternal use and absorption through the skin into maternal and fetal blood.

The cosmetics and personal care product industry, other than relatively small U.S. Department of Agriculture (USDA) certified organic companies, can no longer claim ignorance of the wide range of toxic, and even life threatening, ingredients in products manufactured and sold by multibillion-dollar companies, including those that engage in multilevel marketing.

The FDA is responsible for the regulation of cosmetics and personal care products in the United States. The legislative framework for regulating these products, whether manufactured in the U.S. or imported, is based on the 1938 Federal Food, Drug, and Cosmetic (FFDC) Act, and its amendments.

FDA Regulations stipulate: "Each ingredient used in a cosmetic product and each finished cosmetic product shall be adequately substantiated for safety prior to marketing. Any such ingredient or product whose safety is not adequately substantiated prior to marketing is misbranded unless it contains the following conspicuous statement on the principal display panel: 'Warning: The safety of this product has not been determined.'" This is commonly known as a "Black Box" warning. The Cancer Prevention Coalition further recommends that financial penalties should be imposed on all companies marketing products containing toxic ingredients until they are completely phased out.

Nevertheless, the FDA has rarely exercised its explicit authority over the last seven decades, no matter how dangerous the product and its ingredients.

The minimal exceptions in the decade following the 1938 Act are just the following few ingredients:

- Zirconium—containing complexes in aerosol products, as they can induce granulomas in the lung.
- Hexachlorophene—because of its neurotoxicity; however, this ingredient may still be used in the absence of "an alternative (effective) preservative."
- Mercury compounds—because of their neurotoxicity.
- Chlorofluorocarbon propellants—although they may still be exported.
- Dithionol—as it can cause photosensitivity.
- Halogenated salicylanilides—as they can induce photosensitivity.
- Chloroform—"because of its animal carcinogenicity and likely hazard to human health."
- Vinyl chloride—as an ingredient in aerosol products, "because of its carcinogenic effects on humans and animals."
- Methylene chloride—"because of its animal carcinogenicity and likely hazard to human health."

The Cancer Prevention Coalition emphasizes that the time to require the cosmetics and personal care products industry to phase out carcinogenic and other toxic ingredients is well overdue.

There has been recent progress in one state. Following six decades of the FDA's reckless failure to comply with the requirements of the 1938 FFDC Act, Governor Arnold Schwarzenegger enacted the 2007 California Safe Cosmetics Act. This requires that cosmetic companies disclose to the State Department of Health Services any ingredients in their products that have been identified as causing cancer or hormone disruption. The department can then require the manufacturer to disclose these ingredients and their toxic effects on a Web site for public viewing.

Reflecting concerns at the state, besides federal, levels, this release is being distributed directly to every state governor nationwide.

There is also some recent progress on the federal level. In May 2009, Dr. Margaret Hamburg was appointed as FDA Commissioner by the Senate. Dr. Hamburg is well recognized as a leading public health advocate. As such, she is likely to be highly responsive to concerns on toxic products, and take appropriate regulatory action!

August 14, 2009

How to Sunbathe Safely

Soon we will see summer's fading days and the seasonal end of our culture's annual fixation with slathering sunscreen products on exposed skin in pursuit of 'safety' or vanity.

You have all heard—and probably warned your children—what will happen if they don't use sunscreens. Not only will they get sunburned, their skin will get wrinkled and aged prematurely.

But what if you were warned that the dangers of sunscreens to health, besides the environment, outweigh their proclaimed benefits? Your first response would probably be incredulity. How can a product that's been championed by health agencies the world over possibly be a threat?

The answer hinges on a state of denial, and a false sense of security. This reflects ignorance of the toxic effects of sunscreen ingredients, says the chairman of the Cancer Prevention Coalition, Samuel S. Epstein, M.D.

Sunscreens absorb short-wave ultraviolet light, which is responsible for sunburn. However, they do nothing to block long-wave ultraviolet radiation which is the major cause of a skin cancer, known as malignant melanoma," Dr. Epstein explains.

A Sun Protection Factor (SPF) was introduced in 1962 as an international standard for measuring how much protection sunscreen products are supposed to afford. So a SPF of 25 claims that you can stay safely in the sunshine for 25 times longer than if you had not applied the sunscreen.

However, there are two glaring problems with reliance on the SPF standard, Dr. Epstein warns.

First, swimming and sweating sharply reduce the effectiveness of sunscreens, so they must be applied repeatedly during exposure to sun. How many people actually do this? Second, the SPF number labeled on sunscreens is determined by laboratory tests based on an internationally agreed application rate. However, most people use only a fraction of the required amount—between 10 and 75 percent of the lab test quantity—which renders the listed SPF number meaningless and ineffective.

All this means that people using sunscreens are encouraged to remain in the sun far longer than is safe. This is the reason why, since 1975, the incidence of malignant melanoma has increased by about 200 percent in white men and women, and its mortality has increased by about 10 percent. Dark skinned races are largely protected by pigment, known as melanin, which largely blocks long-wave ultraviolet radiation.

Dr. Epstein cautions that another major and generally unrecognized problem with sunscreens is due to their undisclosed toxic ingredients.

As detailed in Dr. Epstein's most recent book, "Toxic Beauty," (BenBella Books) sunscreen products contain unlabeled dangerous ingredients. These products are also labeled with false and misleading promises about their effectiveness, such as 'all-day protection' and 'blocks all harmful rays.'

Apart from these concerns, he warns, the following common sunscreen ingredients pose toxic effects:

- Benzophenone is a "hormone disrupter" which mimics natural hormones produced by the endocrine system. It is also an allergen, causing allergic reactions, and a "penetration enhancer," which penetrates the skin, and is absorbed into the bloodstream and invades body wide organs.
- Octyl-methoxycinnamate is also a hormone disrupter and penetration enhancer which has been detected in breast milk.
- Oxybenzone, another hormone disrupter, has also been detected in breast milk.
- Parabens are still other hormone disrupters.

These ingredients pose further dangers. Once absorbed through the skin, they generate what are known as "free radicals." "These accelerate skin damage and skin aging, along with sharply increased risks of skin cancer," Dr. Epstein warns.

Some of these ingredients also pose unrelated threats. Once washed off sunbather's bodies, oxybenzone accumulates in sea life and damages their reproductive systems. In 2006, it was found that oxybenzone had transformed the males of coastal fish near California beaches into feminized fish with ovarian tissue.

"Now that you've heard the bad news, you're probably wondering how you can protect your children and yourself from harm," says Dr. Epstein. "Sunblocks containing zinc oxide and titanium dioxide offer protection as they block long-wave ultraviolet light by reflecting the radiation off the skin's surface."

"But beware of recently developed sunblocks," he cautions. "These contains nanoparticles, a technological innovation which reduces ingredient particles to an ultramicroscopic size. These then readily penetrate the skin, invade the blood stream, and pose major toxic threats to distant organs such as liver and bone."

"Fortunately," Dr. Epstein advises, "a new generation of sun-protective natural organic ingredients is on the horizon. These range from SoyScreen, a 'green' sunscreen, based on ferulic acid and soybean oil, to sulforaphane, a broccoli ingredient that significantly reduces ultraviolet light damage."

Until these new natural ingredients, and products based on them, reach consumers and the marketplace, the best advice for self-protection is to limit exposure to the sun, says Dr. Epstein, who asks us to remember the old saying, "Only mad dogs and Englishmen go out in the mid-day sun."

Also, he advises, make sure your children stay in the shade, wear hats, and also special new light sunscreen protective clothing marketed by Solumbra.

Under the explicit provisions of the 1938 Federal Food, Drug and Cosmetic Act, it is anticipated that Dr. Margaret Hamburg, the newly appointed FDA Commissioner and inspiring public health advocate, will prohibit the sale of sunscreens containing toxic ingredients, and also sunblocks based on nanoparticles.

September 4, 2009

The National Cancer Institute Should Delay Its Collaboration with Love/Avon

In August 2009, the National Cancer Institute's (NCI) Cancer Biomedical Informatics Grid (caBIG) and the Love/Avon Army of Women announced that they intended to collaborate. Their objective is to develop a computerized initiative to recruit and study women is order to improve the prevention, diagnosis, and treatment of breast cancer. What could be a more important and worthy objective?

Dr. Susan Love is a well-known and leading national breast cancer surgeon. The Avon Foundation is a non-profit organization of Avon Products, a leading global beauty company. Avon is the world's largest direct seller, which markets to women in over 100 countries through independent sales representatives.

Relating to a November 2008 prominent advertisement by Avon Products in *The New York Times*, I identified a wide range of toxic ingredients in their products:

- Benzophenone-1 (hormonal and penetration enhancer) in Nail Experts Nail Brightener.
- Methylparaben (hormonal), ethylparaben (hormonal), and imidazolidinyl urea (cancer precursor) in Wash-Off Waterproof Mascara.
- Ceteareth-20 (cancer precursor), and disodium EDTA (penetration enhancer) in Advance Techniques Body Building Conditioner.
- PEG-80 sorbitan laurate, and PEG-10 rapeseed sterol (cancer precursors) in Anew Beauty Youth-Awakening Lipstick.

I communicated these disturbing concerns to Avon's Chief Scientific Officer. However, she responded dismissively.

I then informed Dr. Love of these concerns. She replied reassuringly, but non-responsively, to the effect that this information "could be used for future research by Love/Avon."

However, and of major concern, is persuasive evidence that has accumulated over the last decade, that parabens are readily absorbed through the skin, and that they pose powerful hormonal or estrogenic effects even at very low concentrations. Parabens have shown to be readily absorbed through the skin of immature female rodents, and to stimulate premature uterine growth. Parabens have also been shown to stimulate the growth of breast cancer cells in laboratory tests, and incriminated as possible causes of breast cancer.

In should be further stressed that parabens are the commonest of all ingredients in cosmetics and personal care products. As disturbingly, it has been estimated that women are exposed to high levels, as much as 50 milligrams of parabens daily, from cosmetics and personal care products.

Of additional and generally unrecognized concern is that other ingredients, benzophenone, and EDTA, are "penetration enhancers." These facilitate their own absorption, and that of other toxic ingredients in any product, deeply through the skin.

These longstanding public health concerns have been further strengthened by an August 2009 publication in the *Journal of Clinical Oncology*. This warned of the dangers of unknowing exposures, and risks of "estrogenically active compounds" in women using moisturizing creams containing hormonal ingredients.

Based on these considerations, the NCI should insist that Avon reformulate its products to phase out all toxic ingredients and replace them by safe alternatives before proceeding with this important initiative. If Avon is unwilling to do this, the NCI should terminate its relationship with the Love/Avon initiative.

September 15, 2009

Response to Dr. Susan Love's Post on Breast Cancer

Dr. Susan Love is a distinguished breast cancer surgeon who works in close collaboration with the giant Avon cosmetics and personal care products company. Candidly, she claims no expertise for scientific qualifications on the causes and prevention of breast cancer. Nevertheless, in her September 5, 2009 posting, she challenges explicit evidence on the carcinogenicity and hormonal toxicity of ingredients in Avon cosmetics and personal care products, as detailed in my December 18, 2008 e-mail to her.

The great majority of carcinogens, including those in Avon products, have been identified in standard feeding tests in mice and rats by the federal National Toxicology Program (NTP). The results of these tests have been published by the NTP and accepted by the independent scientific community, and federal regulatory agencies, besides by the International Agency for Research on Cancer (IARC).

The scientific evidence on toxic hormonal effects of ingredients in cosmetics and personal care products is based on laboratory tests, and also tests on pregnant rodents. The validity of these tests has also been recognized by Breast Cancer Action, besides other breast cancer activist groups nationwide.

Reflecting this undeniable evidence, it is anticipated that the National Cancer Institute, under its new director, Dr. John Niederhuber, will terminate its prior partnership with the Love/Avon initiative.

September 30, 2009

Talcum Powder: The Hidden Dangers

You've probably used it, or had it sprinkled on you at some time in your life. It's processed from a soft mineral compound of magnesium silicate and is called talcum powder, or just talc.

Talcum powder is manufactured by Johnson & Johnson, among others, and is widely available in drug stores. Women have been persuaded by years of advertisements to dust themselves with talcum powder to mask alleged genital odors.

While the powder has been a symbol of freshness and cleanliness for over five decades, genital talc dusting is a dangerous, but avoidable, cause of ovarian cancer, warns Dr. Samuel S. Epstein, chairman of the Cancer Prevention Coalition.

The first warning of the dangers of genital talc dusting came in a 1971 report on the identification of talc particles in ovarian cancers, a finding sharply contested by Dr. G.Y. Hildick-Smith, who was then Johnson & Johnson's medical director.

A subsequent publication in the prestigious medical journal The Lancet warned that, "The potentially harmful effects of talc . . . in the ovary . . . should not be ignored." This warning was confirmed in a 1992 article in the journal Obstetrics & Gynecology which reported that a woman's frequent talc use on her genitals increased her risk of ovarian cancer by threefold. The talc in question was simple brand or generic "baby powder."

After the 1992 report, at least a dozen other major scientific articles documenting the link between talc and ovarian cancer appeared in leading medical journals such as Cancer, The Lancet, and Oncology. The capstone of this research against talc came in 2003 when the journal Anticancer Research published a 'meta-analysis,' or large scale review, of 16 previous published studies involving 11,933 women. A 33 percent increased risk of ovarian cancer was confirmed, Dr. Epstein points out.

"Not surprisingly," says Dr. Epstein, "the mortality of ovarian cancer in women 65 years of age and older has escalated sharply, especially in black women who have a higher rate of talc use than other races." Nearly 16,000 women in the U.S. die from ovarian cancer each year, which means it is the fourth most common fatal cancer in women. By some estimates, one out of five women regularly applies talc to her genitals. This usage occurs either through direct application, or as a result of tampons, sanitary pads and diaphragms that have been dusted with talc, Dr. Epstein points out.

More acknowledgment of talc's dangers emerged, even from the cosmetics industry. The president of the industry's Cosmetic Toiletry and Fragrance Association, Edward Kavanaugh, conceded in 2002 that talc is toxic and "can reach the human ovaries."

Yet, says Dr. Epstein, "inexplicably, talc manufacturers failed to warn women that the product could be dangerous to their health."

Nor has the Food and Drug Administration (FDA) shown even casual concern about the dangers of talc. The closest admission to this effect came in 1993 when the acting associate commissioner for legislative affairs of the Department of Health and Human Services admitted, "We are aware that there have been reports in the medical literature between frequent female perineal talc dusting over a protracted period of years, and an incremental increase in the statistical odds of subsequent development of certain ovarian cancers."

Dr. Epstein says he was amazed when this official went on to say the FDA "is not considering to ban, restrict or require a warning statement on the label of talc containing products." Aware of talc's extreme dangers and alarmed by continued governmental unresponsiveness, in 1994 the Cancer Prevention Coalition, supported by the New York Center for Constitutional Rights, submitted a Citizen's Petition to the FDA.

This petition requested that talc genital dusting powder be labeled with an explicit warning of the major risks of ovarian cancer. However, says Dr. Epstein, the FDA denied the petition. In May 2008, the Cancer Prevention Coalition submitted another Citizen's Petition to the FDA. This one was endorsed by a range of groups including the Organic Consumers Association, the International Association for Humanitarian Medicine, and Dr. Faye Williams of the National Congress of Black Women.

"We cited new scientific evidence on the dangers of talc, and requested the FDA to mandate that all talc products be labeled with this type of warning: "Frequent application of talcum powder in the female genital area substantially increases the risk of ovarian cancer," Dr. Epstein says.

However, Andrew von Eschenbach, M.D., then Commissioner of the FDA, failed to respond to this petition.

It is anticipated that Margaret Hamburg, M.D., the highly respected new FDA Commissioner, will take prompt regulatory action to protect unsuspecting women from the extreme dangers of talc.

October 6, 2009

Cancer: The Health Risk behind the Cosmeceutical Mask

Anti-aging skin products are known as cosmeceuticals, as they overlap the distinction between cosmetics and pharmaceuticals. These products are the fastest growing sales sector of the entire cosmetics industry, and are widely marketed as being safe. But Cancer Prevention Coalition Chairman Dr. Samuel S. Epstein warns that altering the physical structure of skin with chemicals to look more youthful comes at a hidden price to the skin, and even more so to overall health.

The term cosmeceutical, applied to anti-wrinkle and anti-aging creams, was first adopted by the cosmetics industry in 1984. It was developed as a way to avoid subjecting the industry's claims to the authority of the Food and Drug Administration (FDA). The idea was to create a new category of products that did more than just improve the appearance of the skin, yet do somewhat less than pharmaceutical drugs.

But Dr. Epstein wants to alert consumers to the dangers of cosmeceuticals, including the increased risk of skin cancer.

In addition, he is urging the new FDA Commissioner Margaret Hamburg, M.D. to take "appropriate regulatory action to protect the unsuspecting public from the dangers of cosmeceuticals."

Here is what we know of the overwhelming majority of cosmeceuticals, says Dr. Epstein, based on toxicology and clinical testing.

To increase the permeability of skin, hydroxy acids are widely sold on store shelves and used in cosmetic salons. Both alpha-hydroxy acids (AHA), and beta-hydroxy acids (BHA) are common ingredients in cosmeceuticals.

Worse still, Dr. Epstein warns, AHAs are used in an estimated 5 percent of all products without any labeling to this effect.

Even the industry's Cosmetics Ingredient Review Compendium has admitted that these ingredients strip the skin of its protective surface, which absorbs long-wave ultraviolet radiation from sunlight and tanning salons.

Apart from increased risks of sunburn, exposure to AHAs also increases risks of a dangerous skin cancer, known as malignant melanoma. Although it is one of the less common types of skin cancer, malignant melanoma is responsible for roughly 75 percent of all skin cancer-related deaths.

Reacting to these concerns, in 1992 the FDA issued a consumer warning that products containing these ingredients "could destroy the upper layers of skin, causing severe burns, swelling and pain." However, the FDA took no regulatory action to protect consumers, and the agency still has taken no regulatory action, Dr. Epstein points out.

Bisabolol is another cosmeceutical ingredient which strips off the surface layers of skin. This chemical is also a penetration enhancer, meaning that it increases the absorption of cosmeceutical ingredients through the skin.

Limonene is also a common ingredient in anti-aging products. "Apart from being an irritant, it is a well documented carcinogen," says Dr. Epstein.

Parabens are commonly added to cosmeceuticals as preservatives. However, Dr. Epstein cautions consumers that even when tested at low concentrations on the skin of pregnant rodents, parabens induce toxic hormonal effects in male embryos and infants.

"Nano-particles are more recent and ultra-dangerous ingredients in cosmeceuticals, particularly anti-wrinkle creams," warns Dr. Epstein. "By reducing the size of ingredients to the ultra-microscopic scale, they penetrate readily and deeply through the skin into the blood and organs all over the body."

"Ninety percent of all cosmetics sold in the world today are probably cosmeceuticals," says Dr. Albert Kligman, the dermatologist who first coined the term, in a 2005 interview with the journal Dermatologic Surgery.

"The terminology regarding the distinction between cosmetics and drugs is a marketing game in the U.S.," Kilgman said. "If you reverse aging, you are a drug. If you smooth skin, you are a cosmetic. Categorization depends more on the language on the bottle rather than the product in the bottle."

Dr. Epstein says, "These statements raise troubling concerns regarding the identity and safety of ingredients in cosmeceutical products. So many women, and even some men, slather these products all over their skin, the largest body organ, in the naïve belief that they have nothing to fear but aging."

"The industry markets cosmeceuticals with anecdotal or even wild claims of effectiveness, rather than scientific data, and with reckless disregard for safety," Dr. Epstein cautions.

He points to a 2007 warning from the respected Mayo Clinic that cosmeceuticals have rarely been tested for safety, and also that they may contain "powerful active ingredients that can affect biological processes."

Cosmeceutical manufacturers "make a calculated decision not to make claims that will result in scrutiny by the U.S. Food and Drug Administration of the product as a drug," stated Dr. Mary P. Lupo of the Tulane University School of Medicine in a 2005 issue of Dermatologic Surgery. "Clinical testing could also draw the attention of the FDA, so some manufacturers opt instead to allow the consumer arena to become the test market."

"So there you have it!" Dr. Epstein says, "People who use cosmeceuticals are guinea pigs in reckless and self-serving industry experiments to test whether these products are safe for human health. This should be a loud siren wakeup warning for anyone who still believes that these products have been tested for toxicity by the industry, and approved by the FDA."

In spite of these disturbing concerns, dermatologist Dr. Nicholas Perricone, author of three New York Times best selling books, is an active proponent of a "Men's Skin Care Line," his patented product based on nanoparticles.

Apart from the ineffectiveness of the great majority of cosmeceutical products, most are highly priced. In 2006, Consumer Reports magazine evaluated anti-wrinkle creams on the market, and concluded there was no correlation between price and possible effectiveness. "The best advice is prevent those wrinkles in the first place," read the review. "Stay out of the sun and don't smoke."

Dr. Epstein says that the cosmeceutical product Restylane is an exception to his warnings. "This Swedish anti-wrinkling agent is based on the natural ingredient hyaluronic acid, one of the very few scientifically proven safe and effective cosmeceuticals," he says.

Besides Botox injections, which have been on the market long enough to be accepted as safe, there are emerging green alternatives to the wide range of conventional anti-aging products now on store shelves.

Dr. Epstein says these include natural botanicals, such as date palm oil, which have been found to be safe and effective for certain types of wrinkles, and topical green tea cream, which has proven effective for treating sun damaged skin.

Dr. Epstein anticipates that Dr. Hamburg, the highly respected new FDA Commissioner, will take appropriate regulatory action to protect the unsuspecting public from the dangers of cosmeceuticals.

October 6, 2009

Personal Care Products Pose Unrecognized Toxic Risks to Children

Why has the incidence of childhood cancers increased by about 40 percent over the past three decades? Could it have anything to do with the cancer causing (carcinogenic) ingredients in personal care products targeting infants and children which have crowded supermarket and other store shelves over the same period?

Most of us would like to believe that any products, especially those marketed for infants and children, must be safe or they would never be sold. Surely, the Food and Drug Administration (FDA), the responsible agency of government, besides the industry concerned, must be looking out for the health of our most vulnerable citizens. Right? Wrong!

In fact, babies are about 100 times more sensitive to carcinogens than adults. Infants and young children have immature liver enzymes, which give them only limited ability to detoxify the carcinogens and other toxic ingredients in products which are applied to their skin.

Also, as children's cells divide much more rapidly than those of adults, they are much more sensitive to carcinogens, and more vulnerable to developing cancer later in their lives.

Added to all of that is the fact that the ingredients in the products we apply to the skin of our infants and children are readily absorbed into their bodies. Also, they are retained for much longer than any chemicals absorbed from food or from the air.

So, there is every reason why we should be highly cautious about the personal care products that we buy for our children.

As detailed in my new book, *Toxic Beauty*, most of the infant and childhood products on the market are dangerous. They pose a threat to our children's lifetime health.

Worse still, that threat begins even before birth. Once a pregnant woman absorbs ingredients from the cosmetics and personal care products that she uses, they penetrate through her skin to varying degrees. They then reach the fetus through the approximately 300 quarts of blood pumped daily between the placenta and fetus.

Studies on umbilical and blood cord samples have identified antibacterial ingredients, such as triclosan, often added to deodorants, toothpaste, and cosmetics. Based on rodent tests, triclosan has also been shown to have toxic effects on liver enzymes.

These umbilical and blood cord studies have also identified hormonal ingredients such as phthalates, which are used as solvents in perfumes, lotions and other cosmetics.

Of major concern, exposure to some phthalates has been shown to disturb the hormonal and sexual development of boys, even at relatively low levels.

University of Liverpool toxico-pathologist Dr. Vyvyan Howard describes the significance of these findings for the fetal stage of life, warning, "Changes occur at exposure levels thousands of times lower than the safety limits that were set a few years ago."

"New studies show that many bulk chemicals that we thought were safe are actually biologically active and disrupt human systems. They don't work by having an acute toxicity effect. They work by hijacking development in the uterus. These chemicals can disrupt important cell signaling functions in the developing body," Dr. Howard says.

Once a child is born, this susceptibility to hormonal ingredients in cosmetics and personal care products persists. One of the biggest culprits, incriminated for disrupting sex hormones in boys, is Bisphenol-A (BPA). This is a plasticizer which mimics the effects of the hormone estrogen, and is a common ingredient in cosmetics and personal care products.

Males, both human and rodent, have been shown to be more sensitive to these hormonal ingredients than females. Male rodents exposed to BPA and other related ingredients have developed testicular atrophy, undescended or absent testes, infertility, an absent or malformed prostate and seminal vesicles, and also cancer. Decreased sperm production and a decrease in the distance between the anus and genitals in infant boys have also been documented over the past few decades.

Women are also adversely affected by exposure to BPA. Tests on rodents, as reported in the journal "Reproductive Toxicology" and elsewhere, have revealed that BPA may be responsible for reproductive disorders later in life, decades after their exposure to the chemical in the womb or as infants.

We know that babies being born today have elevated levels of hormonal phthalates in their bodies. A 2008 study in the journal "Pediatrics" confirmed this by testing the urine of babies who had just been shampooed, lotioned or powdered with brand-name baby products. Similar results came from studies done by the U.S. Centers for Disease Control and Prevention.

Based on this disturbing data, in 2008 Health Canada ruled that BPA is a toxic ingredient. However, no such warning has yet come from the U.S. Food and Drug Administration.

Besides toxic hormonal effects, there are other dangers posed by products marketed for infants and children. Here are a few examples:

— Allergens such as benzyl alcohol and lanolin commonly appear.
— Carcinogens such as formaldehyde appears when product ingredients DMDM Hydantoin and Quaternium-15 break down
— Carcinogens found in shampoos and conditioners include the laureths as well as dioxane and ethylene oxide.
— Penetration enhancer ingredients that drive other ingredients deeper through the skin into the body are common. These include sodium lauryl sulfate and EDTA.

Nevertheless, the mainstream cosmetics industry continues to insist that none of their products are harmful, as their levels of toxic ingredients are claimed to be too low to pose any dangers.

Even if this were true, it's a flawed argument. It ignores how infants and children are subjected to multiple assaults of multiple toxic ingredients from a wide range of personal care products applied to their skin each day.

Importantly, we must consider the additive and multiplistic effects of all these chemicals interacting together.

Safe skin products for infants and children are now increasingly available on store shelves for responsible parents. These include USDA certified organic products. These leading products are detailed in the 2009 *Toxic Beauty* book.

Additionally, the Environmental Working Group maintains a database atwww.cosmeticsdatabase.com/special/parents guide/ which provides information on toxic ingredients in children's products, and on safer products.

Under the explicit provisions of the 1938 Federal Food, Drug and Cosmetic Act, it is anticipated that Dr. Margaret Hamburg, the newly appointed FDA Commissioner and inspiring public health advocate, will prohibit the sale of toxic personal care products for children.

October 8, 2009

Unrecognized Cancer and Hormonal Risks of Avon Products

Chairman of the Cancer Prevention Coalition, Dr. Samuel Epstein, is warning women that toxic ingredients in Avon Products put users at risk of cancer and hormonal changes.

For this reason, Dr. Epstein is urging the National Cancer Institute to terminate plans for a joint project with Avon until the company reformulates its products to replace all toxic ingredients with safe alternatives.

A class of ingredients in Avon products, parabens, has been shown to stimulate the growth of breast cancer cells in laboratory tests and parabens have been identified as possible causes of breast cancer, Dr. Epstein points out.

Used as preservatives, parabens mimic the hormone estrogen, which is known to play a role in the development of breast cancers.

Dr. Epstein is concerned about cancer-causing ingredients in all cosmetics and personal care products, but he is particularly concerned about Avon Products because of a newly announced collaboration with the National Cancer Institute, a U.S. government agency.

In August 2009, the National Cancer Institute's (NCI) Cancer Biomedical Informatics Grid (caBIG) and the Love/Avon Army of Women announced that they intend to collaborate. Their objective is to develop a computerized initiative to recruit and study women in order to improve the prevention, diagnosis, and treatment of breast cancer.

Dr. Epstein acknowledges that this is an "important and worthy objective."

Dr. Susan Love is a well-known and leading national breast cancer surgeon. The Avon Foundation is a non-profit organization of Avon Products, a leading global beauty company. Avon is the world's largest direct seller and markets to women in over 100 countries through independent sales representatives.

Relating to a prominent advertisement by Avon Products in a November 2008 issue of The New York Times, Dr. Epstein identified a wide range of toxic ingredients in their products:

- Benzophenone-1 (hormonal and penetration enhancer) in Nail Experts Nail Brightener.
- Methylparaben (hormonal), ethylparaben (hormonal), and imidazolidinyl urea (cancer precursor) in Wash-Off Waterproof Mascara.
- Ceteareth-20 (cancer precursor), and disodium EDTA (penetration enhancer) in Advance Techniques Body Building Conditioner.
- PEG-80 sorbitan laurate, and PEG-10 rapeseed sterol (cancer precursors) in Anew Beauty Youth-Awakening Lipstick.

"I communicated these disturbing concerns to Avon's chief scientific officer. However, she responded dismissively," Dr. Epstein said.

Dr. Epstein then informed Dr. Love of these concerns. She replied reassuringly, but non-responsively, to the effect that this information "could be used for future research by Love/Avon."

However, and of major concern, says Dr. Epstein, is persuasive evidence that has accumulated over the last decade, that parabens are readily absorbed through the skin, and that they pose powerful hormonal or estrogenic effects even at very low concentrations.

Parabens have shown to be readily absorbed through the skin of immature female rodents, and to stimulate premature uterine growth, Dr. Epstein observes.

Parabens have also been shown to stimulate the growth of breast cancer cells in laboratory tests, and incriminated as possible causes of breast cancer, he warns.

Dr. Epstein stresses that parabens are the commonest of all ingredients in cosmetics and personal care products. "As disturbingly, it has been estimated that women are exposed to high levels, as much as 50 milligrams of parabens daily, from cosmetics and personal care products," he points out.

An article in the September 10, 2009, issue of the *Journal of Clinical Oncology* indicates that breast cancer patients may unknowingly be dosing themselves with estrogen by using topical moisturizers. The researchers report that the estrogenically active substances found in laboratory tests of 16 moisturizers were not mentioned in the product ingredient lists. The moisturizers tested were not identified by brand name.

Of additional and generally unrecognized concern is that other ingredients in Avon products, benzophenone, and EDTA, are "penetration enhancers." These facilitate their own absorption, and that of other toxic ingredients in any product, deeply through the skin.

Based on these considerations, Dr. Epstein is urging the National Cancer Institute to "insist that Avon reformulate its products to phase out all toxic ingredients and replace them by safe alternatives" before proceeding with the computerized initiative to recruit and study women to improve breast cancer prevention, diagnosis, and treatment.

If Avon is unwilling to do this, the NCI should terminate its relationship with the Love/Avon initiative, Dr. Epstein says.

The Cancer Prevention Coalition has written to Dr. John E. Niederhuber, the director of the National Cancer Institute, detailing and warning of the risk of cancer, and other risks of Avon cosmetics and personal care products.

Dr. Epstein says products containing these toxic ingredients could be subject to the Food and Drug Administration's Black Box warning as required by the 1938 Federal Food, Drug, and Cosmetic Act.

October 8, 2009

Anti-Aging Creams "Increase Cancer Risk"

Many products claiming to rid skin of wrinkles and fine lines actually strip away the protective top layer and leave it vulnerable to sun damage and dangerous toxins, according to Dr Sam Epstein, chairman of the US Cancer Prevention Coalition.

He said the active ingredient alpha-hydroxy acids (AHAs), found in many leading brands of face cream, were "probably the most dangerous cosmetic products on the market."

Dr Epstein is campaigning for the creams to be regulated in the US and has urged British consumers to be aware of the health risks.

"So many women, and even some men, slather these products all over their skin in the naive belief that they have nothing to fear but ageing," he told the Daily Express.

In Britain there is no requirement for a warning to be placed on creams containing AHAs, but the alleged dangers have already been recognized in the US.

The US Food and Drug Administration has warned consumers that AHAs "could destroy the upper layers of skin, causing severe burns, swelling and pain."

Dr Epstein, who is Professor emeritus of environmental and occupational health at the University of Illinois, added: "Anything that strips the surface of the skin not only risks sunlight penetrating the exposed layer but also allows other toxic products in.

"All of the toxic effects are massively increased by AHAs."

Exposure to the sun's harmful rays can cause skin cancer.

Dr Epstein also expressed concern about other ingredients commonly used in anti-ageing products, such as limonene. "Apart from being an irritant, it is a well documented carcinogen," he said.

Britons spend £673million a year on skin care products, with 42 percent of all moisturizers claiming to combat ageing.

A spokeswoman for the Cosmetics, Toiletries and Perfumeries Association, told the Daily Express that cosmetic firms were not required to warn consumers if their products contained AHAs but only if they contained these ingredients at such high levels they could be dangerous.

She added: "There is a legal requirement for these products to be safe."

November 17, 2009

U.K. Leads the Way in Banning Toxic Ingredients in Cosmetics and Personal Care Products

The Cancer Prevention Coalition commends the UK's largest nationwide chain of health food shops, Holland & Barrett, for its recently announced ban on beauty products containing some toxic ingredients, but warns that products containing a wide range other toxic ingredients remain on the shelves.

On October 6th, Holland & Barrett announced that it would "ban hundreds of leading beauty products over claims they contain toxic ingredients" in their 525 stores nationwide.

Holland & Barrett announced that they have been working over the past year behind the scenes with suppliers to eliminate the use of these chemicals. As a result, they decided to reject certain well-known brands from their stores and reformulate all their own label products.

The main ingredients of concern to Holland & Barrett in this ban are a group of hormonal preservatives known as parabens, and an unrelated harsh detergent known as sodium lauryl sulfate.

Holland & Barrett has additional stores in the Republic of Ireland, in South Africa and in The Netherlands, where they use the trade name "De Tuinen."

Holland & Barrett is the first UK company to take this action, but it is not alone.

In mid-October, the giant retailer Morrisons, one of the nation's leading supermarket chains with over 400 stores, announced that it would shortly review concerns regarding the dangers of parabens.

Cancer Prevention Coalition Chairman Samuel S. Epstein, M.D. warns that numerous published scientific studies over the last two decades have shown that the parabens—methyl, ethyl, propyl, butyl, and benzyl—pose toxic estrogen-like effects.

"These vary widely, from the most potent, butyl, which is hormonal at levels 100,000 times lower than natural estrogen, to the less potent methyl," Dr. Epstein says.

"Parabens readily penetrate the skin of immature female rodents, from where they can pass directly into the blood, and stimulate premature uterine growth," he explains. "Even at very low concentrations, parabens have also been shown to stimulate the growth of estrogen-sensitive breast cancer cells in laboratory tests," Dr. Epstein emphasizes. "Of additional concern, administering parabens to immature male rats decreases their sperm counts and testosterone levels." "Parabens have been identified in the breast tissue of a woman with breast cancer, presumably originating from its presence in a product used as an underarm deodorant or antiperspirant," he cautions, saying, "This incriminates parabens as a possible cause of breast cancer."

Sodium lauryl sulfate is a well-known harsh detergent and a penetration enhancer. Dr. Epstein explains that this chemical damages the superficial layers of the skin and causes prolonged damage to the skin barrier. This allows the ready penetration of carcinogens and other toxic ingredients in cosmetics and personal care products through the skin.

Evidence on the danger of parabens and sodium lauryl sulfate is still denied in the Cosmetic Ingredients Review's annual U.S. Compendium. This document details the industry's claims on the safety of about 1,470 ingredients listed on the labels of cosmetic and personal care products, including parabens and sodium lauryl sulfate.

These two ingredients continue to be claimed "safe" in the 2009 Cosmetic Ingredients Review Compendium, an annual publication of The Personal Care Products Council, formerly The Cosmetic Toiletry and Fragrance Association.

The Council also assures that all products that U.S. consumers buy are safe, and under control. This reassurance remains in the Council's 2009 annual Cosmetic Ingredient Review Compendium.

Dr. Epstein cautions that the Council maintains dozens of full-time lobbyists at the federal and state levels, and pursues an aggressive political agenda against what it considers to be "unreasonable or unnecessary labeling or warning requirements."

"Holland & Barrett is to be commended for its initiative in phasing out parabens and sodium lauryl sulfate," says Dr. Epstein. "However, the company appears strangely unaware of other toxic ingredients. These include a wide range of other hormonal ingredients, such as phthalates and bisphenol, besides a still wider range of carcinogens."

January 12, 2010

Unrecognized Risks of Perricone MD Skin Care Products

The use of nanoparticles in personal care products known as cosmeceuticals poses a generally unrecognized but major public health hazard, warns the Cancer Prevention Coalition. "Nanoparticles, less than 1/10,000 of a millimeter in size, readily penetrate skin, and can invade underlying blood vessels and produce body-wide toxic effects, including brain degenerative disorders, and nerve damage," stresses CPC Chairman Dr. Samuel S. Epstein.

Based on a January 6, 2010 Skin Deep report by the Environmental Working Group, at least 7 of 26 of Dr. Perricone skin products were found to contain nanoparticles, while a total of 25 contain a wide range of other toxic ingredients.

These include carcinogens such as acrylamide, and carcinogenic contaminants such as ethylene oxide, dioxane, nitrosamines and acrylamide, and formaldehyde, Dr. Epstein emphasizes. They also include allergens, and toxic hormonal ingredients. Accordingly, the Environmental Working Group rated 25 of Perricone's products as posing "moderate to high hazards."

Yet, Dr. Nicholas Perricone posted a full page ad on his Cold Plasma product in the December 26, 2009 New York Times Magazine. The ad promised that the product, "gives skin everything it needs," and "works better for skin than anything else ever used."

Dr. Perricone's products, known technically as "cosmeceuticals," promise to rejuvenate wrinkling or sagging skin in aging women.

According to his website, Dr. Perricone is noted for his "holistic approach to aging," and developing a program that "will enhance your life with better overall health and increased energy."

However, Dr. Epstein warns, "His claims are baseless as they are made in the absence of scientific evidence based on double-blind clinical trials." In these, patients are randomly assigned to groups which receive either the test treatment or an alternative untreated control. Neither the patient, nor the dermatologist conducting the study, know whether the treatment or the control has been given to the patient until the trial is completed. This is the standard way of excluding bias or frank misrepresentation.

As detailed in Dr. Epstein's 2009 book Toxic Beauty (BenBella Books, 2009), Perricone's website states, "Dr. Perricone has developed a patented technology excusive to this line, called Fullerene. Fullerenes are highly stable, microscopic hollow spheres that carry the active ingredients into the skin. They bring the intriguing and transformative world of nanotechnology to the fine art and science of high performance skin care."

But these nanoparticles are extremely dangerous and products containing them should be banned, demands Dr. Epstein. "The ultramicroscopic Fullerenes, also known as nanoparticles, have been introduced without any labeling into a growing number of Dr. Perricone's anti-aging products, particularly skin creams and Ceramic Eye Smoother. These are touted as reducing wrinkles and firming up the skin surface.

"Not surprisingly," Dr. Epstein says, "Dr. Perricone has failed to endorse the California's 2007 Campaign for Safe Cosmetics Act. This requires cosmetic companies to disclose all their toxic ingredients on a public website."

In May 2006, the Friends of the Earth, a global network of grassroots groups in 77 countries, published a report "Nanomaterials, Sunscreens and Cosmetics: Small Ingredients, Big Risks." They warned that it is time these high risks products were taken off the market. Two years later, a British Royal Commission report warned that products containing nanoparticles, pose especially high toxic risks.

In November 2009, Dr. Wickson, a researcher with a European Union project on consumer protection laws, raised critical concerns about nanoparticle products, and their environmental accumulation, saying, "In studies of toxicity and exposure, it is crucial to take into account the incredible persistence of carbon nanotubes, which represent one of the most biologically non-degradable man-made materials currently available." Dr. Wickson further warned that the body's response to nanoparticles is similar to that of asbestos.

Although Dr. Perricone touts his website as being the place where "you can get the information and inspiration you need to manage your looks, your health, your weight and your life," his cosmeceuticals are deceptively marketed as safe for the consumer. Nothing could be further from the truth.

March 24, 2010

The Dangers of Triclosan: A Common Anti-Bacterial Ingredient

Triclosan is an anti-bacterial ingredient in many cosmetics and personal-care products. These include nearly half of all commercial antibacterial liquid soaps, cleansers, deodorants, detergents, toothpastes, and mouthwashes.

Water testing studies by the U.S. Geological Survey have found that triclosan is among the top 10 persistent contaminants in U.S. rivers, streams, lakes, and underground aquifers. Of related concern, triclosan persists in the environment, accumulating as it passes up the food chain to our bodies, and contributes to reduced resistance to antibiotics.

Unexpected volatility has been documented when the triclosan in liquid soaps and other household products comes into contact with water, as would happen during common use. At Virginia Tech University, a team of researchers in April 2005 reported that some toothpastes and soaps create a chloroform gas when the triclosan in these products reacts with chlorinated tap water. Triclosan also interacts with free chlorine in tap water and degrades under sunlight to produce chloroform, which is both toxic and carcinogenic following inhalation or skin absorption, particularly while bathing in warm water.

Triclosan, has been shown to produce toxic hormonal effects, known as endocrine disruption, on the development of the thyroid gland in tadpoles, and on sex ratios and fin length in fish. Lab studies on rats have shown that triclosan is toxic to normal liver enzymes. In humans, this preservative has been linked to allergies, asthma, and eczema.

Of further concern, triclosan has been identified as a contaminant in umbilical cord samples collected by Greenpeace International and Britain's World Wifeline Fund. Furthermore, surveys in Sweden have also identified triclosan in the breast milk of 60 percent of women tested.

Based on these concerns, a 2005 advisory panel to the FDA concluded that triclosan posed "unacceptable health and environmental risks." However, the FDA still ignores this warning.

May 7, 2010

Protect Children's Health from Toxic BPA

Chairman of the Cancer Prevention Coalition, Samuel S. Epstein, M.D. is urging public support for the recently introduced Toxic Chemicals Safety Act of 2010, which establishes a program to review and protect children from risks of toxic exposures, including Bisphenol-A (BPA), a common contaminant in consumer goods.

On March 30 this year, Dr. Epstein points out, the Washington Post announced that the Environmental Protection Agency listed BPA as "a chemical of concern." The Post also noted that the U.S. Food and Drug Administration (FDA) previously expressed "concerns about the chemical's hormonal effect on human health." However, the American Chemistry Council claims "that BPA is not a risk to the environment at current low levels."

BPA is widely used in polycarbonate bottles, such as baby products, besides adult personal care and cosmetic products, food can linings, microwave oven dishes, dental sealants, and also medical devices.

Dr. Epstein says there are other recently recognized major sources of BPA such as cash register and credit-card receipts, which are coated with microscopic powdered BPA, and which many of us handle daily.

A 2007 review of about 700 studies on BPA, published in the journal Reproductive Toxicology, found that the fetus and infants are highly vulnerable to the toxic hormonal effects of this ingredient, technically known as "endocrine disruptive."

Dr. Epstein cites an accompanying study by National Institutes of Health researchers in the same journal, reported uterine damage in newborn rodents exposed to levels of BPA comparable with those of normal human exposure. "This finding may also implicate BPA as a cause of reproductive tract disorders in women, after their earlier exposure as fetuses or infants," he warns.

Previous studies in the journal Endocrinology, and elsewhere, reported that BPA masculinizes the brain of female mice and feminizes the brain of male mice. Toxic effects of this hormone disrupter in pregnant women are evidenced in their infant baby boys by the reduction in the normal distance between their anus and genitals. This decrease in anogenital distance is also associated with a decrease in sperm production.

Based on such evidence, Health Canada declared BPA to be a "toxic chemical" in early 2008.

In addition to these toxic effects, exposure of pregnant rodents to BPA, at levels 2,000 times lower than the Environmental Protection Agency's "safe dose," resulted in sexual abnormalities in their offspring. Dr. Epstein warns that these abnormalities include an increased number of "terminal end buds" in breast tissue, which are associated with a subsequent high risk of breast cancer. However, an American Plastics Council spokesman claimed that the human relevance of these findings is only "hypothetical."

Dr. Epstein warns that BPA has also been found in human blood, placental and fetal tissue, and incriminated as a predisposing factor for prostate cancer. "The authors of this study also linked endocrine-dependent human cancers, such as breast cancer, to the minimal levels of BPA to which pregnant women are exposed," he says.

An August 2, 2007, consensus statement by several dozen scientists warned that BPA, even at very low exposure levels, is probably responsible for many human reproductive disorders.

A September 2008 publication, Endocrine-Related Cancer, by Dr. Gail Prins reviewed the substantial scientific evidence on the toxic hormonal effects of BPA, besides other endocrine disruptive chemicals (EDCs) in pregnant women. She concluded that children are highly sensitive to their toxic effects, particularly subsequent risks of prostate cancer.

In October 2008, Science Daily reported on an article on BPA called "A Plastic World," in a then pending special section on Environmental Research. Two other articles reported that fetal exposure to BPA disrupted the normal development of the brain and behavior in rats and mice. Other articles have also reported that BPA is massively contaminating the oceans and harming aquatic wildlife.

The June 2009 Endocrine Disruption Act authorized the National Institute of Environmental Health Science "to coordinate" research on hormone disruption to prevent exposure to chemicals "that can undermine the development of children before they are born and cause lifelong impairment of their health and function."

This bill was supported by public health, consumer and children's advocacy groups, and further strengthened by California's Senator Dianne Feinstein's legislation to ban BPA from food and beverage containers. Of major relevance, this legislation has also been endorsed by the April 2010 President's Cancer Panel On "Reducing Environmental Cancer Risk: What We Can Do Now," 2008-2009 Annual Report. This report further warns that "to a disturbing extent, babies are born pre-polluted."

There are safe alternatives to BPA. As emphasized in the Dr. Sam Epstein's 2009 book Toxic Beauty, the recent development of "green chemistry" has encouraged the phase-out of product packaging that relies on petrochemical plastic containers, particularly those containing BPA. These containers are now being replaced with biodegradable substitutes, including recycled paper. Such "green" packaging reduces energy use, greenhouse gases, and non-degradable or poorly degradable wastes currently disposed of in landfills.

In January this year, the FDA announced an "Update on BPA," with particular reference to its use in food packaging, plastic baby bottles, feeding cups, and metal containers, to avoid childhood exposure. However, FDA has still not taken any regulatory action to this effect. Meanwhile, Dr. Epstein says, the industry's Cosmetic Ingredient Review Panel does not even make any reference to BPA in its annual "safety assessments."

On April 15, Congressmen Bobby Rush and Henry Waxman released a draft of the Toxic Chemicals Safety Act of 2010. The key provisions of this Act include establishment of a program to review and protect children from risks of toxic exposures, including BPA.

Dr. Epstein says, "The passage of this legislation is urgently needed in order to ban BPA from food packaging and other consumer products, especially to prevent any further childhood exposure."

ENDORSER:

Gail S. Prins, PhD
Professor of Physiology and Urology
University of Illinois at Chicago College of Medicine

June 16, 2010

Reckless Failure of the U.S. Food and Drug Administration to Protect against Cancer from Toxics in Cosmetics and GE Milk

The Cancer Prevention Coalition reminds the American public that the 1938 Federal Food Drug and Cosmetic Act explicitly stipulates: "Each ingredient used in a cosmetic product and each finished cosmetic product shall be adequately substantiated for safety prior to marketing."

In the absence of adequate evidence of safety, products must be conspicuously labeled on their principle display panel: "WARNING: THE SAFETY OF THIS PRODUCT HAS NOT BEEN DETERMINED." Furthermore, the Food and Drug Administration (FDA) is authorized to pursue enforcement action after a product containing dangerous ingredients has been marketed.

However, warns Samuel S. Epstein, M.D., Chairman of the Cancer Prevention Coalition, in spite of such explicit pre-and-post-marketing authority, the FDA has taken no regulatory action whatsoever over the last six decades, continuing until today, to protect the public from unknowing exposures to a wide range of toxic ingredients in cosmetic and personal care products. These include allergens, hormones, carcinogens and their precursors, and ultra-microscopic nanoparticles.

On November 17, 1994, the Cancer Prevention Coalition, the Ovarian Cancer Early Detection Prevention Foundation, and the Health and Medicine Policy Research Group filed a Citizens Petition to FDA Commissioner, David Kessler, M.D., on the dangers of talc, based on 17 scientific references dating back to the 1960's. These detailed evidence of major lethal risks of ovarian cancer, particularly in African-American women, from genital dusting with cosmetic grade talc. However, the Petition was rejected.

In May 2008, the Cancer Prevention Coalition, together with directors or representatives of six major national public health organizations, filed a further Petition to FDA Commissioner, Dr. Andrew von Eschenbach, based on additional more recent scientific evidence, "seeking a cancer warning on cosmetic talc products." However, the FDA was again unresponsive.

351

Not surprisingly, on September 10, 1997, Senator Kennedy warned that "the cosmetic industry has borrowed a page from the playbook of the tobacco industry." However, says Dr. Epstein, this is an understatement, as cigarette packs carry an explicit cancer warning, and smoking is uncommon until early adult life. In striking contrast, exposure to cosmetics and personal care products can be lifelong, following their use by pregnant women, and absorption of toxic ingredients through the skin, into the blood and then reaching the fetus.

On May 11, 2007, the Cancer Prevention Coalition, Organic Consumers Association, Family Farm Defenders, and Institute for Responsible Technology, filed a Citizens Petition to FDA Commissioner Andrew von Eschenbach, M.D., on the wide range of undisclosed dangers of genetically engineered bovine growth hormone, commonly known as rBGH, milk.

The Petition detailed the veterinary toxicity of rBGH. It also detailed the wide range of abnormalities in the composition of rBGH milk, particularly the 10-fold or more increased levels of a natural growth factor known as IGF-1, and its ready absorption from the small intestine into the blood; IGF-1 levels in milk are further increased by pasteurization.

"Drinking this milk results in major increased risks of colon, prostate, and breast cancers," Dr. Epstein emphasizes. "Increased IGF-1 levels also block natural defense mechanisms, known as apoptosis or programmed self-destruction, against early submicroscopic cancers. However, the FDA remains recklessly unresponsive to this Petition."

On January 12, 2010, the 2007 Citizen's Petition seeking the withdrawal of Posilac, the brand name under which rBGH is marketed, was re-filed to the current FDA Commissioner Margaret Hamburg, M.D. However, the FDA rejected this Petition, this time on the basis of alleged technical grounds, which had not been previously invoked.

"An even more recent example of FDA's irresponsibility," says Dr. Epstein, "has received prominent emphasis in the prestigious May 6, 2010 President's Cancer Panel (PCP) Report, with illustrative regard to bisphenol-A (BPA)." This ingredient is widely used as an unlabeled plasticizer in baby bottles and food containers, besides in cosmetics and personal care products.

The President's Cancer Panel explicitly warned that BPA "is a chemical of concern," and that "more than 30 studies have linked BPA to breast cancer, obesity, diabetes, and other disorders."

The President's Cancer Panel also summarily rejected, as "incomplete and unreliable," FDA's claims that bisphenol-A is safe, and the FDA's assertion "that neither a ban on the chemical or labeling of BPA-containing products was warranted."

Senator Frank Lautenberg's proposed "Safe Chemicals Act of 2010" would require manufacturers to provide information on "chemicals of concern" in consumer products. To say the least, this is timely, says Dr. Epstein. "Such information would provide the public with critical health and safety information on these products, especially as the FDA has failed to do so since passage of the 1938 Federal Food, Drug, and Cosmetic Act," he says. "Clearly, Congressional investigation and drastic reform of the FDA is decades overdue."

ENDORSERS:

Lennart Hardell, M.D., PhD
Professor, Department of Oncology
University Hospital
Orebro, Sweden

Vicente Navarro, M.D., PhD
Professor of Health Policy
The Johns Hopkins Medical Institutions

Janette D. Sherman, M.D.
Adjunct Professor Environmental Institute
Western Michigan University

Quentin D. Young, M.D.
Public Health Advocate, State of Illinois
Past President American Public Health Association
Chairman, Health and Medicine Policy Research Group

June 28, 2010

Reckless Self-Interest of the Fragrance Industry

People must be protected from exposure to fragrance ingredients that may cause cancer or fetal, hormonal or reproductive toxicity, the Cancer Prevention Coalition warned today. But federal agencies are not regulating these ingredients, leaving the public at risk due to the "recklessly irresponsible" behavior of the fragrance industry, says CPC Chairman Samuel S. Epstein, M.D.

Protection of the public would be implemented by passage of Senator Frank Lautenberg's Safe Chemicals Act of 2010, Dr. Epstein advises. This bill requires manufacturers to provide information on "chemicals of concern" in consumer products.

The bill would provide the public with information on the dangers of these products, especially, says Dr. Epstein, "as the U.S. Food and Drug Administration (FDA) has recklessly failed to do so since passage of the 1938 Federal Food, Drug, and Cosmetic Act."

Perfumes and fragrances are the single largest category of cosmetic and personal care products, especially products used on the hair, face, and eyes. These products represent nearly 50 percent of all prestige beauty dollars now spent in the United States. Fragrances are also extensively used in a wide range of everyday household cleaning products.

Exposure to toxic ingredients in cosmetics and personal care products is predominantly through the skin. In contrast, exposure to toxic ingredients in household cleaning products is predominantly through inhalation.

The FDA has direct authority under the terms of the 1938 Federal Food Drug and Cosmetic Act to regulate toxic ingredients in cosmetics and personal care products. However, seven decades later, it has still failed to do so. Similarly, the U.S. Environmental Protection Agency has also still failed to regulate these toxic ingredients in household cleaning products.

"In the disturbing absence of any federal regulations," Dr. Epstein says, the policies and practices of the cosmetics and personal care products industries are determined by its International Fragrance Association (IFRA). This is an international trade organization of over 100 perfume and fragrance manufacturers, representing fifteen regions including the U.S., Europe, South America, Australia, and the Far East."

The primary objective of IFRA is to protect the self-regulatory practices and policies of the industry by the development of a Code of Practices and safety guidelines, Dr. Epstein says. However, these include maintaining the "trade secret" status of perfume and fragrance ingredients, and pre-empting international legislative labeling and safety initiatives.

Of the more than 5,000 ingredients used in the fragrance industry, approximately 1,300 have so far been evaluated by the industry's International Research Institute for Fragrance Materials. This institute is a "non-profit" organization, created by IFRA in 1966 to conduct research and testing of fragrance ingredients.

"However," Dr. Epstein warns, "this testing is minimal and restricted to local effects on human skin, and short-term toxicity tests in rodents."

Evaluation of ingredient safety is then made by a board of toxicologists, pharmacologists, and dermatologists, identified by the institute as "independent" without disclosure of their qualifications, let alone conflicts of interest.

Their findings are presented to IFRA's Scientific Advisory Board, and then published in its trade journal, Food and Chemical Toxicology. The information reported in this journal is the basis on which IFRA formulates its own "safety guidelines." However, Dr. Epstein points out, due to the "trade secret" status of fragrances, manufacturers are still not required by the FDA to disclose their ingredients on product labels or in any other way.

"These ingredients include a wide range of allergens. They also include synthetic musks, particularly tonalide and galaxolide, designed to mimic natural scents derived from musk deer and ox," Dr. Epstein explains. "They are persistent and bioaccumulate in the body, have toxic hormonal effects, and have been identified in breast milk."

In 1973, in efforts at damage control, IFRA created a Code of Practice listing prohibited ingredients, based on its own safety analyses. This listing has been periodically updated.

In May 1999, in response to repeated complaints of respiratory, neurological, and other toxic effects following the use of Calvin Klein's Eternity perfume, the Environmental Health Network of California hired two testing laboratories to identify the ingredients in the perfume.

Analysis of these results by the Cancer Prevention Coalition, summarized in Dr. Epstein's 2009 book Toxic Beauty, reveal the following:

- 26 ingredients whose "Toxicological properties have not been investigated," or "toxicology properties have not been thoroughly investigated."
- 25 ingredients that are "Irritants."
- 5 ingredients that are "Skin sensitizers," or allergens.
- 3 ingredients that show "Fetal, hormonal, and reproductive toxicity."
- 2 ingredients that "May cause cancer."

In efforts at damage control, IFRA agreed that information on allergenic ingredients in perfumes like Eternity should be made available, but only on request from dermatologists, for diagnostic purposes. "This "Fragrance On-Call List" action denies the public its right to know," Dr. Epstein warns.

More disturbingly, Dr. Matthias Vey, president of IFRA, failed to respond to repeated warnings from August to October 2003 from the Cancer Prevention Coalition. These urged "all fragrance products be labeled to the effect that, apart from the absence of known skin and respiratory allergens, they contain no known carcinogens, gene damaging, hormonal, or otherwise toxic ingredients."

As reported in "What's That Smell," a June 2010 report by Women's Voices of the Earth, faced with continuing criticism of unresponsiveness, IFRA initiated a "compliance program" in 2007. "However," Dr. Epstein warns, "this is based on testing of a mere 50 fragranced products from the global market place to detect prohibited ingredients."

A fragrance may be restricted by IFRA on a variety of grounds. These include: use in products at higher-than-recommended concentrations, sensitization, photosensitization, phototoxicity, allergenicity, neurotoxicity, carcinogenicity, undefined biological effects, and inadequate data.

"This restriction, though, works better in theory than in practice," Dr. Epstein emphasizes. "There is no pre-approval process for ingredient safety other than that claimed by the Research Institute for Fragrance Materials."

January 10, 2011

Unrecognized Dangers of Formaldehyde

The Cancer Prevention Coalition today is drawing public attention to a two-page article in the *New York Times*, "When Wrinkle-Free Clothing Also Means Formaldehyde Fumes," published on December 10, 2010, which stated that "formaldehyde is commonly found in a broad range of consumer products." These include sheets, pillow cases, and drapes, besides "personal care products like shampoos, lotions, and eye shadows."

Samuel S. Epstein, M.D., who chairs the Cancer Prevention Coalition, says, "The dermatologists and other scientists quoted in the Times appear unaware of the longstanding scientific evidence on the carcinogenicity of formaldehyde. However, this had been detailed in five National Toxicology Program Reports on Carcinogens from 1981 to 2004."

The *Times* assured its readers that "most of the 180 items tested, largely clothes and bed linens, had low or undetectable levels of formaldehyde that met voluntary industry guidelines." Accordingly, the *Times* claimed, "Most consumers will probably never have a problem with exposure to formaldehyde," since such low levels "are not likely to irritate most people," other than those wearing wrinkle-resistant clothing.

However, Dr. Epstein points to evidence that links formaldehyde exposure with increased incidence of nasal cancer and breast cancer.

The *Times* article stated that "the U.S. does not regulate formaldehyde levels in clothing . . . . Nor does any government agency require manufacturers to disclose the use of this chemical on labels."

But that could change. On March 5, 2008, Senators Bob Casey, Sherrod Brown, and Mary Landrieu introduced an amendment to the Consumer Product Safety Commission (CPSC) reform bill "that would help protect Americans from dangerous levels of formaldehyde in textiles including clothing . . ."

The senators referred to a 1997 CPSC report on formaldehyde, which admitted that "it causes cancer in tests on laboratory animals, and may cause cancer in humans." Accordingly, the Senators requested the CPSC to "regulate and test formaldehyde in textiles—and protect consumers from this poison."

In August 2010, a Government Accountability Office (GAO) report warned that "a small proportion of the U.S. population does have allergic reactions to formaldehyde resins on their clothes." However, the GAO made no recommendations for any regulatory action.

Dr. Epstein supports both regulatory and legislative action based on scientific evidence in the five National Toxicology Program Reports on Carcinogens that classified formaldehyde as "reasonably anticipated to be a human carcinogen," based on limited evidence of carcinogenicity in humans, and sufficient evidence in experimental animals.

This evidence was confirmed in a series of reports by the prestigious International Agency for Research on Cancer (IARC). Its 2006 and 2010 reports explicitly warn that formaldehyde is "a known cause of leukemia in experimental animals—and nasal cancer" in humans.

"Strong" evidence of the nasal cancer risk was also cited in the May 2010 President's Cancer Panel report, "Environmental Cancer Risk: What Can We Do Now?"

"Nevertheless," says Dr. Epstein, "and in spite of this explicit evidence, a September 2010 Government Accountability Office report attempted to trivialize the cancer risks of formaldehyde on the alleged grounds that exposure levels are low or 'non-detectable.'"

Of further concern, Dr. Epstein warns, "Occupational exposure to formaldehyde has been associated with breast cancer deaths in a 1995 National Cancer Institute report, while environmental exposure has been associated with an increased incidence of breast cancer in a 2005 University of Texas report."

"Disturbingly," observes Dr. Epstein, "none of the dermatologists quoted in the New York Times appear aware of longstanding evidence that most cosmetics and personal care products, commonly used daily by most women, besides on their infants and children, and to a lesser extent men, contain up to eight ingredients which are precursors of formaldehyde."

These include diazolidinyl urea, metheneamine, and quaterniums, each of which readily breaks down on the skin to release formaldehyde, Dr. Epstein explains, warning, "This is then readily absorbed through the skin, and poses unknowing risks of cancer to most of the U.S. population."

January 24, 2011

Danger of Bone Cancer from Fluoride in Toothpaste, Drinking Water

As reported in the January 13, 2011, *New York Times*, Senator James Inhofe (R-OK) warned the U.S. Environmental Protection Agency (EPA) that the move to phase out a fluoride-based pesticide "could create unintended consequences for public health, food safety, and the economy."

Cancer Prevention Coalition Chairman Samuel S. Epstein, M.D. said today that Senator Inhofe may be right about such possible "unintended consequences."

"However," said Dr. Epstein, "he is unaware that these consequences would be clearly beneficial, as they protect against the risks of bone cancer from the use of fluoride in most brands of toothpaste to prevent cavities, and from the fluoridation of drinking water."

In 1977, the National Academy of Sciences expressed concerns on the strong relation between the fluoridation of drinking water and risks of bone cancer to young boys, Dr. Epstein points out.

A decade later, the International Agency for Research on Cancer reported that fluorides in drinking water induced bone cancer in rats. This finding was confirmed by the National Toxicology Program in its 1989, 1990, and 1991 reports.

"Not surprisingly, Procter & Gamble, the leading manufacturer of fluoridated toothpastes, denied that these results were statistically significant," Dr. Epstein said today. "Surprisingly, the Food and Drug Administration (FDA) supported this claim."

Well-documented evidence links bone cancer to fluoride exposure, Dr. Epstein advises.

In 1990, the National Cancer Institute (NCI) reported that, based on an analysis of 1973 to 1987 data, the incidence of a bone cancer, known as osteosarcoma, was increased in males under the age of 20 living in areas where the drinking water was fluoridated. Not surprisingly, this was promptly denied by Procter & Gamble, the major manufacturer of fluoridated toothpaste.

In 1992, the New Jersey Department of Health published a study confirming higher rates of bone cancer in young boys living in fluoridated versus non-fluoridated areas of the state.

A 1993 independent analysis of the 1990 NCI data confirmed excess risks and deaths from bone cancer in young boys exposed to fluoride. These findings were confirmed in a 2001 report by the Harvard School of Dental Medicine. In 2006, a Harvard University team of scientists published a study reporting a five-fold increased risk of bone cancer in teenage boys who had drunk fluoridated water between the ages of 6 and 8. Apart from exposure to fluoride in drinking water, these finding also incriminated fluoride commonly added to toothpaste.

In July 1997, the Washington Post published an article "Toothpaste: How Safe." This noted that the label of Crest toothpaste carried a small print warning: "If you accidentally swallow more than used for brushing, seek professional help or contact a poison control center immediately." Warning labels to this effect had also been required by the FDA in April that year. The *Post* article further warned that children age 4 to 6 usually swallow some toothpaste when brushing, rather than spitting it out and rinsing.

"Concerns on fluoride as a major avoidable cause of bone cancer are further and urgently validated by its unrecognized 20 percent increased incidence in children under the age of 15 over the last three decades," Dr. Epstein warns, "as documented in the 1975-2007 National Cancer Institute Surveillance Epidemiology and End Results (SEER) report."

As currently emphasized by Chris Neurath, research director of the American Environmental Health Studies Project, these concerns are all the more critical as 200 million citizens of all ages are still drinking fluoridated water.

Apart from bone cancer, and as warned by the Fluoride Action Network (FAN) last week, "24 studies have shown an association between exposure to moderate to high levels of fluoride in drinking water and lower IQ (and brain damage) in children."

Dr. Epstein says, "A ban by the FDA on fluoridated toothpaste is well overdue, as is a ban by the EPA on the fluoridation of drinking water."

December 15, 2011

Multiple Carcinogens in Johnson & Johnson's Baby Shampoo

The Cancer Prevention Coalition today congratulated the Campaign for Safe Cosmetics for securing a 11/15/11 agreement with Johnson & Johnson "for reducing or gradually phasing out—trace amounts of potentially cancer-causing chemicals" from Baby Shampoo, "one of its signature products." However, this agreement is limited and restricted to the U.S. market.

"There are two carcinogenic ingredients in Johnson & Johnson's Baby Shampoo, dioxane and quaternium 15," says Samuel S. Epstein, M.D., who chairs the Cancer Prevention Coalition.

"Dioxane is a well-recognized contaminant in alcohol ethoxylates, a group of four ingredients, laureths, oleths, polyethylene glycol and polysorbates," Dr. Epstein explains. "Quaternium 15 is a precursor of two carcinogens, formaldehyde and nitrosamine. Johnson & Johnson has committed to "reducing or gradual phasing out" dioxane and quaternium-15 in their U.S., but not in their international, products."

However limited, Dr. Epstein finds Johnson & Johnson's response to be "in sharp and disturbing contrast to the silence of the Food and Drug Administration (FDA)."

This federal agency has still failed to enforce the explicit requirements of the 1938 Federal Food Drug and Cosmetic Act, Dr. Epstein points out. This directs the FDA to require that "the label of a cosmetic product shall bear a warning statement to prevent a health hazard that may be associated with the product."

The regulatory failure of the FDA extends to its failure to respond to the Cancer Prevention Coalition's extensively documented 1996 Citizen Petition "Seeking A Cancer Warning On Cosmetic Products Containing (the carcinogen) Diethanolamine," says Dr. Epstein.

He says the FDA's regulatory failure extends still further to the Coalition's 2008 Petition, "Seeking A (ovarian) Cancer Warning On Talc Products Used By Premenopausal for Women's Genital Dusting."

Both petitions, endorsed by leading cancer prevention experts, requested the FDA to ban or suspend approval of these products which still pose an "Imminent Hazard," or minimally to require their labeling with a "Caution" or other such warning. However, the FDA has still failed to respond.

"Concerns on the cancer risks of talc, dioxane, formaldehyde, nitrosamine, and ethylene oxide, besides other prohibited and restricted carcinogenic ingredients in cosmetics and personal care products, are not new," Dr. Epstein says. "They were detailed in my 2001 "Unreasonable Risk: How to Avoid Cancer from Cosmetics and Personal Care Products" and 2009 "Healthy Beauty" books."

As published in the February 25, 2011, *Science Insider* editorial, "Advancing Regulatory Science," FDA Commissioner, Dr. Margaret Hamburg, claimed that FDA's regulations must be based on "better predictive models—functional genomics, proteomics, and metabolomics," rather than "high dose animal [carcinogenicity] studies—unchanged for decades."

"Dr. Hamburg's dismissal of standard carcinogenicity tests is bizarre," says Dr. Epstein. "Their scientific validity has been endorsed by other Federal regulatory agencies, the National Toxicology Program, the International Agency for Research on Cancer, besides the April 2010 President's Cancer Panel."

"Furthermore, as stipulated in the 1938 Federal Food Drug and Cosmetic Act, the FDA is charged with regulating food, drugs, and cosmetics based on standard toxicology and carcinogenicity tests. Moreover, the FDA is not charged with, let alone capable of developing irrelevant 'tests that incorporate the mechanistic underpinnings of disease,'" Dr. Epstein points out.

As warned by Senator Edward Kennedy at the 1997 Senate Hearings on the FDA Reform Bill, "The cosmetics industry has borrowed a page from the playbook of the tobacco industry by putting profits ahead of public health."

Dr. Epstein emphasizes, "This warning remains current."

E.

Avoidable Causes of Other Cancers Ignored by the FDA

Avoidable Causes of Other Cancers Ignored by the FDA

February 22, 1994

Notice of Presentation: American Association for the Advancement of Science (AAAS), St. Francis Hilton, San Francisco

- Dr. Samuel S. Epstein condemns the cancer establishment—NCI and ACS—for overwhelming neglect of breast cancer prevention.
- Mounting evidence links women's breast cancer epidemic to avoidable carcinogenic exposures in food, the workplace & environment.
- Not only does the American Cancer Society (ACS) neglect prevention, it recklessly promotes premenopausal mammography, despite its ineffectiveness and excess risk of breast cancer deaths.
- While failing to pursue prevention, the cancer establishment has embarked on Orwellian experiments exposing healthy women to the highly carcinogenic drug, Tamoxifen, which is very likely to cause, rather than prevent, more cancer.
- A new breast cancer risk is women's exposure to the milk from rBGH-treated cows, which contains sustained, elevated levels of IGF-1, a potent growth factor.

Dr. Samuel S. Epstein, the chairman of the Cancer Prevention Coalition, condemns the cancer establishment for its overwhelming neglect of cancer prevention, especially the prevention of women's breast cancer.

Risks that could be avoided are being ignored by the cancer establishment—the National Cancer Institute (NCI) and the American Cancer Society (ACS)—despite their expenditures of more than $1 billion dollars on breast cancer research.

Accumulating evidence links the growing epidemic of women's breast cancer to exposure to avoidable carcinogens in the diet, the workplace and the general environment.

Such avoidable risks include carcinogenic and estrogenic food contaminants, particularly pesticides, some of which induce breast cancer in experimental animals; exposures to known mammary carcinogens in the workplace; and radiation, particularly pre-menopausal mammography.

Dr. Epstein stated, "Instead of promoting prevention, the American Cancer Society is recklessly promoting premenopausal mammography, despite its ineffectiveness and its excess risk of breast cancer deaths."

Dr. Epstein added, "While failing to pursue cancer prevention, the cancer establishment has embarked on Orwellian chemoprevention experiments exposing healthy women to the highly carcinogenic DES-related, ICI-manufactured drug, Tamoxifen. Such treatment is likely to cause more uterine and other cancers, rather than prevent breast cancer. An even more bizarre attempt at breast cancer prevention is the administration of hormonal cocktails designed to block 'incessant ovulation' in healthy young women."

Continued Dr. Epstein, "All women from conception to death will now be exposed to an additional breast cancer risk, the milk from cows treated with recombinant bovine growth hormone (rBGH), also called bovine somatotropin or rBST. Milk from cows injected with this Monsanto drug contains sustained, elevated levels of IGF-1, a potent growth factor which is a potential cause of breast cancer."

Dr. Epstein concluded, "It's time for radical reforms in the leadership and priorities of both the National Cancer Institute and the American Cancer Society, in view of their longstanding, overwhelming neglect of cancer prevention by reducing avoidable exposures to industrial and other carcinogens in air, water, food, and the workplace."

February 6, 1996

Why We Are Losing the War Against Cancer

Americans are being misled by the widespread perception that cancer is a declining public health threat, says a renowned scientist and cancer prevention expert. Even after adjusting for our aging population and smoking, cancer rates are sharply increasing, says Samuel Epstein, M.D. of the University of Illinois Medical Center in Chicago, and Chairman of the Cancer Prevention Coalition.

Recently, Dr. Epstein has gained widespread attention with release of a peer-reviewed publication linking Bovine Growth Hormone milk to risks of breast and colon cancer, and with a "Dirty Dozen" report on carcinogens in food, cosmetics and household products and their link to human cancer.

Epstein contends that government research and regulatory agencies place minimal emphasis on cancer prevention. The costs of cancer, however, are well in excess of $100 billion (two percent of U.S. GNP) and are a major factor in the current health care crisis. The American Hospital Association predicts that cancer will be the leading cause of death and the "dominant specialty" in American medicine within four years.

Epstein asserts that a major cause of cancer—avoidable exposures to carcinogens in food and other consumer products—is underreported due to disinformation by industry and government, besides conflicts of interest in the cancer establishment. Epstein also stresses consumers' right to know so that they can influence the market to produce safer products.

The Food and Drug Administration, Grocery Manufacturers of America and Cosmetics, Toiletries and Fragrance Association declined to participate with Dr. Epstein in this discussion of product safety.

February 4, 1998

New Drug Poses Risks of Ovarian Cancer

On December 10, 1997, Eli Lilly and Company announced FDA's clearance to market Evista(R) (Raloxifene) which has been shown to be effective in preventing osteoporosis, affecting over 20 million U.S. women annually, and in reducing LDL or "bad cholesterol" blood levels. Lilly has submitted applications to market Evista in more than 30 different countries. Surely, this new drug should be welcomed by women worldwide. Unfortunately, this is not the case, as Lilly, with FDA's complicity, has suppressed critical information that this drug poses major risks of ovarian cancer. In a study specifically designed by Lilly to prove the drug's safety, Evista was shown to induce ovarian cancer in both mice and rats. Moreover, carcinogenic effects were noted at dosages extending below the therapeutic. However, the study concluded: "The clinical relevance of these tumor findings is not known." Lilly reached this conclusion despite the scientific consensus that the induction of cancer in well-designed studies in two species creates the strong presumption of human risk. Nevertheless, Lilly failed to disclose this critical information in its "Warning" to women. Furthermore, no reference at all is made to these risks in a Lilly-sponsored publication on Evista in the December 4, 1997, issue of the New England Journal of Medicine. Responding to criticisms on the January 12, 1998, Jim Lehrer Newshour program, a Lilly spokesman claimed that the carcinogenic effects of Evista in the ovaries of sexually mature rodents are irrelevant to such risks in postmenopausal women. However, ovarian cancer is recognized as an uncommon complication of long-term hormone replacement therapy in the post-menopausal.

Ovarian cancer strikes about 24,000 U.S. women every year, accounting for 4% of all their cancers. About 15,000 women die from ovarian cancer annually, making it the most lethal female reproductive cancer. Commenting on these facts, Samuel S. Epstein, M.D., Professor of Environmental Medicine at the University of Illinois Chicago, School of Public Health, stated: "Lilly's suppression of the evidence of ovarian cancer risks from Evista is as reckless as is FDA's marketing approval, conduct which merits congressional and legal scrutiny. This drug should be withdrawn from the world market immediately. As importantly, a 'Cancer

Alert' should be sent to the over 12,000 women who have participated in U.S. and international clinical trials in the absence of informed consent. These women should also be offered lifelong bi-annual surveillance for the early detection of ovarian cancer at Eli Lilly's expense."

April 19, 1998

Chicago Tribune

Failure to Fully Document Risks of Osteoporosis Drug Is "Reckless"

Eli Lilly recently began running full-page color ads for Evista, a synthetic hormone with both estrogenic and antiestrogenic effects, in major national and regional newspapers Tile ads claim that Evista offers "a new way to prevent osteoporosis," but at the same time admit that "its effect on fractures is not yet known." The ads also claim that women taking Evista had no increased *risks* of breast and uterine cancers, in contrast to conventional hormone replacement therapy, and that it reduces LDL or bad cholesterol blood levels. This should be welcome news to women worldwide particularly as osteoporosis has now reached epidemic proportions, affecting 15 million to 20 million American women each year; osteoporosis causes more than a million fractures, including 250,000 hip fractures, and kills some 50,000 elderly women, from complications as a result of their fractures.

While warning of some possible side effects, such as blood clots or hot flashes, Lilly fails to warn of the more serious risks of ovarian cancer. A company sponsored article in the Dec. 4, 1997 issue of The New England Journal of Medicine also ignores this risk. Lilly's pre-market clearance study, however, clearly shows that Evista induces ovarian cancer in both mice and rats. Furthermore, carcinogenic effects were noted at dosages well below the recommended therapeutic level. However, the study concluded: "The clinical relevance of these tumor findings is not known." Lilly reached this conclusion despite the strong scientific consensus that the induction of cancer in well designed tests in two rodent species creates the strong presumption of human risk. Nevertheless, Lilly fails to disclose this critical information in its ads and in its "warning" to patients.

Responding to such criticisms by one of us (Samuel Epstein) during a broadcast of the "Jim Lehrer Newshour" earlier this year [Jan. 12], a Lilly spokesman claimed that the carcinogenic effects of Evista in the ovaries of sexually mature rodents are irrelevant to such risks in postmenopausal women, as their ovaries are inactive, and, therefore, no warning is necessary. Apart from the fact that the rodent studies were specifically designed to evaluate Evista's safely. Ovarian cancer is a scientifically documented complication of long term estrogen replacement therapy in post-menopausal women. Also disturbing is the claim that Evista poses no risks of breast and uterine cancers, based on clinical trials over only some 40 months, a period totally inadequate to possibly measure any such risks.

Ovarian cancer strikes about 24,000 women in the United States every year, accounting for 4 percent of all female cancers. About 15,000 women die annually from ovarian cancer, making it the most lethal of all female reproductive cancers. Lilly's suppression of its own evidence of ovarian cancer risks from Evista is reckless and threatening to women's health and life. Equally reckless is the Food and Drug Administration's December 1997 marketing clearance, especially in the absence of any requirement for warning. Such conduct clearly merits urgent congressional investigation; Evista should be withdrawn from the world market immediately. As importantly, a "cancer alert" should be sent to the more than 12,000 women who have participated in U.S. and international clinical trials, in the absence of fully informed consent. The doctrine of informed consent is ethically and legally protective only when all facts relevant to benefits and risks are affirmatively disclosed. This is clearly not the case with women who have been involved in the Evista trials. These women should be offered semiannual lifelong surveillance for the early detection of ovarian cancer at Eli Lilly's expense.

December 7, 1998

Prestigious International Award for U.S. Expert Who Advocates Emphasis on Cancer Prevention Rather Than Just on Damage Control Diagnosis and Treatment

Prof. Samuel Epstein, M.D., the world-renowned authority on the causes and prevention of cancer and critic of the U.S. cancer establishment, the National Cancer Institute and American Cancer Society, has been named a 1998 winner of the Right Livelihood Award, also known as the "Alternative Nobel Prize."

Dr. Epstein will be presented his award at a December 9 ceremony at the Swedish Parliament, Stockholm, where he will deliver an address "LEGISLATIVE PROPOSALS FOR REVERSING THE CANCER EPIDEMIC." He has been invited subsequently to meet with senior members of the European Parliament and European Commission in Brussels on December 10 and 11 to discuss his proposed legislative initiatives for cancer prevention.

Epstein, Professor of Occupational and Environmental Medicine at the School of Public Health, University of Illinois at Chicago and Chairman of The Cancer Prevention Coalition, will receive the award for his "exemplary life of scholarship, wedded to activism on behalf of humanity." For more than three decades, Epstein has campaigned against environmental pollution from run-away petrochemical and other industrial technologies. He has shown these to be major avoidable causes of cancer, the incidence of which has escalated to epidemic proportions over recent decades. He has argued strongly for strategies based on cancer prevention rather than on virtual exclusionary emphasis on damage control—diagnosis and treatment—particularly as survival rates for most common cancers have not significantly improved for decades. In incriminating environmental pollutants for much avoidable cancer and in campaigning for toxics use reduction, Epstein—and in recent years the Cancer Prevention Coalition which he founded—have pressured governments and corporations to take greater responsibility for product safety and environmental protection. Epstein has thereby made an incomparable contribution to the prevention of a disease that is now responsible for more than a quarter of all deaths in industrialized countries and is increasing worldwide.

Epstein has emerged as the leading international champion for cancer prevention, and for winning the losing war against cancer by preventing or reducing avoidable exposures to industrial carcinogens in air, water, consumer products—food, cosmetics and toiletries, and household products—and the work place.

He has conducted extensive basic and applied research on the carcinogenic and other chronic toxic effects of environmental and occupational industrial pollutants. His some 260 scientific publications date back to the early 1960s. His best known book, *The Politics of Cancer* (1978) won the Notable Book and other awards.

Epstein has played an important role as president or founder of professional societies, especially of the more activist kind and a major role in public interest groups including as president of the Rachel Carson Council. He also has acted as a consultant, including drafting legislation, to a number of congressional committees. His extensive media experience includes contributing editorials for leading newspapers and numerous appearances on major TV and radio programs.

Epstein's most recent surge of activity arose from his precedential February 4, 1992, initiative, when 65 eminent public health experts, including past directors of Federal agencies, joined with him at a Washington, D.C., press conference in releasing a statement on "Losing the War against Cancer: Need for Public Policy Reforms." The statement emphasized that the overall incidence of cancer had increased by 54% since 1950, with increases up to 200% for some cancers, including non-smoking related cancers. The statement blamed this increase on the failure of the "cancer establishment"—the National Cancer Institute (NCI) and the American Cancer Society (ACS)—for their, not always benign, indifference to cancer prevention, and for periodic misleading and exaggerated claims for dramatic improvement in treatment for common cancers which rarely, if ever, have been substantiated. The statement also called for drastic reforms of NCI and ACS policies and priorities. The only response of the cancer establishment was a campaign of personal vilification and scientific "McCarthyism."

Out of this initiative was born the Cancer Prevention Coalition (CPC), which pursues a comprehensive strategy of outreach, education and advocacy to establish prevention as the nation's top cancer policy. The long-term objective of CPC is to reverse modern epidemic cancer rates to their pre-1940 levels. Epstein's book (with Steinman and Levert) "The Breast Cancer Prevention Program," a second edition of which was published by Macmillan in October 1998, details a wide range of scientifically established ways by which women of any age can reduce their risks of breast cancer. This book poses a direct challenge to the NCI and ACS who maintain that there is no way of preventing breast cancer.

In an invited March 1998 submission to Congress, Epstein presented his critique of the U.S. cancer establishment whose failed policies "in no small measure have been critical factors in escalating cancer rates over recent decades." Evidence for these and other charges, including conflicts of interest, have been fully documented in Epstein's November 1998 book, "The Politics of Cancer Revisited." As importantly, the book details practical methods for winning the losing war against cancer based on both personal initiatives for reducing avoidable carcinogenic exposures, and also on political initiatives, particularly the "right-to-know" and toxics use reduction.

March 7, 1999

Human Growth Hormone Antiaging Medication Poses Undisclosed Cancer Risks

Use of the genetically engineered human growth hormone (HGH) for antiaging medication has become a major growth industry. Suppliers of HGH, including those offering mail order prescriptions, are proliferating on websites and the Internet. The Chicago-based seven-year-old American Academy of Anti-Aging Medicine, with over 8,000 members, promotes injectable HGH in programs claiming to stop or even reverse aging, including decreasing body fat, and increasing muscle mass and bone density. However, practitioners of this burgeoning "health" industry are either ignorant of or suppress well-documented information on the grave cancer risks of HGH medication.

HGH induces growth promoting and other effects by stimulating the liver to increase production of the natural Insulin-like Growth Factor-1 (IGF-1) whose blood levels normally decline with advancing age. However, there are numerous publications in prestigious peer reviewed scientific journals showing that elevated IGF-1 levels are strongly associated with major excess risks of colon, prostate, and breast cancers; even minor elevations are associated with up to 7-fold increased risks of breast cancer, risks almost as high as those in women carrying genes (BRCA1 and BRCA2) with the strongest hereditary predisposition. Additionally, IGF-1 inhibits the programmed self-destruction (apoptosis) of cancer cells, thus stimulating the growth and invasiveness of small, undiagnosed cancers, besides increasing the resistance of cancers to chemotherapy. For these reasons, anti-aging HGH medication, compounded by failure to explicitly disclose its grave risks, constitutes medical malpractice.

There are also growing concerns on possible risks from the use of HGH nutritional supplements, including oral sprays. It should, however, be recognized that HGH absorption from the mouth and gut is unlikely to be significant, in striking contrast to complete absorption from injectable medication. Nevertheless, nutritional HGH supplements should be phased out until it can be shown that they do not elevate blood IGF-1 levels.

HGH medication should only be used by qualified endocrinologists for highly restricted medical disorders, such as dwarfism due to pituitary gland deficiency, as approved by the FDA in 1985; anti-aging medication has never received such approval.

April 10, 2000

UIC Cancer Prevention Champion Receives "Alternative Pulitzer Prize" for Investigative Journalism

Samuel Epstein, professor of environmental and occupational medicine at the University of Illinois at Chicago's School of Public Health, will receive what is popularly is known as the "Alternative Pulitzer Prize" for investigative journalism from Project Censored.

Epstein is being honored for his article "American Cancer Society: The World's Wealthiest Nonprofit Institution." The article was published in the fall 1999 issue of the leading peer-reviewed public health journal "International Journal of Health Services."

Project Censored, created by the department of sociology at Sonoma State University, recognizes important news stories that are overlooked by mainstream media. Epstein's article criticizes the American Cancer Society for indifference to prevention, bloated operating budgets, misallocation of funds, as well as links to the cancer drug, mammography and pesticide industries, which, Epstein writes, create conflicts of interest. "My overall objective is to establish prevention as the nation's top cancer policy," Epstein said.

Department of sociology students and faculty at Sonoma begin Project Censored each year by screening thousands of magazine and journal articles and selecting about 100 stories for review by Project Censored judges, nationally-recognized authors, journalists and leaders. The judges select and rank the top 25 censored news stories.

This year's panel of Project Censored judges ranked Epstein's article third. Judges included Howard Zinn, historian and author of the "People's History of the United States," Susan Faludi, Pulitzer-Prize winning author of "Backlash: The Undeclared War against Women," and Rhoda Karpatkin, president of the Consumer's Union.

Seven Stories Press, a publishing house in New York City, published the stories in the recently released "Censored 2000: This Year's Top 25 Censored Stories."

The April 12 Seventh Annual Project Censored Awards, held in New York City at Fordham University, will recognize the authors of the top-10 censored stories. The event is sponsored by Seven Stories Press, Project Censored, the Investigative Fund of the Nation Institute, and the Peace and Justice Studies Program at Fordham University.

Epstein said that he will give a brief presentation on how the "American Cancer Society subverts the democratic process by failing to make available to the public well-documented information on cancer prevention."

"This failure has a tremendous impact on the democratic decision-making process and expresses itself in the fact that one of every two men and one of every three women in America will experience some form of cancer in their lifetime," said Epstein.

The Seventh Annual Project Censored Awards is part of the annual Press Freedom Conference, organized by Fordham and Project Censored. The conference presents panels on journalism, media activism and democracy.

Epstein's presentation, "Failure of the U.S. Media to Cover Important Medical Issues; Needs for an Alternative Press," is part of an investigative journalism panel, from 11:00 a.m. to 12:30 p.m., April 12.

Epstein is a leading international champion of preventing cancer by reducing exposure to industrial carcinogens in the environment, workplace and consumer products including food, household cleansers and cosmetics. He is the founder of the Cancer Prevention Coalition, which aims to influence public policy to place greater emphasis on cancer prevention.

March 23, 2001

"Trade Secrets": The Latest in a Long Line of Conspiracies Charges

Bill Moyers is to be warmly commended for his March 26 program "Trade Secrets." This PBS Special will document the chemical industry's conspiracy in denying information on the grave cancer risks to hundreds of thousands of workers manufacturing the potent carcinogen vinyl chloride (VC) and its polyvinyl chloride (PVC) product.

As newsworthy is the fact that there is a decades-long track record of numerous such conspiracies involving a wide range of industries and chemicals, besides VC. These conspiracies have resulted in an escalation in the incidence and mortality of cancer, and chronic disease, among workers and the general public unknowingly exposed to toxics and carcinogens in the workplace, air, water and consumer products—food, household products, and cosmetics and toiletries.

This misconduct involves negligence, manipulation, suppression, distortion and destruction of health and environmental data by mainstream industries, their consultants and trade associations, notably the Chemical Manufacturers Association (CMA). These practices are so frequent as to preclude dismissal as exceptional aberrations and, in many instances, arguably rise to the level of criminality as illustrated below:

- Suppression of evidence from the early 1960's on the toxicity of VC by Dow Chemical, and on its carcinogenicity from 1970 by the VC/PVC industry and CMA. Based on these findings, a blue ribbon committee of the American Association for the Advancement of Science charged in 1976 that: "Because of the suppression of these data (by the CMA), tens of thousands of workers were exposed without warning—to toxic concentrations of VC."
- Suppression of evidence since the 1930's on the hazards of asbestos, asbestosis and lung cancer, by Johns-Manville and Raybestos-Manhattan, besides the Metropolitan Life Insurance Company. This information was detailed in industry documents dubbed the "Asbestos Pentagon Papers," released at 1978 Congressional Hearings.

- Suppression by Rohm and Haas of information, known since 1962 but not released until 1971, on the potent carcinogenicity of the resin bischloromethylether. This resulted in deaths from lung cancer of some 50 men, many non-smokers and under the age of 50.
- Suppression of carcinogenicity data on organochlorine pesticides: Aldrin/Dieldrin, by Shell Chemical Company since 1962; Chlordane/Heptachlor, by Velsicol Chemical Company since 1959; and Kepone, by Allied Chemical Company since the early 1960's.
- Falsification in the early 1970's of test data on the drug Aldactone and artificial sweetener Aspartame by Hazleton Laboratories under contract to G. D. Searle Company.
- Falsification and manipulation by Monsanto since the 1960's of data on dioxin, and its contamination of products including the herbicide Agent Orange, designed to block occupational exposure claims and tightening of federal regulations. This evidence was detailed in 1990 by Environmental Protection Agency's Office of Criminal Investigation which charged Monsanto with a "long pattern of fraud" and with reporting "false information" to the Agency.
- Fraudulent claims by Monsanto since 1985 that genetically engineered (rBGH) milk is indistinguishable from natural milk. These claims persist despite contrary evidence.
- Monsanto's reckless marketing in 1976 of plastic Coke bottles made from acrylonitrile, a chemical closely related to VC, prior to its testing for carcinogenicity and migration into the Coke. The bottles were subsequently banned after acrylonitrile was found to be a potent carcinogen contaminating the Coke.
- Destruction of epidemiological data on ethyleneimine and other chemicals by Dow and DuPont. This was admitted at 1973 Department of Labor Advisory Committee meetings in response to challenges to produce data on whose basis industry had falsely claimed that these chemicals were not carcinogens.
- Destruction of test data on drugs, food additives, and pesticides as admitted in 1977 by Industrial Biotest Laboratories, under contract to major chemical industries.
- Failure of the mainstream cosmetics and toiletry industries to warn of the wide range of avoidable carcinogenic ingredients, contaminants and precursors in their products used by the great majority of the U.S. population over virtually their lifetimes.

(For supporting documentation of the above charges, see the author's: Testimony on White Collar Crime, H.R. 4973, before the Subcommittee on Crime of the House Judiciary Committee, 12/13/79; The Politics of Cancer, 1979; and The Politics of Cancer, Revisited, 1998.)

Hopefully, the public and the media will be outraged by this longstanding evidence of recklessness and conspiracies, graphically reinforced by Moyers' program. The public and the media should finally hold industry accountable, and demand urgent investigation and radical reform of current industry practices besides governmental unresponsiveness. The Moyers' program has already galvanized formation of a coalition of grassroots citizen groups, "Coming Clean," to demand more responsible and open industry practices, including phasing out the use and manufacture of toxic chemicals.

Criticism should also be directed to the multibillion dollar cancer establishment—the National Cancer Institute and American Cancer Society—for their failure to warn Congress, regulatory agencies and the general public of the scientific evidence on the permeation of the totality of the environment with often persistent industrial carcinogens thus precluding corrective legislation and regulation, besides denying workers and the public of their inalienable right-to-know.

October 10, 2001

American Academy of Pediatrics Guidelines for Treating Behavioral Disorders in Children With Ritalin Ignores Evidence of Cancer Risks

Based on an industry-funded multi-university trial on 282 pre-teen children treated with Ritalin for attention deficit/hyperactivity disorders (ADHD), just published in Pediatrics, the American Academy of Pediatrics has endorsed the use of the drug. However, the Academy ignores clear evidence of the drug's cancer risks of which parents, teachers and school nurses, besides most pediatricians and psychiatrists, still remain uninformed and unaware.

Some 40 years after the drug was first marketed by Ciba Geigy, carcinogenicity tests were conducted at the taxpayers' expense by the National Toxicology Program, the results of which were published in 1995. Adult mice were fed Ritalin over a two-year period at dosages close to those prescribed to children. The mice developed a statistically significant incidence of liver abnormalities and tumors, including highly aggressive rare cancers known as hepatoblastomas. These findings are particularly disturbing as the tests were conducted on adult, rather than young mice which would be expected to be much more sensitive to carcinogenic effects. The National Toxicology Program concluded that Ritalin is a "possible human carcinogen," and recommended the need for further research. While still insisting that the drug is safe, the Food and Drug Administration admitted that these findings signal "carcinogenic potential," and required a statement to this effect in the drug's package insert. However, these inserts are not seen by parents or nurses.

The Physicians' Desk Reference admits evidence on the carcinogenicity of Ritalin, now manufactured by Novartis, qualified by the statement that "the significance of these results is unknown," apparently not recognizing that this is more alarming than reassuring. Apart from cancer risks, there is also suggestive evidence that Ritalin induces genetic damage in blood cells of Ritalin-treated children.

Concerns on Ritalin's cancer risk are more acute in view of the millions of children treated annually with the drug and the escalating incidence of childhood cancer, by some 35% over the last few decades, quite apart from delayed risks of cancer in adult life. These risks are compounded by the availability of alternative safe and effective procedures, notably behavior modification and biofeedback.

There is no justification for prescribing Ritalin, even by highly qualified pediatricians and psychiatrists, unless parents have been explicitly informed of the drug's cancer risks. Otherwise, prescribing Ritalin constitutes unarguable medical malpractice.

May 9, 2002

Escalating Incidence of Childhood Cancer Remains Ignored by the National Cancer Institute

Since passage of the 1971 National Cancer Act, the incidence of childhood cancer has steadily escalated to alarming levels. Childhood cancers have increased by 26% overall, while the incidence of particular cancers has increased still more: acute lymphocytic leukemia, 62%; brain cancer, 50%; and bone cancer, 40%. The NCI, besides by the "charitable" American Cancer Society (ACS), have failed to inform the public, let alone Congress and regulatory agencies, of this alarming information. As importantly, they have failed to publicize well-documented scientific information on avoidable causes responsible for the increased incidence of childhood cancer. Examples include:

- Over 20 U.S. and international studies have incriminated paternal and maternal exposures (pre-conception, during conception and post-conception) to a wide range of occupational carcinogens as major causes of childhood cancer.
- There is substantial evidence on the risks of brain cancer and leukemia in children from frequent consumption of nitrite-dyed hot dogs; consumption during pregnancy has been similarly incriminated. Nitrites, added to meat for coloring purposes, have been shown to react with natural chemicals in meat (amines) to form a potent carcinogenic nitrosamine.
- Consumption of non-organic fruits and vegetables, particularly in baby food, contaminated with high concentrations of multiple residues of carcinogenic pesticides, poses major risks of childhood cancer, besides delayed cancers in adult life.
- Numerous studies have shown strong associations between childhood cancers, particularly brain cancer, non-Hodgkin's lymphoma and leukemia, and domestic exposure to pesticides from uses in the home, including pet flea collars, lawn and garden; another major source of exposure is commonplace use in schools.
- Use of lindane, a potent carcinogen in shampoos for treating lice and scabies, infesting about six million children annually, is associated with major risks of brain cancer; lindane is readily absorbed through the skin.

- Treatment of children with Ritalin for "Attention Deficit Disorders" poses risks of cancer, in the absence of informed parental consent. Ritalin has been shown to induce highly aggressive rare liver cancers in rodents at doses comparable to those prescribed to children.
- Maternal exposure to ionizing radiation, especially in late pregnancy, is strongly associated with excess risks of childhood leukemia.

It is of particular significance that the cancer establishment ignored the continuing increase in the incidence of childhood cancer in its heavily promoted, but highly arguable, March 1998 "claim to have reversed an almost 20-year trend of increasing cancer cases."

The failure of the NCI to warn of these avoidable cancer risks reflects mind-sets fixated on damage control—screening, diagnosis, and treatment—and basic genetic research, with indifference to primary prevention, as defined by research and public education on avoidable causes of cancer.

The minimal priority for prevention reflects mind-sets and policies and not lack of resources. NCI's annual budget has increased some twentyfold since passage of the 1971 Act, from $220 million to $4.2 billion. NCI expenditures on primary prevention have been estimated as under 4% of its budget.

It should be particularly stressed that fetuses, infants and children are much more vulnerable and sensitive to toxic and carcinogenic exposures than are adults. It should also be recognized that the majority of carcinogens also induce other chronic toxic effects, especially in fetuses, infants and children. These include endocrine disruptive and reproductive, hematological, immunological and genetic, for which there are no available incidence trend data comparable to those for cancer.

The continued silence of the NCI on avoidable causes of childhood, besides a wide range of other, cancers is in flagrant denial of the specific charge of the 1971 National Cancer Act "to disseminate cancer information to the public." As seriously, this silence is a denial of the public's inalienable democratic right-to-know of information directly impacting on their health and lives, and of their right to influence public policy.

—

ENDORSER:

Quentin D. Young, M.D.
Chairman of Health and Medicine Policy Research Group
Past President of the American Public Health Association

October 24, 2002

Risks of Ovarian Cancer from the Commonly Prescribed Drug Evista Supported by Recent Evidence

The Cancer Prevention Coalition today warned that women taking the osteoporosis drug Evista (raloxifene), marketed since 1997 by Eli Lilly, are at increased risk of ovarian cancer.

"There is ample scientific evidence that Evista poses risks of ovarian cancer. We also know that the National Cancer Institute (NCI) has ignored these risks," said Samuel S. Epstein, M.D., Chairman of the Cancer Prevention Coalition.

Whether the large-scale treatment of women with Evista since 1997 has resulted in an increased incidence of ovarian cancer cannot yet be determined, as the latest NCI cancer incidence data are now two years old. These reveal an 8 percent increased incidence of ovarian cancer in white females over 65, those most likely to be treated with Evista, from 1997 to 1999.

"This delay in reporting cancer incidence is unacceptable. This is all the more so in view of NCI's admission, in the 10/16/02 issue of the Journal of the NCI, of additional reporting delays, besides underestimating the increasing incidence of cancer," noted Dr. Epstein.

Lilly's own study specifically designed to prove the drug's safety found that the drug was shown to induce ovarian cancer in rats and, at doses well below the therapeutic, in mice. The study admitted, "The clinical relevance of these tumor findings is not known."

However, this conclusion violates the strong scientific consensus that the induction of cancer in well-designed studies in two species creates the strong presumption of human risk.

Nevertheless, Lilly failed to disclose this critical information in the: "Warning" section of the Physician's Desk Reference; a 12/4/97 publication in the New England Journal of Medicine; full page advertisements in major national newspapers; and the drug's label. Even more critical is NCI's continuing silence on this avoidable risk of ovarian cancer despite its annual multibillion-dollar taxpayers' funding.

A study by University of Southern California researchers, presented at the European Society of Human Reproduction and Embryology July 2001 annual meeting, has provided further evidence of Evista's cancer risk. It showed that Evista increases the growth rate of ovarian cancer cells in laboratory studies, and may increase risks of recurrence of ovarian cancer.

These warnings were first raised by Dr. Epstein in a 1/12/98 Jim Lehrer Newshour program and a subsequent 2/4/98 (PR Newswire) press release. That release prompted two women to contact the Coalition saying that they had been diagnosed with ovarian cancer following Evista treatment. The first was a 68-year old Delray Beach, Florida woman, following two years treatment to prevent worsening of her osteoporosis. The second was a 53-year old Chicago woman, treated with Evista for over three years to prevent osteoporosis, and recurrence of her previously treated breast cancer. She was contacted by Lilly about a year ago to obtain information for filing an Adverse Drug Reaction with the FDA. Both women were prescribed the drug in the absence of informed consent with regard to risks of ovarian cancer.

Ovarian cancer strikes about 23,000 women annually, accounting for 4 percent for all of their cancers. About 14,000 women die from ovarian cancer annually, making it the most lethal reproductive cancer.

Commenting on these facts, Dr. Epstein charges that Lilly's suppression of evidence of ovarian cancer risks from Evista is as reckless as FDA's marketing approval.

"The FDA should promptly require "Black Box" warnings on Evista labels to warn physicians and patients of the drug's risks. Additionally, women who have been prescribed the drug (or who have participated in clinical trials) should be offered lifelong surveillance for the early detection of ovarian cancer at Lilly's expense," Dr. Epstein said. "Even more reckless is the continued failure of the cancer establishment, the federal National Cancer Institute and the "charitable" American Cancer Society to warn women of Evista's undisclosed and avoidable risk of ovarian cancer, besides a wide range of other cancers," he added.

Finally, the Cancer Prevention Coalition urges Gilda's Club, The Prevention First Coalition, and other women's reproductive health groups to join the Cancer Prevention Coalition in disseminating information on risks of ovarian cancer from Evista treatment.

May 8, 2003

Public Remains Uninformed of Escalating Incidence of Childhood Cancer and Its Avoidable Causes

From 1975 to 2000, the incidence of childhood cancer has escalated to alarming proportions warns the Cancer Prevention Coalition's new report, "The Stop Cancer before It Starts Campaign." Childhood cancers have increased by 32 percent overall: acute lymphocytic leukemia, 57 percent; brain cancer, 50 percent; kidney cancer, 48 percent; and bone cancer, 29 percent. Childhood cancer is their number one killer, second only to accidents.

The federal National Cancer Institute (NCI) and the American Cancer Society (ACS) have failed to inform the public of the increasing incidence of childhood cancer. Furthermore, the NCI claims that: "The causes of childhood cancers are largely unknown." This is contrary to substantial scientific evidence on their avoidable causes, the wide range of carcinogens to which fetuses, infants, and children are exposed, and their much greater vulnerability than adults. Additionally, most carcinogens cause other toxic effects hormonal or endocrine disruptive, neurological, and immunological.

Avoidable carcinogenic exposures of the fetus, infants, and children fall into three categories:

1. Environmental and Occupational

    *   Pesticides: contaminants in drinking water; urban spraying; uses in schools, including wood playground sets treated with chromated copper arsenate
    *   Petrochemical and other industrial pollutants: atmospheric emissions; contaminants in drinking water
    *   Combustion pollutants: power plants; incinerator stacks; diesel exhaust
    *   Radioactive pollutants: atmospheric emissions from nuclear energy plants; contaminants in drinking water
    *   Occupational carcinogens: parental exposures during pregnancy

2. Domestic/Household

- Pesticides: uses in the home, lawn and pet flea collars; contaminants in non-organic food
- Ingredients and contaminants in lotions and shampoos
- Residence near: hazardous waste sites; chemical and power plants; municipal incinerators

3. Medical

- Radiation: diagnostic x-rays in late pregnancy; high-dose radiation CAT scans of infants and children
- Pediatric prescription drugs: Lindane shampoos; Ritalin, for treatment of attention deficit disorder
- Drugs prescribed during pregnancy: the estrogenic DES; the anti-epileptic Dilantin

NCI's silence on such causes of childhood cancer violates the charge of the 1971 National Cancer Act, launching President Nixon's War Against Cancer, "to disseminate cancer information to the public." This silence is also contrary to NCI's 1998 Congressional testimony that it had developed a public registry of avoidable carcinogens. Not surprisingly, the media remain as uninformed as the public. An April 1, 2003 New York Times article, "Success Stories Abound in Efforts to Prevent and Control Cancer," stated that while amazing progress has been made in treating childhood cancers, "their causes remain a mystery."

Besides the NCI and ACS silence on avoidable causes of childhood cancer, they have failed to provide scientific guidance to regulatory agencies, as reflected in their inconsistent and questionable policies. This is illustrated in the well-intentioned current proposal of the Scientific Advisory Board of the Environmental Protection Agency to develop new guidelines for regulating risks "from Early-Life Exposure to Carcinogens." These proposals, however, are based on attempting to quantify risks from individual carcinogens in air and water, without any recognition of their unpredictable additive or multiplicative effects. These proposals also ignore additional risks from a wide range of other carcinogens, such as those in food and cosmetics, regulated by the Food and Drug Administration, and such, as household products including pesticides, regulated by the Consumer Product Safety Commission. Furthermore, EPA's proposals are flawed by unscientific assumptions, such as that safe levels of exposure to carcinogens can be theoretically quantified, and that risks based on evidence from rodent tests should be downgraded unless their mechanism of action can be shown to be the same as in humans.

The minimal priorities of the NCI and ACS for research and providing the public with information on avoidable causes of childhood cancers reflect imbalanced policies, and not lack of resources. NCI's annual budget has increased some thirtyfold, from $220 million to $4.6 billion, since passage of the 1971 National Cancer Act. NCI expenditures on prevention of avoidable causes of cancer have been estimated as under 4 percent of its budget, while ACS has allocated less than 1 percent of its $800 million revenues, apart from $1 billion reserves, to "environmental carcinogenesis."

Clearly, the time for open public debate, and Congressional oversight of national cancer policy is long overdue.

For further details, see the February 2003 "Stop Cancer before It Starts Campaign" report at www.preventcancer.com; the report has been endorsed by over 100 scientific experts in cancer prevention, and representatives of environmental, consumer, and other activist groups.

August 16, 2004

IBM's Corporate Recklessness: From the Holocaust to Occupational Cancer

It's been long said that history has a way of catching up with all of us. And, in an extraordinary feat of cinematographic come-uppance, IBM's role as puppet master of the Holocaust is dramatically uncovered in the prize-winning documentary, "The Corporation." Featuring Michael Moore, Milton Friedman, and Noam Chomsky, among others, the film is now playing nationwide.

Shortly after Hitler seized power, IBM entered into an alliance with Nazi Germany, continuing well into World War II.

Before the dawn of computers, IBM designed over 200 Hollerith punch card machines, with a unique cross-tabulating technology. These were intended for the comprehensive identification of Jews, ancestral tracing of non-Jews with any Jewish lineage, censusing, and registration. This was the essential prelude for asset confiscation, ghettoization, and the logistics of Reichsbahn railroads, concentration camps, slave labor, and ultimately genocide.

IBM did not just sell the machines, but leased them at high profits. IBM subsidiaries in Berlin and Geneva, and their European surrogates, serviced and maintained the machines, and trained Nazi operators in concentration camps. Meanwhile, the corporation maintained a don't ask, don't tell deniability shield.

One might hope that the revelation of IBM's integral role in the Holocaust would motivate subsequent contrition. But, over recent decades, IBM's deniability shield has extended to America.

Indeed, IBM has assigned its U.S. workers to camps which don't have barbed wire or armed guards. Instead, they are chip-manufacturing plants, where workers have been unknowingly and uncontrollably exposed to well-known cancer causing chemicals. And much the same way as IBM hid its role in the Holocaust, it still is trying to hide the truth about its own plants.

In 1997, former IBM workers and their survivors began suing for work-related cancers. In discovery proceedings from approximately 200 ongoing lawsuits, IBM was ordered to disclose mortality records, detailing the causes of death of over 33,000 former workers over the past three decades. It was also ordered to disclose work history records of over 18,000 workers in its chip-manufacturing plants.

In events unfolding since "The Corporation" documentary was completed, these records were turned over to Dr. Richard Clapp, a distinguished epidemiologist at Boston University School of Public Health. Together with Dr. Rebecca Johnson, an independent statistical consultant, Dr. Clapp analyzed records of cancer deaths in IBM's chip-plant workers. The analysis showed that male workers died from high rates of kidney, brain, blood, and skin cancers, while female workers died from a high rate of kidney cancer.

IBM lawyers fought vigorously to contest the study, and block its publication on spurious legal grounds. The study had been scheduled for publication in a major journal, Clinics in Occupational and Environmental Medicine, published by the Amsterdam-based Elsevier. However, apparently bowing to IBM pressure, Elsevier refused to publish the Clapp-Johnson report, even though it had been approved by the publisher's own scientific reviewers. Nevertheless, the report's results are available in depositions, summarized in a New York Times report last September.

Of course, IBM would have us believe that its World War II history is just that, history. But its actions today show that IBM has learned the wrong lesson. IBM still seems more concerned in protecting its image, rather than human rights.

In stark contrast to IBM, and a wide range of other reckless corporations, there are growing numbers of socially responsible businesses. For instance, the Atlanta-based Interface company leases wholesale carpets, manufactured from non-toxic ingredients, and laid with non-toxic adhesives. After years of use, the carpets are recycled, rather than buried in municipal waste sites, and replaced with new carpets.

The leading specialty retailer, Gap, Inc. recently published a report on corporate responsibility. Far from espousing picture perfect conditions, it openly admits serious deficiencies, and pledges a commitment to making substantive improvements, including environmental concerns, sustainability, and worker rights.

Also, the rise of socially responsible investment funds, like the Calvert Funds or Domini Social Investments, further demonstrates that corporations can behave responsibly, while proving profitable.

Doubtless, some such trends are reactive, resulting from pressure by human rights groups, including The Social Venture Network, the National Labor Committee, the National League of Lawyers, and non-governmental organizations. However, as the documentary emphasizes, corporations' "pathological pursuit of profit and power" can only be halted by drastic constitutional and legislative reform.

March 31, 2005

UIC Professor Receives International Humanitarian Award

Dr. Samuel Epstein, professor emeritus of environmental and occupational medicine at the University of Illinois at Chicago School of Public Health, has received the Albert Schweitzer Golden Grand Medal for Humanitarianism.

The award, given by the Albert Schweitzer World Academy of Medicine, honors Epstein for his "longstanding and pioneering international contributions to cancer prevention."

Epstein is a leading authority and champion of cancer prevention issues. His lifelong work focuses on preventing exposure to environmental carcinogens in air, water, food and the workplace by informing the public of avoidable risks and influencing governmental policies.

The Golden Grand Medal is awarded every other year to individuals who have demonstrated exemplary service to humanity.

"I am just overwhelmed and honored to receive such an outstanding award," said Epstein, who also serves as chairman of the Cancer Prevention Coalition and is author of "Cancer-Gate: How to Win the Losing Cancer War."

The award will be presented to Epstein June 10 at the Royal Castle in Warsaw, Poland, during the International Symposium of the Polish Academy of Medicine.

The Albert Schweitzer World Academy of Medicine, established to promote Albert Schweitzer's philosophies of wisdom, humanity and peace, consists of 256 university professors in 71 countries.

UIC ranks among the nation's top 50 universities in federal research funding and is Chicago's largest university with 25,000 students, 12,000 faculty and staff, 15 colleges and the state's major public medical center. A hallmark of the campus is the Great Cities Commitment, through which UIC faculty, students and staff engage with community, corporate, foundation and government partners in hundreds of programs to improve the quality of life in metropolitan areas around the world. For more information about UIC, visit www.uic.edu.

December 15, 2005

New York Times Whitewashes Environmental Causes of Cancer

New York Times columnist Gina Kolata's article, "Environment and Cancer: The Links are Elusive" (Dec. 13, '05), claims that "cancer statistics do not indicate a cancer epidemic," and that "Rates of cancer have been steadily dropping for 50 years," apart from tobacco-related cancers.

However, these claims are contrary to the National Cancer Institute's (NCI) latest available data in its "Cancer Statistics Review, 1975-2002." During this period, there has been a major decrease in the incidence of lung cancer, the single commonest cancer, due to decreased smoking in men.

Meanwhile, there has been a major increase in the incidence of a wide range of non-smoking related cancers. These include: Non Hodgkin's lymphoma, by 74%; acute childhood leukemia, by 68%; childhood brain cancer, by 52%; acute adult leukemia, by 56%; and testes cancer, by 51%.

Overall mortality rates have remained virtually unchanged, despite $50 billion NCI funding, predominantly allocated to diagnosis, treatment and treatment related research, with only minimal funding for research on cancer prevention.

Contrary to Kolata, there is an extensive body of published evidence on avoidable exposures to carcinogens in the totality of the environment-air, water, the workplace, and consumer products-food, cosmetics and toiletries, and household products. This information has been summarized in the Cancer Prevention Coalition's 2003 "The Stop Cancer before It Starts Campaign," endorsed by over 100 leading scientific experts on cancer prevention and epidemiology. Visit the Cancer Prevention Coalition at: www.preventcancer.com

Further information is detailed in the September 2005 University of Massachusetts review on Environmental and Occupational Causes of Cancer, by Dr. Richard Clapp, a leading international epidemiological expert, and colleagues at the Boston University School of Public Health. Visit: www.sustainableproduction.org

Finally, Kolata's article is consistent with her track record of extreme anti-environmental and pro-corporate bias. Surely, the New York Times could publish a more objective report on such critical national concerns.

September 29, 2006

The Harvard Crimson

Harvard Inquiry into Fluoride Study Problematic

To the editors:

As someone who directed the Laboratories of Environmental Toxicology and Carcinogenesis at the Children's Cancer Research Foundation (now known as the Dana-Farber Cancer Institute), and was a research associate in Pathology at the Harvard School of Public Health from 1960-1970, I am appalled at the controversy surrounding the investigation of Professor Chester Douglass ("HMS Defends Review of Dental School Prof," news, Sept. 19).

First of all, it surprises me that someone from the School of Dental Medicine was put in charge of such a sensitive research issue as the possible connection between water fluoridation and bone cancer. Douglass already had a history of promoting fluoridation and had strong financial ties to Colgate. The issue is actually a medical one, not a dental one. When Douglass' student Elise Bassin found a "robust" relationship between osteosarcoma and young boys' exposure to fluoridated water, it was a finding of monumental importance. If, as charged by the Environmental Working Group (EWG), Douglass concealed these findings from the public and the National Institutes of Health funders of the research for over three years, such behavior is reprehensible. It is therefore baffling that Harvard has exonerated Douglass of all charges without providing any explanation as to why the EWG's well-documented evidence against him should now be ignored.

You report that Harvard claims that the "U.S. Department of Health and Human Services' Office for Research Integrity oversaw Harvard's review of Douglass and determined that no further investigation would be necessary." If so, why can't the public that ultimately funded the Bassin and Douglass research be provided with a cogent explanation of what convinced the investigators that Douglass behaved properly? How did the investigators explain Douglass' written statement to a National Research Council committee saying that his work revealed "an Odds Ratio of 1.2 to 1.4 between fluoride and osteosarcoma that was not significantly different from 1" when his own student, in her PhD dissertation approved by

Douglass, had found a "robust" five to seven fold increase in osteosarcoma rates in young boys exposed to fluoridated water.

I do not believe that the Harvard inquiry has clarified this matter at all, either in Harvard's official Aug. 15 statement or the letter from Dr. Margaret Dale sent out Sept. 7.

Whether or not investigators were somehow influenced by Douglass' million dollar contribution to the new Dental School building, will someone at Harvard please provide a detailed explanation as to why the investigators decided to exonerate Douglass before this matter sullies Harvard's reputation completely? If this cannot be done, then I suggest that President Bok organize a totally independent second inquiry, with a panel drawn from scientists with no affiliation to either Harvard or the U.S. water fluoridation program.

March 17, 2008

New York Review of Books Discredits a New Book on the Cancer War

On March 6, the New York Review of Books published Richard Horton's lengthy review of a new book by Devra Davis on "The Secret History of the War on Cancer." Davis is well recognized as a leading scientific expert on avoidable causes of cancer, besides related public policy concerns.

Nearly a quarter of Horton's review is devoted to complaining of the "quality of vitriol and innuendo that Davis pours on the reputation" of the British epidemiologist Richard Doll, the alleged aristocrat of "modern cancer research." However, these criticisms are factual rather than personal. Moreover, they are widely endorsed by recognized leading scientific experts.

From 1950 to 1970, Doll made major contributions to cancer prevention, with precedential research on smoking, asbestos and radioactivity. However, from the mid-1970's, Doll became a closet industry consultant. In the pay of the asbestos industry, he reassured workers that low-level exposure is safe, and recommended denial of compensation to workers dying of cancer. As a consultant to General Motors, he denied that exposure to automobile exhaust from lead in gasoline is hazardous to children. As a consultant to Monsanto, he trivialized the risks of cancer from exposure to Agent Orange, the defoliant used in the Vietnam War. He also supported Monsanto in rejecting compensation claims of exposed veterans. As a consultant to the Chemical Manufacturers Association, Doll denied well-documented scientific evidence relating occupational exposure to vinyl chloride and brain and liver cancers.

In 2000, Doll admitted to receiving charitable donations from Dow Chemical "in recognition of all the work I had done for them." As evidence of Doll's conflicts of interest finally became common knowledge and unarguable, in 2002, shortly before his death, he belatedly admitted that most cancers, other than those due to smoking and hormones, "are induced by exposure to chemicals often environmental."

Horton charges that, based on the calculations of Davis, Doll "systematically underestimated" the dangers of occupational exposure to hazardous chemicals. However, these dangers, particularly of cancer, have been fully documented in numerous publications in prestigious scientific journals by leading U.S. and international scientific authorities over the past decades.

Despite this well documented information, Horton lobbied for Doll's nomination for the Nobel Prize.

Unfazed by the escalating incidence of a wide range of non-tobacco related cancers over recent decades, Horton criticizes Davis's position that "a worldwide exposure of cancer seems to be taking hold." He also appears strangely unaware that this position is by no means unique. It is widely shared by virtually all leading independent scientists worldwide. Horton also dismisses well documented scientific evidence that, besides smoking, these increases are attributable to "environmental and workplace carcinogens," rather than "the real and more robust dangers that face us every day," particularly obesity.

Finally, it should be noted that Horton's dismissal of the role of environmental and occupational carcinogens reflects the long standing bias of the New York Times leading cancer reporters, compounded by questionable conflicts of interest.

July 27, 2009

Push for New Nuclear Power Sputters, but Old Reactors Still Pose Cancer Risks

Nuclear reactors in the United States should be phased out, and replaced by technologies that don't threaten public health with the emission of radioactive chemicals, urges the Cancer Prevention Coalition.

A recent energy bill sponsored by Congressional Republicans proposed building 100 new nuclear reactors across the United States in the next 20 years.

The proposal, which would double the current U.S. total of 104 operating nuclear reactors, would amount to a nuclear renaissance, as no new reactors have been ordered since 1978.

Concerns about global warming gave utilities the idea for this revival since reactors don't emit greenhouse gases while generating power, and utilities have stopped closing old reactors while proposing 33 new ones to be sited in New England, throughout the South and Southeast, and in Texas, Utah and Idaho.

But this month, two Swedish scientists published an article concluding that a large increase in nuclear reactors will not solve global warming.

The utilities, of course, fail to report that greenhouse gases are emitted throughout the entire nuclear fuel cycle, and operating the reactor itself is the only exception. Both the nuclear reactor industry and its support industries spew radioactive materials into local air and water, posing a serious health hazard, warns Dr. Samuel S. Epstein, chairman of the Cancer Prevention Coalition and Professor emeritus Environmental & Occupational Medicine at the University of Illinois at Chicago School of Public Health.

In the 1970s, Wall Street investors stopped funding new reactor projects due to cost and safety concerns. Today, these issues are unchanged, and private investors again gave a thumbs-down to nuclear power. A 2005 law authorizing $18.5 billion in federal loan guarantees would only cover two reactors.

The Bush administration was a willing partner in the nuclear revival. George W. Bush became the first sitting U.S. president to visit a nuclear plant since a grim-faced President James Carter toured the damaged Three Mile Island reactor on April 1, 1979.

President Barack Obama has poured cold water on the renaissance. He rejected a request for $50 billion in loan guarantees in the stimulus package. Additionally, he rejected further funding for developing the nuclear waste dump at Yucca Mountain Nevada, leaving utilities with no place to permanently store their highly radioactive nuclear waste. It is now being held temporarily at 55 storage sites licensed by the Nuclear Regulatory Commission and at Department of Defense sites and national laboratories across the country.

The major threat posed by nuclear reactors is not the addition of new reactors, but continuing to operate old and corroding ones, says Dr. Epstein. U.S. reactors are granted licenses for 40 years, and many are approaching that mark. Many utilities have asked regulators to extend their licenses for an additional 20 years.

"Each of the first 52 requests has been given a rubber-stamp approval, even though operating a 60 year old reactor would be a huge risk to human health," says Joseph Mangano, MPH, MBA, executive director of the Radiation and Public Health Project.

Notable exceptions are state government officials in New York and New Jersey, who are opposing the attempts to extend licenses for reactors in their states.

About 80 million Americans in 37 states live within 40 miles of a nuclear reactor, including residents of New York City, Chicago, Philadelphia, Detroit, Miami, Phoenix, Cleveland, and Boston. "If a meltdown were to occur, safe evacuation would be impossible and many thousands would suffer from radiation poisoning or cancer," warns Dr. Epstein. "The horrifying specter of Chernobyl, or of terrorists attacking a nuclear plant, is not lost on concerned Americans."

Reactors are a real health threat, not just a potential one, a fact largely ignored by mainstream media, he declares.

To generate electricity, over 100 radioactive chemicals are created—among the most dangerous chemicals on Earth, and the same toxic mix in atomic bomb test fallout. These gases and particles, including Strontium-90, Cesium-137, and Plutonium-239, are mostly stored as waste. But some must be routinely released into air and water. Humans breathe, eat, and drink them—just as they did bomb fallout—raising the cancer risk, especially to children.

Industry and government officials argue that reactor emissions are too small to cause harm. But for years, scientists have produced study after study documenting high cancer rates near reactors. For example, a 2007 review of the scientific literature by researchers from the University of South Carolina found elevated rates of childhood cancers, particularly leukemia and brain cancers, in nearly all 17 studies examined. A 2008 study of German reactors was one of the largest ever done, and it also found high local rates of child cancer.

Mangano and colleagues published a January 2002 article in the journal "Archives of Environmental Health," showing that local infant deaths and child cancer cases plunged dramatically right after shut down whenever a U.S. reactor closed. Because the very young suffer most from radiation exposures, they benefit most when exposures are removed. This research indicated that there would be approximately 18,000 fewer infant deaths and 6,000 fewer child cancer cases over the next 20 years if all nuclear reactors were closed.

Over half the states in the United States, 31, currently host nuclear power plants. Illinois has the most with 11, Pennsylvania has nine, and New Jersey has four.

While waiting for the federal government to phase out nuclear power in favor of safer alternatives, state governments should act to warn and protect their citizens, urges the Cancer Prevention Coalition.

Governors have responsibilities to take whatever political action they can to phase-out nuclear plants. In the first instance, governors should tell their citizens of the danger.

In 1954, Atomic Energy Chairman Lewis Strauss declared nuclear power "too cheap to meter." President Richard Nixon envisioned that the nation would have 1,000 reactors by this time. But the dreams of people like Strauss and Nixon were dashed by staggering costs and built-in dangers.

The attempt to revive this Cold War-era dream has been, and still is, largely talk. While the talk goes on, the nation is fast developing technologies like solar and wind power, which never run out and don't pollute. Putting millions of Americans at risk of cancer by hanging on to old reactors—that produce only 19% of America's electricity and 8% of the country's total energy—is a reckless gamble. Nuclear reactors in the U.S. should be phased out, and replaced by options that don't threaten public health.

ENDORSERS:

Rosalie Bertell, PhD
Founding Member European Committee on Radiation Risk
Founder and President emeritus International Institute of Concern for Public Health

Joseph Mangano, MPH, MBA
Executive Director Radiation and Public Health Project

August 15, 2009

An Overdue Ban on a Dangerous Sweetener

The artificial sweetener aspartame has been shown to cause cancer in lab rats, and should be banned for human consumption, warns the Cancer Prevention Coalition.

Under the explicit provisions of the 1958 Delaney Law, which requires an automatic ban on carcinogenic food additives, the Coalition is calling on Dr. Margaret Hamburg, the newly appointed Commissioner of the U.S. Food and Drug Administration and public health advocate, to promptly ban the continued use of aspartame.

First discovered in 1965 by the pharmaceutical company G. D. Searle, aspartame is an artificial sweetener marketed by Ajinomoto Sweeteners under trademark names including NutraSweet, Equal and Canderel.

Aspartame is the second most widely used artificial sweetener in the world. It is found in more than 6,000 products including carbonated and powdered soft drinks, hot chocolate, chewing gum, candy, desserts, yogurt, and tabletop sweeteners, as well as some pharmaceutical products like vitamins and sugar-free cough drops. More than 200 million people worldwide consume it.

The sweetener has been used for more than 30 years, having first been approved by the FDA in 1974.

After saccharin, aspartame is the commonest sweetener, consumed by over 200 million people worldwide, and represents about 60% of the artificial sweetener market.

Aspartame provides food, soft drinks, candy and chewing gum manufacturers with substantial cost savings compared to sugar, which is 200 times less sweet. Aspartame is a sweetener without calories, which helps people control their weight.

Studies of the carcinogenicity of aspartame performed by producers of the sweetener have been negative.

But Cancer Prevention Coalition Chairman Samuel S. Epstein, M.D., warns that the use of aspartame in foods, vitamins and pharmaceuticals is based on false safety information and political maneuvering going back more than 30 years.

In January 1976, then Food and Drug Administration (FDA) Commissioner Alexander M. Schmidt, M.D., testified before Congress that Hazleton Laboratories, under contract to Searle, had been charged with falsifying toxicological data on aspartame.

The FDA convened a Public Board of Inquiry to review concerns about the sweetener's carcinogenic effects in experimental animals. In 1980, the Board concluded that aspartame could "contribute to the development brain tumors."

Dr. Epstein points out that FDA then recommended that, pending confirmation of these findings, the sweetener should no longer be used.

However, then Searle Chairman Donald Rumsfeld, later Secretary of Defense in the Bush Administration, vowed to "call in his markers," to get the sweetener approved.

On January 21, 1981, the day after Ronald Reagan's inauguration, Searle re-applied to the FDA for approval to use aspartame as a food sweetener, and Reagan's new FDA commissioner, Arthur Hayes Hull, Jr., appointed a 5-person Scientific Commission to review the Board of Inquiry's decision.

It soon became clear that the panel would uphold the ban by a 3-2 decision, but Hull then installed a sixth member on the commission, and the vote became deadlocked. He then personally broke the tie in aspartame's favor.

Hull later left the FDA under allegations of impropriety, and then took a position with Burston-Marsteller, the chief public relations firm for Searle and for Monsanto, which purchased Searle in 1985.

Dr. Epstein is not alone among doctors in his concern about the sweetener.

In a July 25, 2009, letter to the new FDA commissioner, H. J. Roberts, M.D., a Florida internist and diabetes expert, drew her attention to the dangerous health effects of aspartame in foods and other products.

"My own data base encompasses over 1400 individuals who have suffered major disorders that could be directly ascribed to the use of these products, including gum," wrote Dr. Roberts, who authored the books "Aspartame Disease: An Ignored Epidemic," and "Aspartame Disease: an FDA Approved Epidemic."

There have been other calls to ban the sweetener, including one in the UK earlier this year, when Member of Parliament Roger Williams cited "compelling and reliable evidence for this carcinogenic substance to be banned from the UK food and drinks market altogether."

Dr. Epstein says the evidence on the carcinogenicity of aspartame was strongly reinforced in a unique feeding test conducted on rats in an Italian laboratory.

In 2005, based on highly sensitive and life-long feeding tests in groups of about 200 rats and at doses less than usual human dietary levels, the prestigious Italian Ramazzini Foundation confirmed that aspartame is unequivocally carcinogenic. A high incidence of cancers was induced in multiple organs of the lab rats fed the sweetener, including lymph glands, brain and kidney.

Dr. Epstein says rats were fed aspartame beginning in the early fetal stage of life, resulting in their lifelong exposure to aspartame.

"This resulted in a still higher increase in the incidence of cancers at sites, including those previously reported," he says.

The Ramazzini study was reported in the November 2005 issue of "Environmental Health Perspectives," the peer-reviewed journal of the United States' National Institute of Environmental Health Sciences.

"Our study has shown that aspartame is a multi-potential carcinogenic compound whose carcinogenic effects are also evident at a daily dose of 20 milligrams per kilogram of body weight (mg/kg), notably less than the current acceptable daily intake for humans," the Ramazzini authors wrote.

Currently, the acceptable daily intake for humans is set at 50 mg/kg in the United States and 40 mg/kg in Europe.

In April 2007, the results of this study were presented by Ramazzini scientists at the Mount Sinai School of Medicine, New York.

Not surprisingly, says Dr. Epstein, these findings have been sharply challenged by the sweetener industry, major sweetener users, such as Coca-Cola, PepsiCo, Nestle, and Monsanto, and also by the industry-oriented scientific journal "Critical Reviews in Toxicology."

In view of the new scientific evidence of aspartame's carcinogenicity and the political gamesmanship that led to its original approval by the FDA, Dr. Epstein is urging the new FDA Commissioner, Dr. Hamburg, to impose an immediate ban on the use of aspartame for human consumption.

August 20, 2009

A Global Model for Health Care

Imagine a world in which even the remotest inhabitants have access to good health care. That's the vision of Health for Humanity, an international, not-for-profit, Baha'i-inspired organization based in Wilmette, IL. Health for Humanity is founded upon the conviction that humankind constitutes one global family with a common heritage and a collective destiny. The central principles which guide Health for Humanity's mission are inspired by the teachings of the Baha'i Faith.

"Before we can make any progress to address the development challenges in our world, we have to first acknowledge that we are all members of one human family and that the welfare of each of us affects us all," says Dr. May Khadem, assistant professor of clinical ophthalmology at Northwestern University's Feinberg School of Medicine, Chicago ophthalmologist, lifelong Baha'i and founding director of Health for Humanity

Health for Humanity was conceived 17 years ago on January 19th, 1992. On that cold Chicago winter Sunday, about twenty physicians gathered together to make decisions about an initiative many had been discussing for several years. That original group was passionate, unified, and shared an incredibly inspiring vision of an organization that would create effective models for health development that successfully combined best practices with a firm ethical foundation based on universal human values. Their first project was initiated that year at the Albania University Eye Center. The project's goal was to reduce blindness in Albania by improving the capacity for modern eye services, with particular focus on cataract surgery and retina services.

Health for Humanity strives to build the capacity of local partners to improve the health of their populations, while providing opportunities for service for its volunteers. Health for Humanity members are from diverse ethnic, religious and professional backgrounds and membership is open to anyone interested in the Health for Humanity mission. "We were embarked on a different and unique pathway to improve the outcomes of health development by focusing not only on what we do, but how we do it. We might think of what we do as the breadth of our activities based on approaches guided by scientific evidence. How we do it has more to do with the depth of our strategies and the core values we employ. Seventeen years later there is a renewed dedication to explore the depth and learn more about and share the new evolving strategies based on ethics, core human values, and service, in addition to utilizing the best practices espoused by the World Health Organization and the community of non-governmental health development organizations" affirms Khadem.

Health for Humanity works through partnerships with local institutions to identify health problems and implement effective value based interventions through service-oriented leadership training. This unique blend of science and values is Health for Humanity's distinctive contribution to health development. Health for Humanity projects fall under two program areas: technical training and health systems enrichment. The technical training program offers surgical training, clinical training, lectures in various medical specialties, and sponsorship of medical fellowships. Health for Humanity's health systems enrichment program is meant to reinforce and build on the effects of the technical training program. As health care professionals are trained in advanced medical techniques, they acquire skills to facilitate knowledge dissemination, group discussion, and consensus building. Health for Humanity s Values-based Leadership curriculum is the cornerstone of this program and works to encourage the examination of leadership models that incorporate ethical frameworks as a means of improving technical capacity and patient care.

During the last year, Health for Humanity's medical volunteers instructed over 270 doctors and provided over 30 specialized surgical trainings in general cataract surgery, oculoplastics surgery and treatment, pediatric rehabilitation, general pediatrics, psychiatry, HIV/AIDS prevention, mental health issues, pediatric cardiology, and diabetes prevention. Health for Humanity also sponsored fellowships for two Mongolian physicians so that they may have the skills necessary to establish an eye bank and to offer the most modern glaucoma treatments. Additionally training was provided in the field of Values-Based Leadership for health care professionals. Health for Humanity's current projects include working with healthcare providers in Mongolia to help prevent avoidable blindness, in China to improve the quality of life for children with disabilities, and with hospitals in China and Mongolia to improve their continuing medical education programs.

Recently, after 17 years Dr. Khadem stepped down as its volunteer executive director. Her passion and commitment carved an illustrious history of successful international partnerships. While her contributions are considerable they can be perhaps best summed up by a quote from the head surgical nurse in ophthalmology, Vincenc Gjergji, whom Dr. Khadem worked with in Albania for 13 years. "I thank you that you gave us value. It helped us to appreciate ourselves . . . For me the moral leadership workshop was the most helpful. This was the first time that we had anything like this in our clinic . . . After that, I changed my style of communication with those under me. They saw a difference in me and they liked it. It changed them too. They work differently now. The way we organize our work changed completely . . . We never used to prepare the patients for surgery. We never said anything to them. Now we explain to the patients what kind of surgery they are having and for what reason. The patients feel much better and the nurses feel much better. We talk to patients now . . . We appreciate so much everything you did for us. You gave us a new vision of ourselves and it is only growing as we learn more . . ."

Health for Humanity envisions a world in which all members of the human family, even in the most remote regions, have the resources and educational opportunities to address the health challenges of their communities and is then able to shoulder the leadership for their own progress. These values, found in all cultures, nations, and faiths are what unite humanity into one family and constitute the essence of humanity's common heritage and future.

January 6, 2010

A Dangerous Spin on the Cancer Risks of a Sugar-Free Sweetener

The Cancer Prevention Coalition notes with alarm that on January 2 this year, in a heavily advertised special health-theme issue of *People Magazine*, Kraft announced a new campaign on Crystal Light, a sugarless powdered drink mix which can easily be poured into tap and bottled water drinks. Crystal Light's ingredients include the artificial sweetener aspartame, under the trademark names of NutraSweet and Equal, besides citric acid and sodium citrate.

Cancer Prevention Coalition Chairman Dr. Samuel S. Epstein warns that, based on scientific evidence published in peer-reviewed journals and presented to the U.S. Congress, aspartame is both toxic and carcinogenic. The coalition is calling upon the U.S. Food and Drug Administration (FDA) to ban all dietary uses of aspartame.

Crystal Light was first marketed in 1982 to "make drinking water more enjoyable," and much less caloric than fruit juices. Aspartame, 200 times sweeter than sugar, is also widely used as a sweetener in tea and coffee, especially by the weight conscious.

Aspartame was synthesized by G. D. Searle in 1965 after its strong sweet taste was first noted.

Subsequent toxicology tests by Searle revealed brain damage in mice, and cancer in the liver, testes and thyroid of rats. However, the results of these tests were never published nor reported to the FDA.

After saccharin, aspartame is the second most widely used artificial sweetener in the world. It is found in more than 6,000 products including carbonated and powdered soft drinks, hot chocolate, chewing gum, candy, desserts, yogurt, and tabletop sweeteners, as well as some pharmaceutical products like vitamins and sugar-free cough drops.

Aspartame is consumed by over 200 million people worldwide and represents about 60% of the artificial sweetener market.

Aspartame provides manufacturers of food, soft drinks, candy, and chewing gum with substantial cost savings compared to sugar, which is 200 times less sweet. Aspartame also is a sweetener without calories, which helps people control their weight.

In 1975, a FDA Task Force conducted a comprehensive review of the scientific literature on the toxicity of aspartame. This revealed gross abuse in Searle's claims which trivialized or suppressed evidence on the toxic and carcinogenic effects of aspartame.

In January 1976, then FDA Commissioner Alexander M. Schmidt testified before Congress that Hazleton Laboratories, under contract to Searle, had been charged with falsifying toxicological data on aspartame.

The FDA convened a Public Board of Inquiry to review concerns about the sweetener's carcinogenic effects in experimental animals. In 1980, the Board concluded that aspartame could "contribute to the development brain tumors." The FDA then recommended that, pending confirmation of these findings, the sweetener should no longer be used.

Evidence of these toxic effects was subsequently confirmed by leading independent U.S. scientists. Reacting to these concerns in 1976, Senator Edward Kennedy warned, "This extensive nature of the almost unbelievable range of abuses in several major Searle products is profoundly disturbing."

At invited 1979 testimony before the House Committee on the Judiciary, apart from other examples of corporate crime, Dr. Epstein detailed evidence on Searle's criminal denial of the carcinogenicity of aspartame. This evidence was subsequently posted in the Congressional Record.

In 1996, based on a comprehensive review of the scientific literature, Dr. John Olney, a leading independent U.S. scientist, confirmed that aspartame caused brain cancer when fed to rodents.

A decade later, Dr. Epstein points out, the prestigious Italian Ramazzini Foundation, based on large scale life-long feeding tests in large numbers of rats, commencing in infancy, confirmed that low levels of aspartame induced brain cancer and cancers at other sites. The Ramazzini study was reported in the November 2005 issue of Environmental Health

Perspectives, the peer-reviewed journal of the United States' National Institute of Environmental Health Sciences.

"Our study has shown that aspartame is a multi-potential carcinogenic compound whose carcinogenic effects are also evident at a daily dose less than the current acceptable daily intake for humans," the Ramazzini scientists warned.

Of further significance, these conclusions were endorsed by the Federal National Toxicology Program, says Dr. Epstein. "Nevertheless, and not surprisingly, Searle and its consultants still attempt to challenge these conclusions, and persist in their reckless claim that aspartame is safe."

"In view of the unequivocal scientific evidence of aspartame's carcinogenicity, besides the political gamesmanship that led to its original approval by the FDA," Dr. Epstein says, "it is anticipated that Dr. Margaret Hamburg, the new FDA Commissioner, will ban all dietary uses of aspartame."

March 9, 2010

Malignant Melanoma: How to Avoid A Lethal Cancer

On February 23 and 24, the *New York Times* published two full page articles on experimental drug trials on malignant melanoma, respectively titled "After Long Fight, Drug Gives Sudden Reprieve" and "A Drug Trial Cycle: Recovery, Relapse, Reinvention."

As stated in the February 24 article, at an international oncology meeting, Dr. Keith Flaherty described "the extraordinary recovery of the melanoma patients in the experimental drug trials he was leading." However, he frankly admitted "The drug's ability to stop the melanoma, on average appears to be approximately six months."

Malignant melanoma is the fastest rising cancer in the world. Since 1975, its incidence in white men and women has increased by about 240 percent and 170 percent, respectively, while its mortality has increased by 55 percent and 24 percent, respectively. In sharp contrast, malignant melanoma is virtually unknown in black men and women.

All these articles focused on efforts to treat this lethal cancer. However, exclusive emphasis was directed to a specialized experimental treatment known as "targeted therapy," strongly promoted by the cancer drug industry—notably its two giant companies, Roche and Glaxo. Emphasis was also directed to clinical trials by two patient "advocacy groups," the Melanoma and Melanoma Research Foundations. However, minimal or no reference was made to the obvious fact that malignant melanoma, just like lung cancer, is essentially avoidable.

A 1992 publication by Dr. Garland in the *American Journal of Public Health*, "Could Sunscreens Increase Melanoma Risk" documented the scientific evidence that sunscreens protect against sunburn due to short-wave ultraviolet (UV-B) radiation. However, sunscreens give no more than two hours protection, no matter how high their sun protection factor (SPF) is rated. Also, sunscreens wash off readily following even a short swim.

More seriously, Dr. Garland emphasized the alarming evidence that sunscreens do not protect against long-wave (UV-A) radiation. This penetrates deeply into the skin, and is responsible for the lethal malignant melanoma, now the fastest rising cancer in the world.

Prolonged exposure to sun is particularly dangerous during childhood and adolescence. Years of research data has clearly shown a strong relationship between the number of sunburn episodes before the age of fifteen, and the subsequent development of malignant melanoma later in life.

Since 1975, its incidence in white men and women has increased by about 240 percent and 170 percent, respectively, while its mortality has increased by 55 percent and 24 percent, respectively. In sharp contrast, malignant melanoma is virtually unknown in black men and women. This reduced cancer risk is due to the fact that skin contains high levels of melanin, the natural black pigment, which is very effective in blocking the dangerous long-wave radiation.

In a sharp contrast to sunscreens, sunblocks, based on zinc oxide and titanium dioxide, are highly protective and long-lasting. They act by reflecting radiation off the skin surface. However, sunblocks are generally unfavored as they whiten the skin. Far more seriously, unscrupulous manufacturers have increased their effectiveness, by incorporating unlabeled ultra-microscopic particles known as "nanoparticles." These are ultra dangerous as they can penetrate deeply through the skin and even invade small blood vessels, with poorly predictable body wide toxic effects.

Fortunately, as emphasized in my 2009 book *Toxic Beauty*, there are safe alternatives to sunscreens. These include Soyscreen, based on natural plant ingredients, which is long acting and does not wash off in the sea. They also include Solumbra, a highly effective sun-protection brand of light clothing, particularly for children.

Surely the Melanoma foundations will support these and related initiatives for reducing exposures to long-wave UV radiation, and thus eliminate the only known and well-documented cause of the malignant melanoma, apart from a possible role of ozone depletion.

May 20, 2010

President's Cancer Panel Warns of Bisphenol—a Toxic Effects

Cancer Prevention Coalition Chairman Samuel S. Epstein, M.D. is drawing public attention to the 2010 President's Cancer Panel report which explicitly cited Bisphenol-A (BPA) as a "chemical of concern," and warned that "more than 130 studies have linked BPA to breast cancer, obesity, and other disorders."

Bisphenol-A is widely used as a plasticizer in polycarbonate baby bottles, besides adult personal care and cosmetic products, food can linings, microwave oven dishes, dental sealants, and also medical devices. Other recently recognized major sources are cash register and credit-card receipts, which are coated with microscopic powdered BPA, and which many of us handle daily.

The Panel rejected the March 2009 Food and Drug Administration (FDA) safety assessment of BPA as "incomplete and unreliable because it failed to consider all the relevant scientific works." The Panel also warned that FDA's "safety assessment on BPA" had been rejected by a March 2009 consortium of independent experts from academia, government, and industry. The Panel report further emphasized that "science at the FDA is deficient, and the Agency is not prepared to meet regulatory responsibilities."

The scientific evidence on the toxic effects of BPA is extensive, Dr. Epstein emphasizes. A 2007 review of about 700 studies on BPA, published in the journal Reproductive Toxicology, found that the fetus and infants are highly vulnerable to the toxic hormonal effects of this ingredient, technically known as "endocrine disruptive." An accompanying study by National Institutes of Health researchers reported uterine damage in newborn rodents exposed to levels of BPA comparable with those of normal human exposure. This finding may also implicate BPA as a cause of reproductive tract disorders in women, after their earlier exposure as fetuses or infants.

Previous studies in the journal Endocrinology, besides elsewhere, reported that BPA masculinizes the brain of female mice and feminizes the brain of male mice. Toxic effects of this hormone disrupter in pregnant women are evidenced in their infant baby boys by the reduction in the normal distance between their anus and genitals. This decrease in anogenital distance is also associated with a decrease in sperm production. Based on such evidence, Health Canada declared BPA to be a "toxic chemical" in early 2008.

In addition to these toxic effects, exposure of pregnant rodents to BPA, at levels 2,000 times lower than the Environmental Protection Agency's "safe dose," resulted in sexual abnormalities in their offspring. These include an increased number of "terminal end buds" in breast tissue, which are associated with a subsequent high risk of breast cancer. However, an American Plastics Council spokesman claimed that the human relevance of these finding is only "hypothetical."

Dr. Epstein warns that BPA has also been found in human blood, placental and fetal tissue, and incriminated as a predisposing factor for prostate cancer. The authors of this study also linked endocrine-dependent human cancers, such as breast cancer, to the minimal levels of BPA to which pregnant women are exposed. An August 2, 2007 consensus statement by several dozen scientists warned that BPA, even at very low exposure levels, is probably responsible for many human reproductive disorders.

A September 2008 publication, Endocrine-Related Cancer, by one of us (Dr. Gail Prins) reviewed the substantial scientific evidence on the toxic hormonal effects of BPA, besides other endocrine disruptive chemicals (EDC's) in pregnant women. She concluded that infants and children are highly sensitive to their toxic effects, particularly subsequent risks of prostate cancer.

In October 2008, Science Daily reported on an article on BPA called "A Plastic World," in a then pending special section on Environmental Research. Two other articles reported that fetal exposure to BPA disrupted the normal development of the brain and behavior in rats and mice. Other articles have also reported that BPA is massively contaminating the oceans and harming aquatic wildlife.

The June 2009 Endocrine Disruption Act authorized the National Institute of Environmental Health Science "to coordinate" research on hormone disruption to prevent exposure to chemicals "that can undermine the development of children before they are born and cause lifelong impairment of their health and function." This Bill was supported by public health, consumer and children's advocacy groups, and further strengthened by California's Senator Dianne Feinstein's legislation to ban BPA from food and beverage containers. Of major relevance, this legislation has also been endorsed by the April 2010 President's Cancer Panel On "Reducing Environmental Cancer Risk: What We Can Do Now," 2008-2009 Annual Report. This further warns that "to a disturbing extent, babies are born pre-polluted."

Dr. Epstein stresses that there are safe alternatives to BPA. As emphasized in the author's 2009 Toxic Beauty book, the recent development of "green chemistry" has encouraged the phase-out of product packaging that relies on petrochemical plastic containers, particularly those containing BPA. These containers are now being replaced with biodegradable substitutes, including recycled paper. Such "green" packaging reduces energy use, greenhouse gases, and non-degradable or poorly degradable wastes currently disposed of in landfills.

In January this year, the FDA announced an "Update on BPA," with particular reference to its use in food packaging, plastic baby bottles, feeding cups, and metal containers, to avoid childhood exposure. Nevertheless, FDA has still failed to take any regulatory action to this effect. Meanwhile, the industry's Cosmetic Ingredient Review Panel does not even make any reference to BPA in its annual "safety assessments."

In March this year, Congressmen Bobby Rush and Henry Waxman released a draft of the Toxic Chemicals Safety Act of 2010. The key provisions of this Act include establishment of a program to review and protect children from risks of toxic exposures, including BPA. The passage of this legislation is urgently needed in order to ban BPA from baby bottles, food packaging and other consumer products, especially to prevent any further childhood exposure.

One month later, Senator Lautenberg introduced the "Safe Chemicals Act of 2010," aimed at revamping the 34 year-old Toxic Substances Control Act. This is intended to ensure that "those who make the chemicals— ought to be responsible for testing them before they are released to the public." This surely should be the case for BPA.

ENDORSER:

Gail S. Prins, PhD
Professor of Physiology and Urology
University of Illinois at Chicago College of Medicine
Chicago, Illinois

July 16, 2010

Reflecting on the 65th Anniversary of the First A-Bomb

July 16 marks 65 years since the first atomic bomb explosion, known as Trinity. It is a date that changed world history forever, and created new health and security threats that still plague the planet.

Details of Trinity have been documented before, but merit a recap, since memories may fade with the passage of so many years. The collision of two forces—the discovery of atomic fission and the rise of Nazi Germany—in the creation of the Manhattan Project in late 1942. Fearful that the Germans would develop and use a nuclear weapon, President Franklin D. Roosevelt directed the U.S. army to develop such a weapon first. Working furiously, scientists had developed enough nuclear material for a bomb in less than three years. By then, Germany had been defeated, but American forces were still engaged against Japan.

Before a nuclear weapon could be used in war, a test was needed. Manhattan Project directors considered 11 locations, and selected the White Sands Bombing Range in southern New Mexico. The site was a remote location, relatively close to the Los Alamos National Laboratory, where the project's scientists were based. Soldiers prepared a 100-foot tower for the bomb and two trenches for observers. The trenches were 10 and 17 miles away, as nobody really knew how powerful the blast would prove. The bomb, nicknamed "Gadget" was assembled and readied.

At 5:29 a.m. local time, the Trinity explosion occurred and the atomic age officially began. The test succeeded, putting to rest any doubts harbored by Manhattan Project team members. A deafening roar went up, and a blinding flash illuminated the desert, visible 200 miles away. A gaping crater 10 feet deep and 1100 feet in diameter was formed. The shock wave from the explosion could be felt for more than 100 miles. The yield of the plutonium-based bomb was estimated at 23,000 tons of TNT. To maintain secrecy, the Army issued a press release, stating that an "ammunition magazine" had exploded, without anyone being injured.

The 260 observers present were awed. Dr. J. Robert Oppenheimer, who directed the team that created the bomb, later remembered that the blast brought to mind a passage from the Bhagavad-Gita:

If the radiance of a thousand suns
Were to burst at once in the sky
That would be like the splendor of the Mighty One . . .
I am become Death
The shatterer of Worlds

The cloud from Trinity quickly rose 35,000 feet into the air, and moved northeast with prevailing winds. Scientists didn't track the fallout with much precision, but the cloud traveled an extensive distance. That fall, Eastman Kodak labs discovered imperfections in x-ray films. Time magazine reporter Lansing Lamont, in his 1965 book *Day of Trinity* related that Kodak officials traced the imperfections to radioactive cerium in strawboard—from Trinity—produced with river water from Indiana, over 1,000 miles from the Trinity site.

Today, Trinity is a National Historic Landmark, a quiet spot in the desert, only open for public visits twice a year. A 12 foot lava obelisk stands on the site of the blast. Residual radiation at the site is still about 10 times higher than normal.

Current public policy issues that began with Trinity (and the Hiroshima and Nagasaki bombs several weeks later) are multiple. The test stands as the first "weapon of mass destruction" in history, proving that large-scale casualties could occur in just seconds. It also was a prototype for subsequent atom bomb tests; the U.S. and former Soviet Union conducted 422 atmospheric tests—with the equivalent yield of 40,000 Hiroshima bombs. Not until the 1963 treaty signed by President John F. Kennedy and Premier Nikita Khrushchev were all tests consigned to below ground locations. Although virtually all tests worldwide ceased two decades ago, concern of a resurgence of nuclear tests and subsequent use in war by nations that do or don't have atomic weapons is still prevalent.

Another legacy of Trinity is nuclear waste. To produce material for the bomb, massive efforts to convert uranium to bomb-ready material took place at facilities in Oak Ridge Tennessee and Hanford Washington. These operations generated enormous amounts of over 100 radioactive chemicals, not found in nature, which served no purpose other than waste. The critical need to produce the bomb as fast as possible for national security purposes relegated safety and health to a secondary role, and large airborne releases of radioactivity were vented. Workers at Oak Ridge and Hanford also were exposed. While production of new nuclear weapons halted after the Cold War, the problem of safely storing waste from reactors is still a major concern.

The Trinity bomb also helped usher in an era of increased electricity generation from nuclear reactors, which use a controlled version of an atomic bomb explosion. With fears of nuclear war growing, President Dwight D. Eisenhower's 1953 "Atoms for Peace" speech at the United Nations spawned the drive to build nuclear power reactors. Promises like that of energy "too cheap to meter," as stated by Atomic Energy Commission head Lewis Strauss, could be created by reactors initially caused a rush of construction. President Richard Nixon predicted the U.S. would eventually have 1,000 reactors. But extremely high costs of construction and operation, plus safety concerns epitomized by the Three Mile Island and Chernobyl meltdowns, took the momentum from the nuclear expansion. Today, 104 reactors in the U.S. produce just 19 percent of the nation's electricity. No new reactors have been ordered since 1978.

The decades-long effort to reduce nuclear weapons stockpiles has received considerable support from both democrats and republicans. Both are also committed to ensuring the control of nuclear materials to keep them out of the hands of "rogue" states that might otherwise develop, test, and employ atomic weapons.

But nuclear reactors are another story. Capitalizing on environmental concerns caused by carbon emissions, nuclear industry leaders have spent the better part of a decade pushing to keep aging reactors operating and to build new ones for the first time in over three decades. Finding little interest from Wall Street financiers for these projects long before the current economic downturn, these leaders turned to Washington instead.

And leaders of both parties have responded. The administration of George W. Bush proved very sympathetic, and did much to promote nuclear power. At Bush's urging, Congress passed a law in 2005 allotting $18.5 billion in federal loan guarantees to underwrite the cost of construction new reactors. But since last year, President Barack Obama—who repeatedly cautioned about nuclear environmental and health issues in his 2008 campaign—has jumped on the bandwagon. Perhaps the most blatant of the Obama administration's efforts is his Energy Department's proposal to add another $36 billion in loan guarantees.

The same cocktail of 100-plus radioactive chemicals in the Trinity blast—Strontium-90, Cesium-137, Iodine-131, and Plutonium-239—is produced by nuclear reactors. Each causes cancer, and is most harmful to the fetus, infant and child. The average nuclear plant stores the equivalent of hundreds of Trinity bombs as nuclear waste, and this waste must be kept out of the environment for thousands of years. President Obama should be applauded for his efforts to reduce nuclear weapons proliferation, but he shouldn't make a distinction between weapons and reactors. Both are children of that tremendous blast in New Mexico 65 years ago, and both must be controlled in the name of health and safety.

ENDORSER:

Joseph Mangano, MPH, MBA
Executive Director of the Radiation and Public Health Project
Author of the 2007 *Radioactive Baby Teeth: The Cancer Link*
New York

August 2, 2010

Nuke Accident Would Dwarf Oil Spill

Bob Herbert's July 19 *New York Times* column rightly states that the harm from a meltdown at a nuclear power plant "would make the Deepwater Horizon disaster look like a walk in the park." Herbert also warns that systems needed to prevent a meltdown are not well developed. "Right now, we're not ready," he says.

The damage from the April oil well rupture which spewed into the Gulf of Mexico is still being calculated. It killed 11 workers and thousands of aquatic creatures. Recovery workers have become ill attempting to cap the damaged well. The ecosystem of a large body of water and coastline has been damaged. The economic losses are staggering.

But the Deepwater disaster still can't hold a candle to a nuclear accident.

Understanding why a meltdown would be so devastating is possible only after recognizing that nuclear reactors produce the same radioactive chemicals in atomic bomb explosions. Splitting uranium atoms produces a cocktail of 100-plus chemicals that are radioactive waste products, including Cesium-137, Iodine-131, and Strontium-90.

If water cooling a reactor's core or waste pools was removed, from mechanical failure or act of sabotage, huge amounts of toxic gases and particles would be released and breathed by humans. Many thousands would be stricken immediately with radiation poisoning, and subsequently with cancer. Infants and children would suffer most.

From 1945 to 1963, atom bombs were tested in the atmosphere in remote areas of the south Pacific and Nevada. But still, the fallout drifted long distances and contaminated the diet of all Americans. In 1999, the National Institute of Medicine concluded that up to 212,000 Americans developed thyroid cancer from the Nevada tests.

But reactors are not in remote locations. Most are near highly populated areas. One example is Indian Point, which is just 23 miles from the New York City border. The plant has three reactors; one has shut down, but the other two have been operating since the mid-1970s. Its aging parts are corroding, and several "near miss" meltdown situations have occurred in the past decade, according to a 2006 Greenpeace report.

If Indian Point experienced a meltdown, and an evacuation was attempted, New York area traffic would be far worse than its usual crawl. Radioactivity, carried by winds, would reach 21 million people living within 50 miles of the plant. Even among those evacuated, many would not be able to return to their homes, since their environment would remain contaminated.

Indian Point may be the worst case scenario for a meltdown, as New York is the most populated city in the U.S. But nuclear plants are situated on the outskirts of virtually every major metropolitan area in the nation.

Bob Herbert's warning that systems to prevent meltdowns at nuclear plants are insufficient was also a conclusion of the 9/11 Commission. One of the hijacked planes headed for Manhattan flew directly over Indian Point. Had the plane crashed into Indian Point's core or waste pools, the consequences would have been far worse than the loss of nearly 3,000 lives at the World Trade Center.

Safety systems exist at nuclear plants, but anything less than 100 percent effectiveness is dangerous. One flaw came to light in 2002 at the Davis Besse plant near Toledo Ohio. Boric acid had eaten through nearly all of an 8-inch a steel beam in the plant's ceiling, reducing it to less than half an inch at its thinnest part. Disturbingly, the problem was discovered accidentally, not from any routine safety procedure.

The meltdown scenario is disturbing, but there is more to the nuclear threat. Most radioactive waste is stored, but some is routinely or accidentally released into air and water from all 104 U.S. nuclear reactors. These enter our bodies through breathing, and also the food chain.

No government program has ever measured how much radioactivity from reactors enters our bodies, as officials call these amounts "negligible." But a landmark study, whose results have been published in five leading medical journals, has provided evidence to the contrary. Levels of Strontium-90 in nearly 5,000 baby teeth are 30 to 50% greater in children living closest to nuclear plants, and are rising over time. In the 1950s and 1960s, Strontium-90 was often cited as one of the most toxic chemicals in bomb fallout.

Tooth study results raise the question of whether reactor emissions have raised cancer rates near nuclear plants. Again, government officials dismiss this possibility. But near nuclear plants in New York and New Jersey, increases in Sr-90 in teeth were matched by similar increases in local childhood cancer rates a few years later.

Children suffer the greatest damage from radiation exposure, but adults are not exempt. Thyroid cancer is one of the most radiation-sensitive cancers, because radioactive iodine in bomb fallout and reactor emissions seek out the thyroid gland and destroy its cells. A 2009 scientific article reported the highest U.S. thyroid cancer rate in a small 90-mile radius. This encompassed eastern Pennsylvania, central New Jersey, and southern New York, where 16 reactors are located.

Other scientific reports have documented evidence that nuclear plant shut downs are followed immediately by dramatic reductions in local infant deaths and child cancers. This is similar to what happened nationally following the 1963 ban on above-ground atomic tests.

Proposals to build new reactors to replace carbon-producing coal plants are accompanied by claims that nuclear power is "clean." This could not be further from the truth. We should never forget that nuclear reactors are essentially controlled atom bombs.

As lessons of the Deepwater fiasco are learned, we must understand the hard truth that certain energy sources pose very high risks to our security and health. We must do all we can to prevent another massive oil spill, or a nuclear meltdown. But we should go further, by developing energy sources that are safe. Solar panels need no security precautions. Wind mills don't cause environmental catastrophes. We must be proactive and safe.

ENDORSER:

Joseph Mangano, MPH, MBA
Executive Director of the Radiation and Public Health Project
Author of the 2007 *Radioactive Baby Teeth: The Cancer Link*
New York

December 6, 2010

Evista: A Prevention Drug That Has a Fatal Risk

Eli Lilly's full page advertisement in the October 18 New York Times offered post-menopausal women a free trial month voucher for the prescription drug Evista, with the trade name Raloxifene. This has been widely promoted and marketed since 1997 for preventing and treating osteoporosis, affecting over 20 million women annually.

The ad warns that the side effects of Evista may include "hot flashes and joint pain, blood clots in the legs and lungs, and dying from stroke." What the ad particularly fails to warn is Evista's risk of ovarian cancer, which strikes about 24,000 women each year, accounting for 4 percent of all their cancers, according to the Cancer Prevention Coalition.

Based on the latest National Cancer Institute data, ovarian cancer death rates have increased dramatically in white and African American women over the age of 65 by 15 percent and 36 percent, respectively. There are now about 15,300 deaths from ovarian cancer each year, making it the most lethal cancer in women after colon, breast and lung.

On December 10, 1997, pharmaceutical company Eli Lilly announced the FDA's clearance to market Evista. This had been claimed to be effective in preventing osteoporosis, affecting over 20 million U.S. women annually, and in reducing LDL or "bad cholesterol" blood levels. Lilly also submitted applications to market Evista in more than 30 different nations.

"Surely, this new drug should have been welcomed by women worldwide. Fortunately, this was not the case," says Cancer Prevention Coalition Chairman Samuel S. Epstein, M.D.

"With FDA's complicity, Lilly has attempted to suppress explicit evidence that Evista poses major risks of ovarian cancer on the alleged grounds that the 'clinical relevance of these tumor findings is unknown,'" asserts Dr. Epstein.

In Lilly's November 21, 1997, Pharmacology Review, designed to prove the drug's safety, Evista was reported to induce ovarian cancer in both mice and rats, Dr. Epstein points out.

"Moreover," he explains, "the carcinogenic effects in mice were noted at dosages extending down to one-third less than the recommended standard treatment dose."

"This critical information never made it to the drug label warning," Dr. Epstein warns.

Furthermore, he says, the pharmaceutical company's own data revealed an 8 percent increased incidence of ovarian cancer in white females over 65, those most likely to have been treated with Evista, from 1997 to 1999.

"Responding to my criticisms of Lilly on a January 12, 1998 Jim Lehrer Newshour program debate, a company representative claimed that carcinogenic effects of Evista in the ovaries of rodents are irrelevant to any such risks in postmenopausal women," Dr. Epstein says. "However, these claims were critically discounted by Jim Lehrer."

Of further and related concern, Dr. Epstein points to a July 2001 study by Dr. David Taurgeman, of the University of Southern California School of Medicine. He reported that Evista, alone or in combination with estrogen, increased the growth rate of ovarian cancer cells, and could increase the risks of recurrence of ovarian cancer.

Dr. Epstein warns, "The October 18, 2010 New York Times advertisement shows reckless disregard for women's health and lives."

December 23, 2010

Did the Atom Bomb Test Fallout Cause Cancer?

The huge mushroom clouds from atom bomb tests of the 1950s and 1960s are an unforgettable part of the American saga. The tests were cloaked in rhetoric typical of the Cold War, i.e., they were needed to achieve "superiority" over the Soviets in the event of a nuclear war.

But all the patriotic nuclear talk couldn't prevent widespread concern that nuclear war would kill tens of millions. But many were also troubled by fallout in the mushroom clouds, which contained huge amounts of over 100 deadly radioactive chemicals that traveled through the air across the continental U.S. Precipitation brought this fallout back to earth—and into the food chain and human bodies.

Concerns became so great that scientists and citizens began calling for studies of how much fallout was entering people's bodies, and how much harm it was causing—especially to the highly-sensitive fetuses, infants, and children. Dr. Herman Kalckar of the National Institutes of Health published an article in August 1958, calling for a baby tooth "census"—a program of collecting teeth and testing them in laboratories for fallout levels. In particular, Kalckar suggested that Strontium-90 be measured.

Of the more than 100 radioactive chemicals in fallout, Sr-90 was the most feared. Chemically similar to calcium, it attaches to bone and teeth, where it attacks cells, causing cancer. It can penetrate into the bone marrow, where the red and white blood cells so important to the immune response are formed. In 1956, Presidential candidate Adlai Stevenson made a speech singling out the potency of Sr-90:

"This radioactive fallout, as it is called, carries something that's called strontium-90, which is the most dreadful poison in the world. For only one tablespoon equally shared by all the members of the human race could produce a dangerous level of radioactivity in the bones of every individual."

In December 1958, a group of visionary scientists at Washington University in St. Louis, working with the citizen group Committee for Nuclear Information, began collecting baby teeth, locally and across the country. They obtained federal grants to cover their costs, and generated large numbers of volunteers to help with tooth collection. Schools, PTAs, churches, scout groups, dental societies, libraries and clinics all took part. Children were rewarded for donating teeth with a small button bearing a likeness of a boy with a gap in his front teeth, with the phrase "I Gave My Tooth to Science."

A staggering total of about 320,000 teeth were collected over the next dozen years. Lab tests found that children born in 1963 had about 50 times more Sr-90 in teeth than those born in 1950. Washington University officials used their results in testimony to the U.S. Senate leading to the Partial Test Ban Treaty signed by President John F. Kennedy, ending all above-ground atom bomb tests.

Testing had ended, but the thorny question of health hazards to Americans—especially children—remained. U.S. childhood cancer rates had climbed in the 1950s and early 1960s, but scientists were stumped as to why. Studies of the fallout-cancer link were only conducted after the Cold War had ended. A 2002 U.S. Centers for Disease Control report calculated that fallout caused 15,000 U.S. cancer deaths, a figure some believed was a gross underestimate. The following year, a blue ribbon European panel reported 61,600,000 cancer deaths worldwide from fallout.

The St. Louis tooth study was seemingly headed for the history books, until 2001, when Washington University officials stumbled upon 85,000 teeth not used in the study in a remote storage area. The school donated the teeth to the Radiation and Public Health Project (RPHP), a research group conducting its own study of Sr-90 in baby teeth, near U.S. nuclear reactors. Each tooth is enclosed in a small envelope attached to a card identifying the tooth donor.

RPHP scientists recognized that these teeth could help answer the long-awaited question of fallout's harm to the health of Americans. The tooth donors, now in their 40s and 50s, could be tracked at current addresses or through death records. And Sr-90 could still be measured in each tooth, as the chemical decays very slowly.

Earlier this month, the first results of the RPHP health study were released in an article in the International Journal of Health Services. Baby teeth of St. Louis baby boomers who died of cancer by age 50 had more than double—122 percent more—the Sr-90 concentration than did Boomers who are alive and healthy. This research, known as a case-control study, is the first evidence that bomb tests harmed Americans using actual levels of fallout in human bodies. It is not yet possible to estimate the number of cancer victims from fallout, but it appears that the CDC estimate of 15,000 deaths is too low.

Bomb testing into the atmosphere ended in 1963, and even below-ground tests stopped in 1992. The study of fallout's impact on cancer, however, is not an idle look into history, but has much current relevance, namely:

1. With 150 million Americans alive who were exposed to above-ground bomb tests, and with 40% expected to be diagnosed with cancer at some point, it is important to understand causes of the disease.
2. The Comprehensive Test Ban Treaty of 1996, which proposes to end all atom bomb tests, has been ratified by 153 nations—but not the U.S. President Obama has pledged to convince the U.S. Senate to ratify the treaty, and information on health risk is an important aspect supporting the Treaty.
3. The 104 nuclear power reactors in the U.S. produce the same mixture of chemicals as atom bomb tests. Most of this toxic mixture is stored as high level nuclear waste, but some is emitted into the air and water, and enters human bodies. The RPHP study of baby teeth showed that Sr-90 levels in children near reactors were 30-50 percent greater than children in distant areas, and that levels were rising sharply over time, as aging reactors corrode.

Studying health risks of radioactive emissions from both weapons and reactors has been a highly politicized issue, as the military and industries producing these chemicals are not eager to present findings of harm. However, the only way to truly reduce cancer rates is to understand causes and take preventive actions. Baby teeth, even those from half a century ago, hold the clues to one such cause.

November 4, 2011

Cancer Risks of Dental Radiation

The well-documented evidence on the dangers of premenopausal mammography is persuasive, although belatedly recognized. In striking contrast, the evidence on the dangers of routine and highly profitable dental radiation, particularly in children, is still virtually unrecognized, warns the Cancer Prevention Coalition.

However, these concerns are not new, says Samuel S. Epstein, M.D., Chairman of the Cancer Prevention Coalition. He points to a 2001 report by Dr. John Gofman, a leading international authority on the dangers of radiation, which published well-documented evidence on the cancer risks of "low dose medical x-rays," especially to children.

A July 2006 publication by Dr. Ruth Kleinerman in Pediatric Oncology, "Cancer Risks Following Diagnostic and Therapeutic Radiation Exposure in Children," warned that the most radiosensitive organ in children is the thyroid gland.

This report also noted that "although thyroid cancer is rare, 6 other large studies had previously confirmed its relationship with prior radiation for treatment of enlarged tonsils or other head, face, or neck concerns."

Dr. Epstein cites a report in the June 2010 MailOnline newspaper published in the U.K., which warned that "Ten dental x-rays raise cancer risks—by at least ten times." This article cautioned that "x-rays should not be given at checkups or when registering new patients, despite these practices being common in many dental surgeries.

The MailOnline report also cited a 2010 collaborative study between the U.K. National Health Service and the universities of Brighton and Sussex which reported that "multiple exposures to dental x-rays may be associated with increased risks of developing thyroid cancer—particularly in children and adolescents."

The report further noted that these findings were consistent with previous warnings of increased risks of thyroid cancer in dentists and dental assistants.

Dr. Epstein finds further evidence in a November 22, 2010, *New York Times* article, "Radiation Worries for Children in Dentists' Chairs," which warned against risks of radiation from a new scanning device, known as a cone-beam CT scanner.

Cone-beam CT scanners are continually generating x-ray images, while rotating around the patient. They emit much higher levels of radiation than do conventional dental x-rays.

"Not surprisingly," says Dr. Epstein, "the incidence of thyroid cancer has escalated by 168% since 1975. The past and continuing practice of routine dental radiation, especially in children, is flagrant malpractice, if not criminal."

Dr. Epstein quotes Ralph Nader, who urged at 1979 hearings on the Corporate Criminal Liability Act by the Crime Sub-Committee of the House Judiciary Committee, "Jail for crime in the streets, but bail for crime in the suites."

INDEX

A

AAAS (American Association for the Advancement of Science), 369, 383

ACD (allergic contact dermatitis), 283-84

ACS (American Cancer Society), xiv, 12-13, 15, 30-31, 33, 38, 42, 56, 63-64, 66-68, 70-71, 74-78, 80-83, 369-70, 381-82

ADI (Acceptable Daily Intake), 177-78, 198-99, 202, 414, 421

AHAs (alpha-hydroxy acids), xxii, 329-30, 340-41

American Chemistry Council, 288-89

American Public Health Association, xi, 148, 151, 181, 206, 210, 235, 247, 307, 310, 390

anti-aging medication, 117-18, 380

antibiotics, xxix, 22, 90, 94, 96, 99, 104, 106, 108, 114-15, 120, 122, 124, 127, 131

apoptosis, 91, 108, 111, 115, 121-22, 125, 137, 158, 160, 352, 379

aspartame, 412-15, 419-21

a-tocopherol, 252

Avon, 78, 83, 323-24, 337, 339

B

baby teeth, 433, 437-39

benzophenone, 321, 323-24, 338-39

Bertell, Rosalie, 54, 65, 69-72, 74, 79, 303, 307, 411

BGH (bovine growth hormone), xxvii, 20, 62, 89, 91, 93-100, 104, 106, 117, 119, 124, 127, 130-31, 156, 370-71

BGH milk, 94, 96, 98, 117

bone cancer, 361-62, 388, 394, 404

BPA (Bisphenol-A), 334-35, 348-50, 352-53, 424-26

brain cancer, xxvii, 168, 245, 260, 388, 394, 410, 420

breast cancer, 11-18, 20-21, 25, 30-36, 38-39, 41-43, 47-49, 51-52, 57-59, 61-64, 66-68, 70-72, 74, 76-77, 81-82

Breast Cancer Action, 325

Breast Cancer Coalition, 10-12, 14

Breast Cancer Prevention Program, xvii, 378

Breast Cancer Unawareness Month, 30, 76

breast implants, 5-8, 12, 25, 28, 31, 36, 41, 45-46

www.ingramcontent.com/pod-product-compliance
Lightning Source LLC
Chambersburg PA
CBHW020719180526
45163CB00001B/38